© **Haffenreffer Museum of Anthropology**

Brown University, 1986

Library of Congress Cataloging-in-Publication Data

Haffenreffer Museum of Anthropology.
 Costume as Communication.

 (Studies in anthropology and material culture; v. 4)
 Bibliography: p.
 1. Indians of Mexico—Costume and adornment—Catalogs. 2. Indians of Central America—Costume and adornment—Catalogs. 3. Indians of South America—Andes Region—Costume and adornment—Catalogs. 4. Haffenreffer Museum of Anthropology—Catalogs.
 I. Schevill, Margot. II. Franquemont, E.M. III. Title. IV. Series.
 F1219.3.C75H34 1986 391'.008998 86-26958

COSTUME AS COMMUNICATION

Distributed by

Haffenreffer Museum of Anthropology, Brown University, Mount Hope Grant, Bristol, RI 02809

and

The University of Washington Press
PO Box C 50096
Seattle, WA 98145

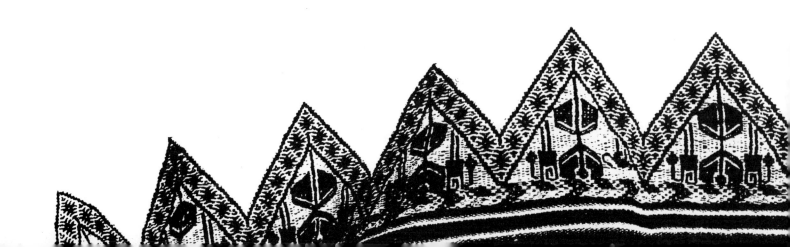

Honorary Board of Governors · Friends of the Haffenreffer Museum

MR. CARTER Y. BUCKLEY

MR. BARNET FAIN

MR. AND MRS. ROBERT E. GRANT

MRS. SIDNEY GREENWALD

MR. AND MRS. CARL HAFFENREFFER

MR. AND MRS. RUDOLF HAFFENREFFER 3RD

MR. DONALD HALL

MR. ROGER HIRSCHLAND

MR. AND MRS. JAMES HOUSTON

MR. ROBERT KILMARX

MRS. HAROLD NACE

MR. WATSON SMITH

Staff of the Haffenreffer Museum of Anthropology

Barbara A. Hail, Executive Director and Curator

Douglas Anderson, Curator of Research

Thierry Gentis, Assistant Curator

Joyce Smith, Conservation Technician, Exhibits/Preparator

Lyn Udvardy, Programs Specialist

Patsy Sanford, Education Specialist

Margot Blum Schevill, Research Associate

Bets Giddings, Curator Emerita

Danielle Toth, Photoarchivist

Alexandra Allardt, Conservator Consultant

Ethel Rudy, Secretary

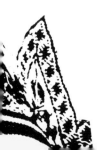

Studies in Anthropology and Material Culture: Volume IV

COSTUME AS COMMUNICATION

ETHNOGRAPHIC COSTUMES AND TEXTILES FROM MIDDLE AMERICA AND THE CENTRAL ANDES OF SOUTH AMERICA

in the collections of the Haffenreffer Museum of Anthropology, Brown University, Bristol, Rhode Island.

by Margot Blum Schevill

E.M. Franquemont, Andean consultant and essayist

The publication of this catalogue was supported by grants from the National Endowment for the Arts, Haffenreffer Family Fund, Rhode Island State Council on the Arts, Rhode Island Foundation, and Mr. and Mrs. Bruce M. Docherty.

Catalogue design by Todd Cavalier Design, 1986

typeset by Typesetting Service

printed by Mark-Burton, Inc.

Table of Contents

Foreword

The fourth volume in the Haffenreffer Museum's "Studies in Anthropology and Material Culture" describes the Museum's collections of twentieth century textiles from Middle America and the Central Andes of South America, two areas in which cloth has long been of primary importance. For the most part these textiles represent ordinary wear. As such, they are eminently suitable for interpretation in an anthropological context, that is, for what they tell us about their makers and wearers.

Margot Schevill, the Museum's research associate, recognized the unique value of this collection and its capability for communicating cultural mores. She invited Edward Franquemont to contribute to the analysis and discussion of the textiles because he, like herself, is an anthropologist and a textile specialist, with a working knowledge of the techniques used in traditional clothmaking and a strong interest in the societal role of costume. Franquemont's discussion covers the Andean collections; Schevill's the Middle American. Both scholars have apprenticed with traditional weavers in their respective areas of expertise. Together they provide new insights into the various attitudes of these native peoples toward costume, and help to explain where and to what degree traditional costume has resisted change.

I wish to express grateful recognition to editor Margot Schevill who has lovingly guided this work from its original conception. She has been responsible both for the theoretical framework and the technical organization of the book, as well as overseeing its production. Through her careful scholarship the research potential of this area of the Museum's collections has been fully utilized.

The publication of this catalogue is made possible through funding generously provided by grants from the National Endowment for the Arts and the Haffenreffer Family Fund, with additional monies for color plates provided by The Rhode Island State Council on the Arts and The Rhode Island Foundation. Their support is gratefully acknowledged. I would also like to thank Mr. and Mrs. R.F. Haffenreffer, 3rd, and Mr. and Mrs. Carl W. Haffenreffer for their continued enthusiasm for the Museum's diverse programs in research, education, exhibition, acquisition and publication.

Barbara A. Hail
Executive Director and Curator

Acknowledgements

I am grateful to all those who participated in this catalogue project and would like to acknowledge their contributions. Suzanne Baizerman, Susan Bean, Janet Catherine Berlo, Ned Dwyer, Ed Franquemont, Barbara Hail and James Schevill read all or parts of the manuscript in various stages. Mary Troeger and Barbara Hail served as able, alert editors.

Andean consultants Irene Saletan and Ed Franquemont contributed their knowledge to the catalogue section. Irene commented on the knitted textiles and Ed analyzed and commented on all of the Andean textiles, in addition to his fine essay.

Danielle Toth patiently photographed each textile listed in the catalogue and provided the prints. Catherine Allen, Marilyn Anderson, Ed Franquemont, Carl W. Haffenreffer and Barbara and Justin Kerr allowed me to use their fine photographs. Brooke Hammerlee and Richard Hurley contributed their photographic expertise. Many of the historic prints appear courtesy of the John Carter Brown and John Hay Libraries of Brown University or are in the Herbert J. Spinden Photo Archives at the Haffenreffer Museum.

The catalogue sections contain comments from many sources: thanks to Jeff Appleby, Barry Bainton, Barnet Fain, Olga A. Geng, Cynthia LeCount, Walter F. Morris Jr., James Plunkett and Ann P. Rowe. Fine textile analyses were provided by Betty Kennedy, Cheri Weitman, and especially Annie Fisher, who prepared the first draft of the Andean section.

Todd Cavalier is responsible for the book design while Tad Hanna and Syd Bauman utilized the Brown University mainframe computer to typeset the text.

I deeply appreciate the support I have received from the Haffenreffer Museum staff and especially Ethel Rudy. I wish I could thank personally each weaver whose textile art appears on these pages. For it is the determination of these indigenous peoples to persist in the production of traditonal cloth and costume, in spite of internal and external social and economic pressures, that created the primary motivation for this catalogue.

Margot Blum Schevill
Research Associate

Preface

The organization of this catalogue follows from the fact that the two largest ethnographic costume and textile collections from areas outside of the United States presently in the Haffenreffer Museum of Anthropology were gathered in the Central Andes and Middle America. The combination of costumes and textiles from two distinct and geographically distant areas under the cover of one catalogue suggests that complementary relationships and inferences may be drawn from the essays, costumes, and textiles presented. Research on possible connections between Middle America and the Andes has been pursued by archaeologists (Lathrap 1966, Badner 1972) and linguists (Olson in Kaufmann 1973–1974). Similarities in costume between Ecuador and West Mexico as seen on pre-Columbian ceramic figures (Anawalt in Conte 1984:13) have reinforced the still controversial suggestion that there may be a link between the Quechuan language of the Andes and the Tarascan language of Southwest Michoacan, Mexico (Kaufmann 1973–1974:961). Further culture contacts between these areas include the probable importation of maize from Mesoamerica to the Andes and peanuts, metallurgy, and hammocks in the opposite direction.

Indigenous peoples of these areas retain many culture traits including religion, costume, and costume technology, which have their roots in the pre-Columbian past. Moreover, the Spanish Conquest and occupation of Middle America and the Central Andes has left an indelible mark. The major indigenous groups – the Aztec, the Maya, and the Inca – reacted in different ways to the Spanish regime. The Aztec and the Maya, who had a highly developed cosmological system that was open to innovative ideas and styles, syncretized Christianity and native religions. The Inca accepted Christianity, blending the new rituals with those already in use, but rebelled against the civic authority because the good order of the Supreme Inca was not in force under Spanish rule.

Occupation and habitat link these groups as well. Indigenous peoples of both Middle America and the Andes are farmers and herders, living in remote rural areas, often accessible by foot only. The geographical areas under consideration share still another trait. While costume as communication is a theme that informs the study of costume in general, this theme is particularly provocative when analyzing layers of meaning embedded in costume and cloth from Middle America and the Central Andes of South America over centuries of Spanish, then national, rule.

The Collectors and the Collections

Over four hundred costumes and textiles from Latin America have been acquired by the Haffenreffer Museum of Anthropology over the past twenty-five years. Systematic field-collecting by students and teaching staff of the Department of Anthropology along with textiles acquired for the Museum's Education Program by the Friends of the Haffenreffer Museum and interested travelers account for the majority of the collections. Museum purchases from importers who wholesale native arts and from dealers who specialize in the unique, unusual item have been made possible by the Haffenreffer Special Fund. These purchases have enriched the collections with unusual rare textiles such as the late nineteenth- and twentieth-century Peruvian and Bolivian ponchos, shoulder and skirt cloths, and complete female costumes. In 1961 Professor Dwight Heath of the Anthropology Department and Anna M. Cooper made the first large collection, over two hundred and ninety-two items, as part of a *Meso-American Ethnographic Survey*. Textiles account for sixty of the total. The purpose of the expedition was to gather representative samples of crafts to use in exhibitions and material culture studies. Heath selected objects that might soon be replaced by commercial goods. A small grant from Brown University and the commitment from the Museum to reimburse out-of-pocket expenses made possible this expedition. The itinerary developed out of a limited prior knowledge of the areas visited. Chiapas, Mexico and the highland villages of Guatemala proved to be fertile collection grounds. Local specialists were sought out and many items were purchased in native markets. A return trip four years later provided confirmation that many traditional costume elements were becoming obsolete: for example, palm leaf raincoats had been replaced by plastic ones. Detailed field notes, covering three-fourths of the items, accompanied the collection.

Carl W. Haffenreffer traveled to Middle America on two occasions, in 1967 and in 1971. On the first trip, Haffenreffer photographed the Mayan ruins in Copan, Honduras (see fig. 3) and the Quiché Mayan town of Chichicastenango, Guatemala. Both a man's costume (112, 113, 125, 126, 128, 131) and a woman's costume (114, 123, 130, 132) were purchased directly from the owners

The second trip included a sojourn with the Tarahumara who inhabit the Copper Canyon of the Sierra Madre of Chihuahua, Mexico. The Reverend Luis G. Verplancken, S. J., hosted the Haffenreffers at the Tarahumara Mission in Creel. Twenty-five objects were collected, including a woman's costume and other textiles (2–7, 9, 10). Upon request, Verplancken sent seventy-seven slides of Tarahumaran life which show the objects in context (see fig. 18). A recent donation of Tarahumaran material gathered by Gino Conti from 1940–1970 has enriched these collections still further (8).

Clare and Burges Smith, importers of crafts of native peoples, have increased the Middle American textile collection with items purchased in Mexico and Guatemala since the 1970s. The Guatemalan pieces were produced before the earthquake of 1976. The collectors' criteria were the beauty of the object and the fact that the items had been produced by a living artist. Clare Smith, a professional photographer, focused on textiles, costume, and weavers during her field trips. In 1985, the Smiths donated thirty textiles from their collections, most of them *huipiles*. They have also made their photo-archives available for study and use (see figs. 16, 19).

In 1978, I received a grant from the Haffenreffer Special Fund to collect Mayan ethnographic textiles. I was a graduate student in anthropology working with Jane Powell Dwyer, who also was director of the Museum. For my field work I had elected to study with a Mayan weaver in order to gather data for a master of arts thesis (Schevill 1980). Thirty-two weavings were systematically gathered and documented, including seven complete costumes.

During this same period, a collection of twenty contemporary Guatemalan textiles was purchased from Fern Sandhouse, a student at the Rhode Island School of Design, who had traveled in Guatemala. In 1985 I had the opportunity to purchase well-documented contemporary textiles of highland Chiapas, Mexico from Walter F. Morris, Jr., who had worked extensively with Tzeltal and Tzotzil weavers, helping them to form the cooperative, Sna Jolobil. These textiles complemented the Heath collection. A final donation by New York collector Ron Podell of sixteen *huipiles* and one sash from Mexico and Guatemala, woven from 1940–1980, completes the Middle American textile collection.

Twenty-nine textiles collected by a Brown University graduate, Barry Bainton, form the earliest accessioned Central Andean textile collection. Bainton, an anthropology major who worked at the Museum under the guidance of the first director and chairman of the Anthropology Department, J. Louis Giddings, joined the Peace Corps after his 1963 graduation. He was assigned to the Central Andean area of Peru. Bainton became involved with AID-sponsored, community-based activities in various mountain villages located in the departments of Cuzco, Puno, Ayacucho, and Apurimac. Familiarity with local products, such as textiles, pottery, and farm implements, convinced Bainton that he should collect for the Museum, an offer that was readily accepted by Mrs. Ruth Giddings, curator. The Museum acquired Bainton's collection and his notes in 1966. Since then Bainton has amplified his field notes with additional information.

Dwight Heath served as Director of the Research Institute for the Study of Man in Bolivia in the mid-1960s. As an adjunct to his epidemiological investigations among the Aymara, he collected two hundred and twenty objects during this period of time, including fifty-nine textiles. As in Middle America, Heath purchased directly from native peoples, when possible. Heath's excellent field notes contain provenience of the purchase and origin (if different) of the item, anecdotal information, and descriptive data. The Heath and Bainton collections complement each other and reflect the distinct perspectives of the collectors, allowing the viewer to experience textiles and accessories from the Central Andes of the 1960s.

During the late 1960s and 1970s, collections were made for the Museum's Education Program by Mr. and Mrs. Edward Hail and Mr. and Mrs. Sidney Greenwald. Objects that could be handled by children were selected from aspects of Andean indigenous life (see Appendix). Jane Powell Dwyer, the third director of the Haffenreffer Museum, and Edward Dwyer contributed to the Museum's collections during the 1970s. Collecting was done on an informal basis during sojourns in Cuzco and Lima and travels in the Andes. Ethnographic textiles were obtained through the Dwyers' personal contact with native peoples. Money was left with *compadres*, parents of their godchild, in Cuzco who would purchase textiles for the Dwyers in local markets. The Dwyers became interested in unusual weavings from Q'ero (303), an isolated village where traditional costume is still worn and unusual spinning practices distinguish the textiles. The child's costume (277, 280, 286, 287) is an example of the syncretization of traditional and generalized Cuzco costume elements with commercially produced trims such as rickrack. The Dwyers collected objects such as dolls to be used for demonstrating costume and custom of the Andes to New England school children (311). Additional Andean textiles were donated by a Providence importer, Jone Pasha, and purchased from other sources.

One dealer in Andean cloth played an important role from 1980–1985 in rounding out the Museum's collection. Two complete female costumes, a group of late nineteenth- and early twentieth-century ponchos, shoulder and skirt cloths, and other fine examples were purchased with funds from the Haffenreffer Special Fund. Some collection material was provided, but not with the accuracy of detail or what E. M. Franquemont calls "the anthropological insistence" of Heath's field notes (see VI).

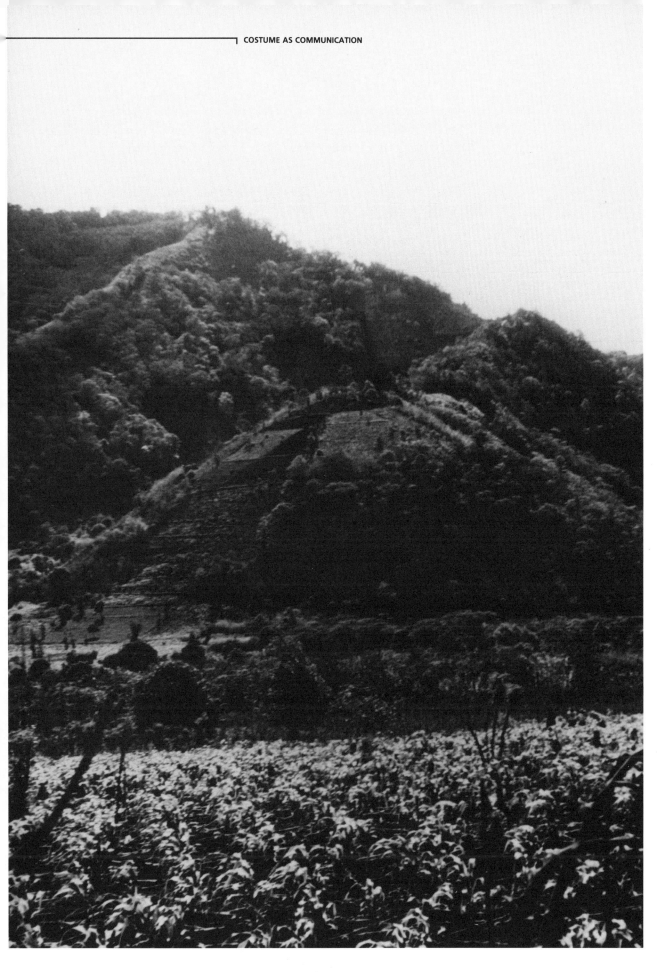

Guatemala. 1978. Photo by Margot Schevill

1 Costume as Communication

Costume is the mode or fashion of personal attire and dress (including the way of wearing the hair, style of clothing and personal adornment) belonging to a particular nation, class or period. There is always a certain pleasure in contemplating the costume of a distant nation (Murray, *A New English Dictionary on Historical Principles*).

Clothing, costume, and cloth all serve as cultural artifacts or signs, speaking in a silent language and communicating information visually without benefit of words. Scholars have viewed cloth as "an economic commodity, a critical object in social exchange, an objectification of ritual intent, and an instrument of political power" (Schneider and Weiner 1986:178). Commenting on the *huipiles* or blouses worn by Mayan women, Guatemalan poet Miguel Angel Astúrias wrote:

tantos símbolos, cábalas, sabidurías,
astrales y cálculos se urden en sus telas (1974)

so many symbols, spells, sayings,
stars and conjectures are warped in their cloth

Anthropologists, semioticians, and others have studied costume as a form of symbolic communication that can convey rank, class, status, region, religion, or age. Costume can satisfy practical, aesthetic, erotic, and magical functions required by a community. Focusing on these broad levels of analysis, Petr Bogatyrev wrote of folk costume in Moravian Slovakia. He defined the communicative event (wearing the costume) and analyzed the communicative hierarchy. What elements of costume are most powerful? What does color communicate? Dina and Joel Sherzer and Mari Lyn Salvador have studied the *mola* or blouse of the Kuna Indians who occupy the San Blas Islands of Panama. They found that an overlapping series of interdependent systems in *mola* making is reflected in social, economic, and aesthetic criteria practiced throughout Kuna life.[1]

1 Petr Bogatyrev, 1971; Mari Lyn Salvador, 1978; Dina and Joel Sherzer, 1976.

Other scholars have viewed costume in a less global way, focusing on more discrete elements of the costume itself. French theoretician Roland Barthes, writing in *The Fashion System*, offers another perspective for looking at the communicative potential of costume. He organizes garments into three categories: "image clothing," that which is photographed or drawn; "written clothing," that which is described with words; "real clothing," that which is technically described in relation to construction, materials, and other elements (1983:3–5). "Real clothing" serves as the source or mother tongue from which the iconic or "image" and verbal or "written" structures derive. Barthes utilizes scientific terminology, such as "genera" (type of fabric utilized, colors) and "species" (costume elements and ensembles), to find the "signifying unit," such as "this wrap-around skirt" or "that blouse with a floral embroidered neck" (ibid.:7).

Barthes' system is particularly appropriate when dealing with hundreds of costume items in a museum catalogue. When studying ethnographic textiles, a multilevel approach is imperative, for "real" clothing is presented out of context, accompanied by technical analyses based on "genera" and "species." The garments are capable of speaking for themselves. "Image" clothing is presented through photographs of prehistoric and historic images. Ethnographic notes of collectors combined with documentary sources describe the "written" garments.

In addition to the global perspectives of costume's communicative power and the more focused one of Barthes, one finds in the literature a wide variety of ways dress may serve to communicate. A fiber artist may create wearable or portable art in which the decorative becomes functional and the functional becomes decorative.

It is art moved out of the gallery onto the street. It moves the man or woman into a painting. The walls of the gallery are replaced by men and women. They move, they change, the forms change. The performance becomes a spontaneous combination of the colorful, the decorative, the bizarre (Westphal 1980).

How we feel about ourselves and our environment can be conveyed by how we dress. Long after the Maya ceased painting codices (illustrated books) or murals, some of their artistic traditions persisted in their costume. Luis Cardoza y Aragón, Guatemalan writer, stated: "their cloths recollect the fields, they are covered with them, they dress themselves with skies, birds, flowers, mountains, and butterflies" (Foppa 1976).

Costume may signal ethnicity to a knowing receiver of such signals. Handwoven cloth in the Andes is integrated into a distinctive fiesta dress worn in folklore competitions. Groups, like the Calcha of Bolivia who continue to maintain an ethnic identity, use dress along with music and dance as a form of communication to defend and define their ethnicity in relation to other participating groups in these competitions. E.M. Franquemont describes eloquently the role of cloth in the Andes (see V), which is part of an "ethnic code" communicating village identity. The cloth of Calcha is unique to Calcha, and although older weavings have been sold and thereby are lost to the community, weavers are still producing their strongest emblem of ethnicity, cloth (Medlin 1983:290–291; **370–378**).

Research by Pamela Hearne at the University Museum, University of Pennsylvania, Philadelphia, provocatively suggests that there is a connection between clothing and language itself and that cultural cohesion is broader than community affiliations. Applying Barthes' terminology, forty "species" of "real" clothing (that which is technically described in terms of construction, materials, and other elements) were analyzed. In this case, two hundred and forty *huipiles* or blouses were the subject of a computerized study. "Genera," such as the construction or pattern, design elements, the positioning of these designs on the *huipil*, colors, thread count, and fibers, from a geographical cross section of highland Mayan towns, were isolated for comparative study. Hearne found that in spite of the Mayan woman's tradition of distinctive clothing, shared characteristics exist which can be related to linguistic group affiliation (Hearne 1985:54–57).

In an agricultural society of indigenous peoples, designs of costumes and cloth often are believed to have the power to protect one from supernatural harm. The layout of the design field of a *huipil* can be viewed in a symbolic manner (see fig. 1). The head hole becomes the sun, and four cloth medallions affixed to the *huipil* represent the four cardinal points of North, South, East, and West. Double-headed eagles, the tree-of-life, or small animals relate the wearer to clan images and the natural world, so important to agrarian peoples. The *huipil* forms a cross, and the wearer is placed in the center of the universe, surrounded by levels of meaning and family symbols (Sayer 1985:227; Rodas, Rodas, and Hawkins 1940:124).

In the Andes, handwoven coca cloths called *unkhuñas* are an important component of ceremonial bundles, treasured and handed down over generations (see pl. 17). The community uses these textiles in annual ceremonies to "mark" and to ensure the fertility of their herds. These cloths are sometimes spoken of as being "restless," a response generated by the unbalanced layout of the design areas (Zorn 1985). Miniature cloths serve as mediators of spiritual forces when offered by pilgrims to the Shrine of El Señor (Isbell in Schneider and Weiner 1986:180).

While the preceding examples show costume used to nourish, strengthen, or protect, it could be used as well to terrify. The Aztec intimidated their enemies in battle by their dress. Costume represented economic power and signaled elaborate sacrificial rites that were dreaded by the conquered. Totemic animal images related to warrior clans were visible in combat (Pasztory 1984:21–22). Probably it seemed as if symbolic eagles and jaguars were fighting because actual animal skins provided the cloak or mantle for the warrior. Upon viewing an advancing army of magnificently costumed,

Fig. 1
Chichicastenango blouse or *huipil*. **117**.

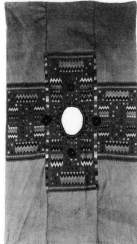

Fig. 2
Village *poblanas* smoke and talk with a sarape-clad horseman. Lithograph by Carlos Nebel. 1836. Courtesy of the John Hay Library, Brown University.

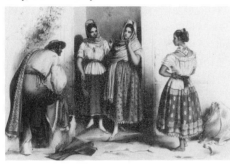

2 ¡Vivan Las Fiestas!, an exhibition at the Museum of International Folk Art, Museum of New Mexico, Santa Fe. Summer, 1985.

animal-like men, the morale of the opposition must have been stunned, if not severely shaken.

Barthes gives us insight for following costume innovations when he discusses "the transformational myth which seems attached to all mythic reflection on clothing" and the "multiplication of persons in a single being" (1983:256). Quoting Sartre, he lists three levels: "(1) a popular and poetic conception: the garment (magically) produces the person; (2) an empirical conception: the person produces the garment, *is expressed* through it; (3) a dialectical conception: there is a 'turnstile' between person and garment" (ibid.:fn. 256).

As a result of contact with missionaries and traders at the end of the nineteenth century, the Seri, Tarahumara, and Navajo adopted a Victorian-style costume. The traditional blanket dress of the Navajo was retained for ceremonial purposes, while the pelican-skin robe of the Seri disappeared entirely (1, 3, 9, 10). Did these native peoples believe that, as Sartre implied, one "is" what one wears, or that because they dressed like the intruders, they would be more readily accepted?

Other contemporary examples of costume transformations include the Aztec-style feathered *huipil* and the *China Poblana* costume. The former has been transformed into the wedding costume of the Zinacantán in Chiapas, Mexico (see 83 and pl. 2, 84). The *China Poblana* was considered the national costume of non-Indian or *Mestizo* Mexico until the 1950s (see pl. 10, fig. 2). Origin myths vary. The etymology – China (maid), Poblana (village) – reflects the idea that it originated in the nineteenth century and was worn by maids who came from the country to work in the houses of the rich. A caption or label associated with this costume on exhibition stated that the *China Poblana* was "fabled to have originated with the dress of a Chinese princess in Puebla, Mexico, but was probably adapted from Mexican peasant dress."[2] By the early twentieth century, this costume was used widely for fiesta or fancy dress balls in Mexico City and Santa Fe, New Mexico, but was worn by the mistresses, not the maids. This transformation suggests an example of Sartre's dialectical conception of a "turnstile" relationship between person and garment. For in the late nineteenth century, wealthy women loved this costume, but could only don it on outings to the country, certainly not at dress balls in the capitol. The message signaled by this lovely costume today is one of exoticism and magic, the idea of more than one person in one single being, mistress and maid together. One is reminded of the exchange of character by means of costume which transpires in the fourth act of Mozart's *The Marriage of Figaro* between the maid, Susanna, and her mistress, the Countess.

An issue that relates to this kind of transformation concerns the effect of historical events on costume evolution, a theme that will be noted in some of the catalogue citations in response to the hybrid nature of Middle American and Central Andean costume elements. Barthes suggests that fashion (costume) remains outside of history. History cannot act on forms analogically, but it can certainly act on the rhythm of forms, to disturb or to change it (1983:256). Barthes allows that old forms can persevere while utilizing new materials and cites the example of ancient African societies in the process of development. They maintain traditional costume but "submit it nonetheless to variations in Fashion (yearly changes of fabrics, prints, etc.): a new rhythm is born" (1983:297).

Not all costume researchers are in accord with Barthes. H.H. Hansen and J. Laver have endeavored to establish analogic relationships between the clothing and the architecture of an epoch (1956, 1949). Schevill has traced evolution of textile design present in the male headdress or *tzute* from Chichicastenango, Guatemala, over an eighty-five-year span. Relationships seem to exist between internal and external events and social pressures on

Mayan weavers and the acceptance of innovation in motifs, techniques, materials, and function of their weaving (Schevill 1986).

The Southwestern United States textile scholar, Kate Peck Kent, explored the relationship between the changing Navajo aesthetic, reflected in their weaving, and the historical events that were affecting their lives. She follows this theme over a three-hundred-year period from 1650 to present times as the weavers move from accepting innovation voluntarily to the imposition of trader influence upon their design, color, and materials (Kent 1985).

Similarly in Middle America, some say the visit of the French Navy to the Pacific coast of Guatemala in the mid-nineteenth century left its mark on the male costume of a remote village in Huehuetenango, Todos Santos Cuchumatán (**98, 99, 103–106**; Bell, pers. com. 1978). In the Central Andes, European-style bowler or derby hats, and helmet-style headgear modeled after those worn by the *Conquistadores* have been adopted by Quechuan and Aymara women of the Andes (see **247** and pl. 6, **347, 393**).

Costume seems to be the last artistic element of ancient heritage to be totally abandoned. However, when costume becomes a symbol or ethnic marker that divides progressive from nonprogressive members of a community, traditional clothing slowly gives way to commercially produced costume elements. For example, in Middle America, homogeneous work clothes that indigenous males adopt when going to work on large plantations do not signal village, religion, or age. School uniforms, enforced by the predominantly Catholic schools in Mexico and Guatemala, eliminate the possibility of pride in being an *indigena*. To those who have chosen to leave their villages to work in the cities, village styles seem uncivilized, a reminder of the "old ways" left behind.

In recent times another activity has affected the symbolic communication of cloth and costume. In the Andes, since the 1970s, certain older costume elements and ceremonial cloths have been marketed by dealers abroad with considerable financial success. These textiles are often purchased in remote villages by middlemen to sell to dealers in the big cities. Cloth now signals monetary profit, the ritual significance being superceded by the demands of poverty. The Andean people, needful of this additional income, relinquish their treasured and revered cloth for which there can be no replacement. In 1986, one dealer offered thirty thousand dollars for a nineteenth-century hoard of textile ceremonial bundles; another offered two tractors. The outraged village elders asked the National Archive of Bolivia for protection of their ritual bundles, and the textiles were deposited there for safekeeping (Murra, pers. com. 1985; Davis, pers. com. 1986).

Another example of the increasing demand for textiles as an economic commodity comes from Guatemala. Over the past ten years, dealers have been selling what appeared to be older ceremonial textiles for large sums of money to collectors and other clients. They sent photographs of available textiles to clients in the United States and Europe, and, in effect, mail orders were placed. Eventually, it was discovered that these textiles were imitations of older styles valued by collectors and had been commissioned from Mayan weavers by entrepreneurs and dealers (Berlo and Senuk 1985:84). In the past repeating older styles has been a way that fine weavers pass on textile traditions and history from one generation to the next. These replicated textiles are highly valued by the community, as are fragments of those that have worn out. In the situation cited, the weavers were receiving better than normal compensation for producing these textiles, but the dealers were the real financial beneficiaries. The result is that the integrity of some of these fine "textile artists" has been seriously questioned by those who eventually buy the weavings, be it a museum or private collector. In addition, the power of symbolic meanings embedded and encoded in the iconography of the older costume pieces has been diluted, as streamlining of materials and techniques, in what is often called "quality-controlled" textiles, is expected by entrepreneur and client. If cloth and costume come to function only as economic commodities, how will the ritual and symbolic qualities of the art of weaving be affected?

II Cloth and Costume in Middle America

Introduction

Mexico and Guatemala are the sources for two hundred and fifty indigenous costumes and textiles in the Haffenreffer Museum of Anthropology. Most were gathered in the "heartland regions" of Southern Mexico and Guatemala, known as Mesoamerica where the great pre-Columbian indigenous civilizations flourished (Helms 1975:xi). There is also a small sampling from the northwestern Mexican frontier states of Sonora and Chihuahua.

Middle America encompasses cool temperate highlands, warm tropical lowlands, and a series of microenvironments that provided the setting for early plant domestication and the cultivation of maize. The great northern desert is intersected by the Sierra Madre that extends into Southern Mexico and Guatemala and forms the highlands, an extension of the Andean "cordillera." Volcanoes, dense tropical jungles, a limestone peninsula, long stretches of beaches, and fertile mountain valleys form the "heartlands," an area that shares a cultural history dating from 1500 B.C. to A.D. 1519, over 3000 years. Great cultural centers flourished and then were replaced by new regimes, traditions, and architecture. Trade networks connected remote geographical areas of Middle America to fulfill the ruling elite's requirements for exotic goods.

Today Mexico and Guatemala occupy over 800,000 square miles, separated by a border from the Carribean Sea to the Pacific Ocean, created in part by the Usumacinta River as it winds its way through the Mexican states of Campeche, Tabasco, and Chiapas and the Peten of Guatemala. Ruins of ancient Mayan cities survive amid the dense hardwood forests of this region.

The indigenous population of Mexico, living mainly in rural areas, numbers six million. They are identified by language, customs, and their political affiliation with indigenous communities. The two and one half million Maya of Guatemala live primarily in the western highlands. Throughout Middle America nonindustrialized areas are covered with *milpas* – fields of corn, beans, and squash – tended by these agrarian peoples, dependent on the labor-intensive swidden or slash-and-burn farming practiced since earliest times. In southern Mexico and northern Guatemala, the Mayan land and water management was very sophisticated. Recent excavations at the Classic Period site, Rio Azul, Guatemala, revealed a carefully controlled landscape with cultivated fields and water-filled canals (Adams 1986:445). As a result of the conflicts between the army and the guerrilla movement over the past ten years, many *milpas* in northwest Guatemala, on which rural Maya are dependent, have been destroyed, forcing migration across the border to Mexico and into refugee camps.

The dominant class of Guatemalans and Mexicans are *Ladinos* (in Guatemala) or *Mestizos* (in Mexico), those of mixed European and Indian descent who have renounced traditional indigenous customs known as *costumbre*, and who speak only Spanish, the lingua franca. Despite this, seventy Indian languages are still in use in Middle America. In Mexico, forty-six indigenous languages are spoken. The Maya continue to speak twenty-four distinct languages. Costumes of twenty-two linguistically differentiated ethnic groups are represented in the Haffenreffer collections.

Mexico and Guatemala have shared a recent as well as an ancient history.

The Aztec empire fell to Cortes in 1521, and the Maya were overwhelmed by Alvarado in 1524 (see time line). The period of colonial occupation gave way to independence from Spain in 1821. From this time on, Mexico and Guatemala have gone in different directions. In recent times, an intense and accelerated period of change has affected all of Middle America. Traditional life of indigenous peoples has been seriously threatened. Will the art of weaving and, as a result, costume cease to exist in the future? The Haffen-reffer Museum collection offers a look at the past and allows one to experience visually the resilience and creativity of the indigenous artistry of Mexico and Guatemala.

Post-Conquest Time Line for Mexico, Guatemala, Peru, and Bolivia

MEXICO

1519	Arrival of Cortes
1521	Fall of Aztec empire
1528–35	Mexico ruled by royal *Audiencia*; called New Spain
1535–1821	Colonial period
1767	Jesuits expelled
1821	The *Plan de Iguala* proclaims Mexico's independence from Spain
1824	Creation of Federal Republic
1857	Benito Juárez becomes president Separation of church and state
1864	Maximilian becomes emperor of Mexico
1867	Maximilian executed; Juárez reelected
1876–1911	Presidency of Porfirio Díaz
1910–20	Mexican Revolution
1921–40	Reformist period
1929	Creation of PRI (Partido Revolucionario Institucional)
1949	Creation of the Instituto Nacional Indigenista

GUATEMALA

1523	Invasion by Alvarado
1524	Conquest
1523–1821	Colonial period; Guatemala part of Central America
1767	Jesuits expelled
1821	Independence from Spain
1823	United Provinces of C.A., abolished in 1823; a succession of dictators rule the country
1917	Germans dominate Guatemalan highlands
1934	President Ubico promulgates Vagrancy Law, requiring Indians to work on plantations for at least 180 days per year
1945	President Juan Jose Arévalo abolishes law; unused land to be leased to peasants. Arbenz follows Arévalo
1954	Overthrow of Arbenz by CIA; Colonel Castillo Armas becomes president. Reforms overturned. Guerrilla movement starts that continues today

PERU/BOLIVIA

1532	Pizarro arrives in Peru and captures Inca Atahualpa
1533	Execution of Atahualpa. Spanish arrive in Cuzco and crown Manco Inca
1536–39	Rebellion of Manco Inca. Inca exile government by regents in Vilcabamba continues to 1572
1572	Vilcabamba captured by Spanish. The Inca Tupac Amaru executed in Cuzco
1570–81	Viceroy Toledo "vista general" reorganization of Spanish/Indian relations
1613	Guaman Poma's *El Primer Nueva Corónica y Buen Gobierno* describes Inca history from the native perspective to the Spanish king. Many drawings of native costumes (see fig. 30)
1779–83	Inca rebellions of Jose Gabriel Tupac Amaru and others. Movement to establish an independent Peruvian Indian state is crushed
1820–24	Wars of Independence in Peru. Battle of Ayacucho (Dec. 1924); final defeat of the Royalists. "Henceforth the aborigines shall not be called Indians; they are the children and citizens of Peru and they shall be known as Peruvians." S. Bolivar
1879–83	Wars of the Pacific. Chile defeats Peru and Bolivia; realignment of national boundaries
1924	Establishment of the APRA (Alliance for Popular American Revolution) by Victor Raul Haya de la Torre. Call for land reform and Indian rights
1968–75	Revolutionary government of Juan Velasco Alvarado established massive land reforms and peasant cooperatives. Nationalization of all large land holdings
1970	Establishment of the *Sendero Luminoso* as a Marxist-Leninist-Maoist party. Call for Indian/peasant revolution led by Abimael Guzman
1980–86	First armed attack of *Sendero Luminoso* at Chuschi, Ayacucho. Armed struggle continues in much of the central highlands. Massive dislocations of native population

3 Mary Elizabeth King shows how Paracas clothing "spoke" to both its wearers and viewers. She successfully translates this "language" utilizing Barthes' semiotic system to analyze "image clothing" and "real clothing." For pre-Columbian Peruvian textile studies, "written clothing" does not exist (1986).

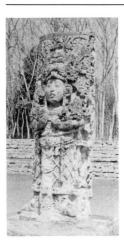

Fig. 3
Stela H. Copán, Honduras. 1967. Photo by Carl W. Haffenreffer.

Male	Female
loincloth, *maxtlatl*	skirt
hip-cloth	hip-cloth
cape	cape
kilt	rounded poncho, *quechquémitl*
sleeveless jacket, *xicolli*	triangular poncho, *quechquémitl*
robe	blouse, *huipil*
open quilted armor	
closed quilted armor	
short tunic, *ehuatl*	
warrior ceremonial costume	
ceremonial costume	

Male	Female
cloak, *manta, tilma* (short, long)	blouse, *huipil, pot* (long, short)
kilt	skirt, *utz* (tied around waist)
loincloth	head cloth
cotton quilted armor	
sleeveless jacket, *xicolli*	

Before the Conquest

No complete pre-Columbian costumes have survived in Middle America because of climate and ancient burial methods. Textile fragments and a few ritual garments, what Barthes designates as actual or "real" clothing, give some insight as to the technical and stylistic aspects of costume. It is by means of visual material or "image clothing," such as murals, painted ceramics, figurines, and sculpture, that the power of pre-Hispanic costume before the arrival of Cortes is projected[3] (see fig. 3).

Further visual representation of pre-Columbian costume is provided by painted codices of pictorial writing. These renderings were set down in books of bark paper or deer skin. Fortunately, some survived the impetuous book-burning periods carried on in post-Conquest times by Catholic bishops determined to christianize the New World "pagans." Such books codified information about secular and sacred life and were used primarily by elite scribes. In them occur hundreds of detailed descriptions of costume and textiles (Anawalt 1981).

Sixteenth-century missionary accounts of native life describe costume before the Conquest as well. Fray Bernardino de Sahagún's encyclopedic coverage of Aztecan society is presented in twelve volumes known as the *Florentine Codex*. Illustrations and descriptions rendered by elderly Indian informants include, among other subjects, information about costume, textiles, and the weaving process. Inferences about the costume of the less well-documented highland Maya have been posited from this wealth of visual information (Anawalt 1974).

In the Mayan region, ceramic figurines and codex information are augmented by Classic Period, large-scale, three-dimensional sculptures from a host of Mayan sites. These sources allow us to trace aspects of costume evolution from pre-Hispanic to contemporary times. The *quechquémitl* or shoulder poncho (**27, 28**), the *huipil* or blouse (see **59** and pl. 1), and the *manta* or cloak (**50**) are but a few examples of pre-Columbian dress form survivals. Information provided by "image clothing" has been derived primarily from pictorial sources in Mexico and lowland areas of Guatemala and Honduras. As of the 1980s, little visual information pertaining to the costume of the highlands of Guatemala exists. Native documents such as the *Popol Vuh* (Tedlock 1985, Edmonson 1971), *The Annals of the Cakchiquels* (Recinos and Goetz 1953), and *Title of the Lords of Totonicapán* (Chonay and Goetz 1953) give some costume information from the sixteenth and seventeenth centuries. Since highly evolved societies were in existence in Guatemala at the time of the Conquest, overall Mesoamerican cultural features such as costume elements must have been shared by the highland Maya.

Patricia Anawalt has codified all information available, gleaned from visual material ("image clothing"), published sources ("written clothing"), and archaeological textiles and ethnographic cultural survivals ("real clothing") (1981). She has assembled a pan-Mesoamerican costume repertory for male and female costume based on six Mesoamerican groups or areas for which there is Late Post-Classic–Early Contact period data: Aztec, Tlaxcala, Tarascan, Mixtec, the Borgia Group, and Lowland Maya. Underlying this organizational pattern is the principle of construction utilized, and Anawalt presents five categories: draped, slip-on, open-sewn, closed-sewn, and limb-encasing garments.

To Anawalt's basic male repertoire, skirts of various lengths, belts (perhaps not woven), stoles (perhaps *quechquémitls*), and headbands could be added (Mahler 1965:583–586; Schele and Miller 1986:68).

Anawalt has inferred the nature of pre-Columbian highland Mayan costume and proposed the following male and female costume repertoire based on extrapolation from pan-Mesoamerican garment patterns (1974).

One could surmise that jewelry, headbands, other accessories, and perhaps belts were also part of highland Mayan costume.

Cloth in Trade, Tribute, and Worship

In the *Codex Mendoza*, a pictorial Aztecan manuscript from 1325–1521, images present costume and textiles paid as tribute to Tenochtitlán, the Aztecan capitol, by the many provinces that made up the powerful Aztecan empire. "Image clothing" of feather warrior outfits, dresses, and mantles appear. Each drawing bears a symbol for a numerical unit and by deduction one learns that three thousand six hundred mantles were sent in tribute. Currency in the form of gold or silver coins did not exist. Finely drawn illustrations indicate the complexity and beauty of these highly valued textiles (see fig. 4). Costume and cloth were part of a communication system that signaled wealth, religious rituals, and political power.

An Aztec could recognize the rank and military exploits of a man by his dress, and at a glance evaluate the power of a city, and its gods and rulers by its temple and sculptures (Pasztory 1984:21).

Cloth was an important trade item. Columbus encountered the Maya in 1502 off the island of Guanajo near Honduras on a trading expedition. Goods included "bells, razors, knives…and chiefly draperies and different articles of spun cotton in brilliant colours" (Sayer 1985:30).

As with the pre-Columbian peoples of coastal Peru, textiles may have served as offerings, evidenced by the more than six hundred fragments dredged from the Sacred Cenote of Chichén Itzá, Yucatan, in the late nineteenth century by Edward H. Thompson. Speculation concerning these fragments suggests that they might be pieces of clothing worn by sacrificial victims or wrappings for ceremonial objects. Another explanation supports the belief in the animate nature of textiles, for they may have been ceremonially "killed" or torn up as were other objects that were thrown into the well, a ritual of the Cenote cult in Post-Classic Mayan times. Another view is that these fragile cotton and agave weavings were torn while being extracted from the "muck" near the bottom of the well (Lothrop n.d.; Coggins 1984:143).

Votive offerings of whole garments have been found in the dry caves of Mixteca Alta, Oaxaca. They include two plain-woven *huipiles* with weft cording and *kelim*-slit neck openings. There is evidence of red coloring. Two tiny plain-weave *quechquémitls* and a slightly larger *huipil* are finished with a twined weft fringe. Accompanying these textiles were several webs of cotton cloth (Johnson 1967:179–190). In the high-status burial at Altun Ha, Belize, known as "The Sun God's Tomb," the entire crypt seemed to have been covered with cloth; much of the preserved cloth was of a red color (Pendergast 1969:22). Post-Conquest writings attest to the continuing use of finely woven textiles and bolts of cloth as offerings to male and female deities.

Costume as Status Symbol

Some costume elements were given by the Aztecan ruler as rewards for memorable deeds in battle and were not available for sale in the market. If one chose not to go to war, one could be deprived of lip-plugs, golden garlands, many-colored feathers, earplugs, armbands, shields, weapons, insignia, mantles, and loin-cloths (Durán 1971:197–200).

In both Aztecan and Mayan society, emblems of dress and adornment indicated class and occupation. The size of a headdress or the length of the skirt indicated authority or status. Eighth-century Mayan murals at the site of Bonampak offer information on costume specialization. Warriors and priests had distinctive garments and accessories. Musicians wore long skirts, sashes, and towering headdresses (see fig. 5). Animal headdresses and

Fig. 4
Codez Mendoza. 1673. Courtesy of the John Carter Brown Library, Brown University.

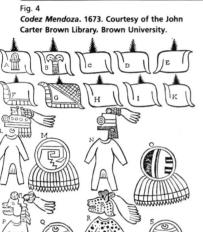

Fig. 5
Performers and musicians on the stage, Room I, Structure I, Bonampak, Mexico. Painting by Antonio Tejada. Courtesy of the Carnegie Institution of Washington.

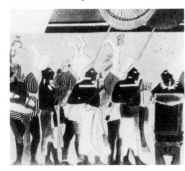

other accoutrements transformed dancers into mythic beings (Mahler 1965:588).

Sumptuary laws imposed by the ruling class denied the use of cotton to the lower class as a means of control. While common fibers such as agave, yucca, or palm were woven or netted into cloaks and other garments by the ordinary people, the laws could not repress the people's use of clothing as expression. Some cloaks were "burnished with a stone"; others were painted with whirlpool designs like eyes or an ocelot design (Sahagún 1950–1969:Book 10:63). These garments could have been an imitation of the ornate clothing of the nobility. Anawalt commented:

Authoritarian efforts to govern artistic expression as reflected in dress have seldom been successful and personal adornment irrepressibly appears to be people's favorite art (Sayer 1985:73).

The *Conquistadores* recognized the value of cloth, also highly valued in Spain, to the conquered peoples of New Spain. Among the first treasures sent to Charles V, king of Spain and the Netherlands, cloth was well represented. In 1520 the German artist, Albrecht Dürer, visited Brussels to view the first dispatch of tribute and wrote in his diary:

I also saw things that were brought to the king from the New Land of Gold...strange garments, mantles, and all sort of strange objects for human use, all of them so beautiful that they are a marvel and were valued at a hundred thousand ducats. In all my days I have never seen anything equally enchanting to my heart as these things and I marveled at the subtle genius of men in distant lands (Keleman 1942:36).

This dazzling display increased the emperor's desire to conquer the "golden" land. The metal work was melted down for bullion, and the textiles disappeared without a trace. Only one item of "real clothing" remains, a green quetzal feathered headdress on view in Vienna's Museum für Völkerkunde, sent to Spain between 1519 and 1524. (Feest, pers. com. 1986).

Post-Conquest to the Twentieth Century

The Conquest once begun was viewed by the indigenous peoples of the New World as a world cataclysm; one world was over and the second had begun. One-third to one-half of the native population was eliminated by disease. Many natives were forced into the *encomienda* system, controlled by the Spanish settlers who demanded tribute and labor. The southern half of Middle America, less densely populated, was deprived of its indigenous peoples who were enslaved and sent to work in mines or on plantations. Considering the fate of Indian Middle America, it is a wonder that any pre-Columbian dress forms survived. But cloth and clothing continued to be used as tribute. Introduction of new materials, techniques, and styles from Spain were gradually absorbed and fused into costume.

Over the next three hundred years, European-influenced costume elements were adapted, transforming or replacing pre-Columbian dress forms. Chloë Sayer has traced costume in Mexico during this period with considerable detail (1985). For Guatemala, information has not been easy to find. As Ann P. Rowe states:

Unfortunately, there is also a dearth of information on textile innovations and costume changes of the Colonial period. When the lacuna ends and information becomes available for the late 19th century, it is clear that the male costume has been almost completely changed but that the female costume retained many pre-conquest elements. The only way to date these changes is by comparison with dated European antecedents. Unfortunately, few such antecedents are datable; some appear to have been derived from Spanish peasant dress, which in itself is poorly documented (1981:15).

Colonial influence in Chiapas is discussed briefly by Walter F. Morris, Jr. (1984). The Spaniards were not the only occupants of *Ciudad Real*, the polit-

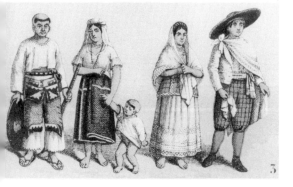

Fig. 6
Zoque Indians of Tuxtla Gutiérrez, Chiapas.
Ordinary and wedding costumes. Plate by An-
tonio García Cubas. 1876. Courtesy of the
John Hay Library, Brown University, Church
Collection.

Fig. 6
Zoque Indians of Tuxtla Gutiérrez, Chiapas.
Ordinary and wedding costumes. Plate by An-
tonio García Cubas. 1876. Courtesy of the
John Hay Library, Brown University, Church
Collection.

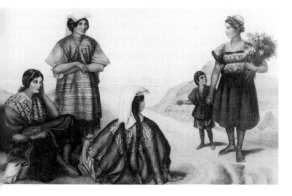

Fig. 7
Huipil-clad Indian women from the mountains
of the southeast. Lithograph by Carlos Nebel.
1836. Courtesy of the John Hay Library,
Brown University.

Fig. 8
Indians from Santa María de Tlapacoya, Puebla. Lithograph by Carlos Nebel. 1836. Courtesy
of the John Hay Library, Brown University.

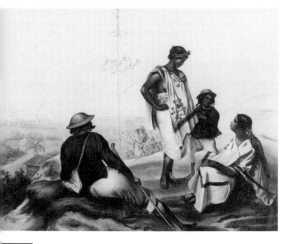

ical, economic, and religious center of the highlands. Mexicas and Tlaxcalans from Central Mexico, Mixtecas from Oaxaca, and Quichés from Guatemala all helped to settle the city, which became San Cristóbal de las Casas. European as well as pre-Columbian influences are present in costumes worn today (83, 84).

"Image clothing" of 1836 appears in lithographs by German architect, Carlos Nebel. Plates from Mexican artist and writer Antonio Garciá Cubas' *The Republic of Mexico in 1876* (see figs. 6, 7, 8) and photographs from other nineteenth-century publications by travelers, such as Alfred P. and Anne Cary Maudslay, provide additional information about the styles of this period. By the twentieth century, a costume had evolved that could be regionally or locally defined. European costume elements coexisted with pre-Columbian dress form survivals, and new styles were created, embued with levels of symbolic meaning.

The Twentieth Century

Traditional costume has survived in many parts of Middle America. Of the fifty different Indian groups living in Mexico, many have continued to produce and wear their own typical clothing or *traje*. When Donald and Dorothy Cordry were collecting material for their monumental 1968 publication, *Mexican Indian Costumes*, a culmination of research that began in the 1930s, they focused on twenty-eight linguistically distinct groups, never claiming to have studied all existing indigenous costumes and textiles. Even most recent research does not present a comprehensive listing of village and language group in relation to costume (Lechuga 1982; Sayer 1985).

This is not so in Guatemala where anthropologists and costume historians have been studying evolution in style, techniques, and materials since the 1930s (Osborne 1935; O'Neale 1945; Start 1948). By the mid-1960s, two hundred recognizably different costume styles could be identified in a country no larger than New York state. If substyles within a village were to be included in the total number, then five hundred would be more accurate (Osborne 1965:9). In the mid-1970s, the total number of documented styles had shrunk to one hundred and forty-eight (Pancake 1976). Many concerned researchers warned of the possibility of total extinction of costume due to upheavals experienced by the indigenous population of Middle America. "When Indians are being absorbed into the national culture, costume is often one of the first aspects of their indigenous culture to disappear" (Sayer 1985:10). To the contrary, as the Middle American collection in the Haffenreffer Museum reveals, costume and textiles are still being produced, especially by the Maya for whom "costume is a visual representation of a community and in abstract it incorporates certain ideas the inhabitants hold about themselves, their relationship to the universe and the world around them" (Lathbury 1974:5).

For those men who must work on plantations or in mines, costume has proven to be a source of embarrassment and alienation. Only the use of sandals and a shoulder bag connect the migratory worker, otherwise dressed in western-style work clothes, to his heritage. When a worker's family joins him, on the other hand, traditional clothing is worn by the women and girls. In contrast, the Huichol men (12, 13, 14) and the Mayan men of Chiapas (81, 85–91), to mention only a few examples, persist in wearing typical clothing, not only within their villages, but when visiting nearby cities. It is an indication of the symbolic power and pride invested in the way in which they are viewed by *Mestizos* and *Ladinos* with whom they interact regularly.

The contemporary male and female costume repertory is made up of pre-Columbian dress form survivals and those that have been adapted from clothing worn by the Spanish and subsequent travelers to Middle America.

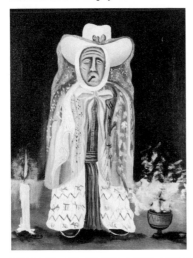

Fig. 9
Maximón. 1978. Painting by Juan Manuels.

Fig. 10
Fiesta in Comalapa. 1978. Painting by Samuel
Soz.

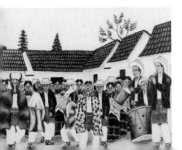

The following list of costume elements has been extrapolated from textiles in the Haffenreffer Museum collection.

For some twentieth-century costume elements, handwoven cloth has been replaced by commercial cloth, but the form of the "image clothing" has been retained (**14**). Other adaptations include adorning the *huipil* with embroidery instead of weaving in the patterns (**40**).

Male shoulder bags or *morrales* represent a pre-Columbian survival in form, technique, and material. Single elements of agave and cotton are knotted or interlocked to form netted bags (**63**). Other bags made by men use the European-introduced techniques of knitting or crocheting. A curious blending of pre-Columbian and Hispanic clothing can be seen in the long cape or *capixay* worn by the Mayan men of San Martín Sacatepéquez (Chili Verde), Quezaltenango, Guatemala (see pl. 16). Some researchers claim that it is modeled after the priest's robe. Others state that the model is the Spanish riding coat. It is a tailored garment with sleeves, a collar, and wide cuffs. However, the garment is worn as a cape, with the sleeves tossed over the shoulders revealing a decorative fringe.

The *sombrero* is a powerful symbol of male dignity, similar in function to the elaborate headdresses worn by the Aztec and Maya that signaled authority and status. Palm leaf or agave is manipulated by men as it was in pre-Columbian times for cloaks of the Aztecan lower classes. Then it is plaited into strips and sewn together to form various shapes (**13, 16, 47, 81**). One's state and linguistic affiliation can be perceived by the style of and adornment on the hat (**13**). The complement of trims on the Huichol hat indicates that the wearer has been on peyote pilgrimages (Sayer 1985:203). The Mayan men of Chiapas sew their own hats which are decorated with brightly colored commercial ribbon. As in pre-Columbian times, women's sashes serve decorative and practical functions. Pregnant women bind themselves for support with wide sashes which also hold their wraparound skirts in place.

The use of textiles in religious contexts persists in Middle America. In the Mayan highlands, replicas of saints and the Virgin Mary are dressed in specially woven garments which are replaced periodically with fresh new ones. Sometimes layers of *huipiles* adorn the statues (Morris 1986:52). In Magdalenas, Chiapas, the village commissions from the best weavers textiles, which are owned by the community and rented by village dignitaries for ceremonial occasions. In the Guatemalan village of Santiago Atitlán, *Maximón* is a religious icon to whom offerings are made and who serves as an intermediary between supplicants and their patron saints or deities. In this traditional village, he is dressed in a combination of Mayan and Spanish-influenced clothing, including a white *sombrero*, backstrap-woven pants and shirt. A cigar is placed in his mouth. In a *Ladino* village, he wears western-style clothing. The hat and cigar are symbolic of his *Ladino* nature, a reminder of Barthes' idea of "the multiplication of persons in a single being" (Barthes 1983:256; fig. 9).

The use of costume in dance continues to provide a transformational experience for the wearer and viewer. In *La Danza de los Conquistadores*, as enacted in Comalapa, Chimaltenango, animals that Alvarado encountered on his march through Guatemala in the early 1500s are represented by means of masks and costume elements (see fig. 10). The conqueror himself with his golden hair and white skin and sixteenth-century-style costume of velvet is also portrayed. The animals are endowed with special power and conquer Alvarado at the end of the dance, a victory for the Maya and a reversal of the events of 1524. The Spaniards transposed their victory over the Moors into the dance, *The Conquest of Mexico*, where costume elements include armor, helmets, and velvet breeches. Another popular dance, *Danza de los Quetzales*, reminds the viewers of the male glory of

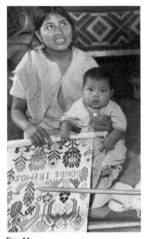

Fig. 11
Where shall we go? 1980. Photo by Marilyn Anderson.

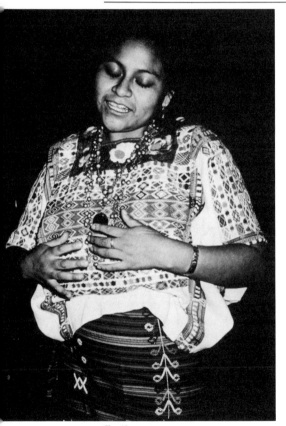

Fig. 12
Rigoberta Menchú. 1985. Photo by Margot Schevill.

pre-Columbian times and of the Spanish Conquest, for the dancers wear immense and colorful headdresses combined with European-style trousers and satin capes.

The last three decades have been a period of great turbulence and unrest for the indigenous peoples of Guatemala, particularly in the northwestern highlands. Large numbers have been forced to leave their villages. Some have been involuntarily relocated in "model camps" by the army; others have fled to refugee camps in Chiapas. Some have been able to take their costume and traditions with them as in the case of the Quiché and Mam speakers who left their villages seventeen years ago because of the lack of work and land. They settled a camp which they named *Manos Unidas* on the Pasión River in Guatemala. In spite of the tropical climate and loss of community, typical highland clothing and customs are still in use (Wilkerson 1985:527).

For those in refugee camps, costume has taken on a political dimension for, in the minds of the Guatemalan military, it associated them with the guerrilla movement, and thus these Maya became targets for violent government reprisals. As a result, costume was abandoned by indigenous peoples who were trying to cross the border into Chiapas. Nevertheless, weaving continues but the communicative message has changed (see fig. 11). Textiles made in refugee camps and in cooperatives within Guatemala are being imported into the United States by religious and charitable organizations in an effort to raise money for these dispossesed peoples and to communicate abroad what disasters have befallen much of the Guatemalan indigenous population.

An example of the multilayered power carried by costume can be found in Tecpán, Chimaltenango, during the most violent period of Guatemalan government repression in the early 1980s. A traditional Maya was the first Indian to be ordained by the Catholic Church. For his ecclesiastical robe he commissioned a native weaver to produce brown cotton cloth made of the highly valued *ixcaco* or *cuyuscate* which is tawny, short-staple cotton used in the ceremonial *huipil* of this area. Then he took it to a *Ladina* embroiderer who decorated it with traditional Catholic iconography (Hendrickson 1985). The message was one of subtle syncretism, a coexistence of Mayan and Catholic meanings, understood and maintained by the Maya since the Conquest (Tedlock 1983:243).

The Mayan people want to maintain their traditions of which costume is an integral part. As Rigoberta Menchú, a Quiché Mayan woman in exile, wrote: "In the eyes of our community, the fact that anyone should ever change the way they dress shows a lack of dignity. Anyone who doesn't dress as our grandfathers, our ancestors, dressed, is on the road to ruin. The ancient Mayan text, the *Popol Vuh*, exhorts: 'Children, wherever you may be, do not abandon the crafts taught to you by Ixpiyacoc because they are crafts passed down from your forefathers. If you forget them, you will be betraying your lineage' " (Burgos-Debray 1984:37,59). Dressed in traditional Mayan costume, Rigoberta realizes that she has become a symbol for her people abroad and gives them courage and belief in the future. "We are weavers of stories and we are weaving a new history for our country as well as our own clothes" (pers. com. 1985; see fig. 12).

III The Art of the Weaver

Before the Conquest, a woman was expected to weave for herself and her family and to produce ceremonial clothes for use in temples and as offerings. A fine weaver had status in the community. During the early years of the Conquest, the *Recopilación de leyes de los reynos de las Indias*, **Book VI, Chapter 10, Law 15 of November 9, 1549, stated:**

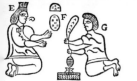

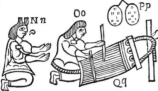

Fig. 13
Codez Mendoza. 1673. Courtesy of the John Carter Brown Library, Brown University.

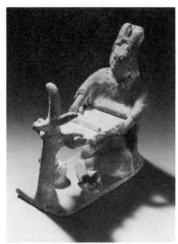

Fig. 14
Backstrap weaver, figurine from Jaina Island, Mexico. Photo by Barbara and Justin Kerr.

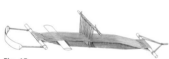

Fig. 15
a. Backstrap weavers. Santa María de Jesús, Guatemala. 1978. Photo by Margot Schevill.
b. Drawing of backstrap loom by Lucretia Nelson (O'Neale 1945).

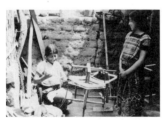

Fig. 17
Plying yarn into balls. Santa María de Jesús, Guatemala. 1978. Photo by Margot Schevill.

Fig. 18
Tarahumara staked loom. Creel, Chihuahua, Mexico. 1971. Photo by Rev. Luis G. Verplancken.

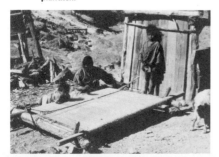

No *encomendero* or other person shall in any case force Indian women to be shut up in corrals or elsewhere to spin and weave the clothing that they are to give as tribute, and they shall have freedom to do this in their houses so that they will not be exploited (Cordry 1968:1).

A fine weaver today has the respect of her village and often contributes extra income to her family through her weaving.

Children learn by imitation, watching their mothers spin, prepare yarn, warp the loom, and weave (see fig. 13). By the age of twelve, they are expected to take weaving seriously. Before that it is like a game, and children are given yarn and weaving implements to play with. One must be accomplished in weaving by the age of sixteen since that is the time for marriage. Rituals accompany the beginning of a new weaving. Women in San Pedro Chenalhó, Chiapas, measure the warp yarns for the loom, and then symbolically "feed" them with beans or maize to ensure that they will not run out (Sayer 1985:152). One mother scolded her daughter who was afraid and trembling at the idea of weaving. She was told that this was women's work and her mother offered candles to the Virgin, asking her to put the art of weaving into her daughter's heart (ibid.:151).

The Loom

The backstrap loom has been in use in Mesoamerica since 1500 B.C. (Conte 1984:13). Among the objects excavated at Chichén Itzá was a loom which may have been ceremonially offered as part of the Cenote cult rituals. Sticks associated with ornamentally incised spindle whorls and textile fragments were also dredged from the well (Lothrop n.d.). Classic Mayan figurines from Jaina Island show the weaver at her backstrap loom (see fig. 14). This loom is sometimes called the hip-loom or stick-loom, and both male and female indigenous weavers produce cloth on this simple apparatus (see fig. 15; 206, 207). A strap is required for support around the waist or hips of the weaver. The other end is attached by rope to a tree or post. Tension in the warp or vertical threads is created by leaning back and forward. This movement allows the creation of sheds so that weft or horizontal threads can be inserted to create cloth. A warp can be woven into a four-selvedge cloth, or, more rarely, cut into smaller pieces depending on the required function of the textile.

In Oaxaca, female weavers use a backstrap loom with a rigid heddle to produce wide, ornamental belts for sale (see fig. 16). In contrast to the labor-intensive warping and weaving process required by the string-heddled loom, the rigid heddle allows the weaver to move ahead more rapidly. Weaving implements utilized for backstrap weaving are few in number. The most important is a finely crafted sword or batten which creates the open shed and can be used as a beater. Other implements include various sticks, shuttles (sometimes of bamboo), and a bone needle to use for picking up threads. Warping can be done on a board with wood pegs or simply on sticks pounded into the earth. Swifts are used for holding yarn while plying or making balls, a job that is relegated to the young or the old who can no longer weave competently (see fig. 17).

Other weavers such as the Tarahumara of Chihuahua utilize a staked, horizontal loom (see fig. 18). Weavers produce a textile with fringe at both ends. By A.D. 700 this loom had been adopted by the Hohokam in the Southwest of the United States and was the precursor to the upright tapestry loom used today by Pueblo and Navajo weavers. The Tarahumara also produce wide sashes and belts on a smaller version of the horizontal loom.

The Spaniards introduced the floor or treadle-loom into the New World. Weaving on this type of loom, usually done in a small workplace, was a male-oriented task in Spain and was taught to indigenous males who soon learned how to produce yardage, a requisite for the cut-and-sew tailored fashions of the Spanish. Today, Zapotec male weavers in Teotitlán del Valle,

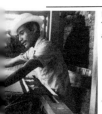

Fig. 19
Treadle loom weaver. Teotitlán del Valle, Oaxaca, Mexico. 1973. Photo by Clare Brett Smith.

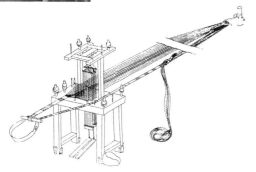

Fig. 20
Combined treadle and backstrap loom for weaving hair ribbons. Drawing by Lucretia Nelson (O'Neale 1945).

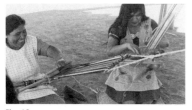

Fig. 16
Rigid heddle loom weavers. Santo Tomás, Oaxaca, Mexico, 1977. Photo by Clare Brett Smith.

4 In the Andes, eucalyptus is burned and textiles are held over the fire to absorb the smoke given off, which produces a dark, black color as well as a refreshing odor (Sakiestewa pers. com., 1985).

Oaxaca, use treadle looms to produce lightly textured woolen rugs that are a popular export (see fig. 19). Weft-, complex-, and double-ikat cloth is woven on treadle looms in Salcajá, Quezaltenango, for sale to highland Maya for use as wraparound skirts. *Ladinas* also weave on the treadle loom, even though this occupation has been stereotyped as predominantly male (Schevill 1980:11). A unique loom is used to create hair ribbons or *cintas* in Totonicapán. It combines features of both the backstrap and treadle loom (see fig. 20). Two other imports, the draw loom and the jacquard loom, can produce yardage of great complexity.

Materials

Cotton has been the most important fiber for weavers since pre-Columbian times. In 1566, Bishop Landa noted its characteristics in *Relación de las cosas de Yucatán*.

Cotton is gathered in wonderful quantity and grows in all parts of the land and there are two kinds of it. One they sow every year and its little tree does not last more than a year and is very small. The stalk of the other lasts five or six years and bears its fruit every year, which are pods like walnuts with a green shell which opens in four parts in due time and contains the cotton (Tozzer 1941:200).

These two varieties are *Gossypium hirsutum*, a long-staple white cotton, and *Gossypium mexicanum*, a short-staple, tawny-colored cotton known as *ixcaq*, *ixcaco*, or *cuyuscate*. The longer stapled white cotton became the most popular with weavers for it was more easily spun than *cuyuscate*. Both are still in use. *Gossypium hirsutum* is now factory-spun, while hand-spun *Gossypium mexicanum* is reserved for ceremonial garments, as in the *sobre-huipil* of Comalapa, Chimaltenango, Guatemala.

Agave, yucca, and other vegetal fibers were in use at the time of the Conquest. Dyed rabbit hair and feathers were integrated into Aztec weavings. With the introduction of sheep by the Spanish in the sixteenth century, wool was readily adopted by native weavers for its warmth, its sturdy and thick texture, and its ability to take dye. These fibers are still utilized along with imported silk floss, pearl cotton, assorted embroidery cottons, and synthetic yarns.

Attempts have failed to detect the presence of dyes on cloth fragments from the Sacred Cenote of Chichén Itzá. However, information derived from historical sources and Mayan dictionaries gives an idea of the range of colors available to sixteenth-century Mayan peoples. Indigo or *chot* produced a blue dye or paint that was considered ceremonial. Brazil wood or red wood was "good for house beams...cut up fine and thrown into water, it turns to blood." It was known as *chacte* or *palo colorado*. Red worm or cochineal was used for medicinal purposes, but its value as a dye could hardly have gone unnoticed. *Palo de tinta* or *Ek*, known as logwood, gave forth black, blue, and purple dyes. *Kuxub*-can or coral was an herb whose berry yielded a red dye. *Tzitz* or *Bailey*, a perennial, also gave a purple dye used in ceremonial contexts. *Zabac-che*, *falso quina*, or Princewood was burned[4] and the smoke produced a dark dye (Lothrop n.d.).

To this repertoire, one might add red-brown. Research carried on by Robert Carlsen of the University of Colorado Museum on the cotton shroud excavated from Tomb 19 at Rio Azul, Guatemala, revealed the possiblility of cinnabar as a colorant. It is believed that this tomb dates from between A.D. 450 and 500, seven hundred and fifty years before the Cenote rituals of Chichén Itzá (Adams 1986:445).

Additional information about coloring techniques derives from "image clothing" on the Bonampak murals and codices (Miller 1986). These images suggest that textiles were painted with designs and that tie-dye and ikat techniques were known. Ikat or *jaspeado* is a flourishing textile art practiced by contemporary textile makers in Mexico and Guatemala, using both wool and cotton (154, 211).

Certain colors projected symbolic meanings as Sylvanus Morley, an expert on the ancient Maya, postulated. Blue was associated with sacrifice, black for weapons and war, red for blood. Yellow was the color of corn and represented food. Colors were also related to the four cardinal points: red for East, white to the North, black to the West, and yellow for the South. Green was the *axis mundi* that served as a central pole that pierced the layers of the universe (Morley 1956:383).

Synthetic dyes became available in the Southwest of the United States by the 1860s and probably traveled quickly to Middle America. In 1876, an electric mill was in operation in Cantel, Quezaltenango, which produced pre-spun and pre-dyed yarn for highland Mayan weavers. In the early twentieth century weavers used a few natural and synthetic dyes in a way that gave only a limited color range (Schevill 1986:35). As the availability of brightly colored yarn increased, the palette of indigenous weavers expanded rapidly. Rainbow coloring is a predictable and enjoyable aspect of mid-twentieth-century costume and textiles.

Since the 1970s, external pressure from dealers, tourists, and other interested persons has been exerted on some weavers to try natural sources for dyes. The most successful venture of this kind is taking place in Chiapas, under the guidance of Walter F. Morris, Jr., with Tzeltal and Tzotzil weavers. A cooperative, Sna Jolobil, was formed and weavers are experimenting with natural dyes and older textile designs with satisfying results (see 59 and pl. 1, 60).

Techniques and Iconography

The Cenote Fragments

Over six hundred textile fragments recovered from the Sacred Cenote of Chichén Itzá provide greatest insight into the technical accomplishments of the pre-Hispanic weavers. Single cotton fibers were always spun in a Z or right-to-left direction, and when two-ply yarn was desired, two Z-spun yarns were plied in the S or left-to-right direction. Agave and bast fibers were spun in an S direction. These spinning practices have persisted to present times.

In pre-Columbian times, basic cloth or plain weave was produced with a numerical dominance of warp over weft threads (O'Neale 1942:4). The Cenote fragments were woven with predominantly single warps while the weft could be singles or pairs. The following list presents the techniques noted in the Cenote fragments (Lothrop n.d.).

warp, weft stripes	embroidery
plaids	tufted cloth (pile of looped wefts)
twills (compound, diamond, broken)	tapestry (slit, wrapped)
	transposed warps
supplementary weft inlays	gauze with weft inlays
supplementary warps (few)	open work (weft wrapped, woven slit, bound warp)
warp floats	knotted warps

It is interesting to note that the Rio Azul shroud, referred to earlier, was woven with an open-work or gauze-weave construction, similar to some of the Cenote fragments and to open-work, white-on-white weaves being produced today in Alta Verapaz, Guatemala, and Chiapas and Oaxaca, Mexico (Adams 1986:436; 27, 139–141).

Textile trims included individually constructed borders, tassels, and braids that were affixed to the textile. No examples of netting or double cloth were found among the Cenote fragments, but an example of the latter was discovered at the Post-Classic site of Mayapán.

Techniques of Today

All the techniques present in the Cenote fragments are still being produced by Middle American weavers. Many are present in the Haffenreffer Museum collection as will be noted. Warp-predominant cloth with supplementary weft brocading is the most frequently represented combination. It is a technique for decorating cloth while still on the loom. Three types of brocading are in use. Single-faced produces a pattern recognizable on only one side. In two-faced brocading, the yarn floats on the reverse side be-

Fig. 21
a. single-faced brocading. b. Two-faced brocading. c. Double-faced brocading.

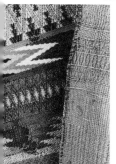 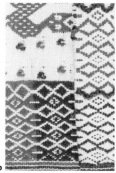

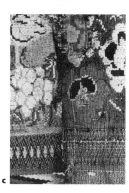

tween pattern areas forming an inverse of the design. Double-faced brocading presents a nearly identical pattern visible on the front and back of the weaving (see fig. 21).

The existence of double-faced brocading is mentioned in a story found in the *Popol Vuh* relating to clan images assigned to the lords by the gods. The lords, who founded the three leading matrilineages, wore cloaks with animals represented on them that were woven into the cloth. The figures were placed *chuwach*, "on the face," or single-faced brocading. Elsewhere in this story these images are described as being *chupam*, "on the inside," or double-faced brocading (Tedlock and Tedlock 1985:124).

Weavers may also add a mark into the cloth, a substitute for the initials or names which sometimes appear. These marks may be weft or warp stripes, animal or bird images, or some other imaginative sign (see 111, 183, 203, and pl. 14, 220, 224).

Iconography is varied. Geometric shapes, plants, animals, and other realistic images are woven in a representational, stylized, or abstract fashion. The precise meaning of these designs to the weavers may never be known, but textile researchers frequently pursue this topic. In his analysis of highland Mayan weaving from Chiapas, Morris suggests that a mythical history is woven into textiles, and that a weaver's world vision can be deciphered by the organization of designs on her *huipil*. From Morris' standpoint, for the Maya, costume is memory (Morris 1984:55).

Hearne has related design motifs, among other stylistic elements, to four major language groupings in the Guatemalan highlands: Mamean, Kanjobal, Pocom, and Quichean. She found an affinity for certain design combinations within a linguistic grouping even though the speakers may not live in close geographic proximity to each other (Hearne 1985:84–87).

Muestras or samplers are another means for sharing designs for weaving or embroidery (71). Worn-out fragments of cloth also perpetuate design traditions.

Additional techniques used to adorn and create textiles include beading, embroidery, knitting, and crocheting. Two copper bells and some shells were found in context with the Cenote fragments, suggesting a type of surface decoration similar to beading (11). Pre-Columbian weavers were already skilled in embroidery, but new techniques such as cross-stitch were taught by the Spanish nuns. Crocheting and knitting were taught to Mayan men by the Spaniards (Conte 1984:19). Bags, *bolsas* or *morrales*, are still being knitted, crocheted, beaded, and cross-stitched by males (11, 12, 98, 175). The Mayan men embroider designs on their costumes and on their wives' belts (see 126, 130, and pl. 13). Commercial trims replace what was formerly accomplished by hand.

IV The Middle American Textile Catalogue

Catalogue data will follow this format:

Native name
Object

Entry number

> **Department: Town or village**
> **Linguistic affiliation**
> **Source**
> Dimensions: inches and centimeters
> • Yarn make-up
> Fabrication
>
> **Iconography**
> **Comments**
> Haffenreffer Museum number
> References cited
> See **Internal References** to textiles in the collection

Entry number is the catalogue number and the textile referred to by this number within the text.

Object is identified in English and in Spanish.

Department is the state in which the village or town is located.

Town or village is where the textile was purchased or manufactured.

Source indicates the name (if there are only a few donations) or the initials of the donor, the collection date if known, and the museum accession date, which often postdates the acquisition.

Dimensions are presented with the length first, then the width, sleeve measurements not included. For *hats*, the length refers to the depth of the crown, the width relates to the diameter of the brim. For *skirts*, the measurement of the waist is the width even though some are a flexible gathered style. For *ponchos*, the length from shoulder to hem is recorded, or one-half of the actual length of the textile.

Yarn make-up includes several indices: the type of yarn, ply, spin, color, and warp and weft count. Cotton is used most in Middle America. The most common is mercerized, factory-produced, called *mish* which comes in two- and three-ply. Embroidery yarns of a wide variety include *artisela* (artificial silk), *sedalina* (pearl cotton), *manchada* and *ombra* (space-dyed cotton), and *lustrina* (multicotton threads unplied). All yarn is machine-spun unless otherwise indicated. *Color* is created by synthetic dyes unless otherwise noted; cochineal and indigo are natural dyes still utilized. The word natural has not been included for the color of wool since primarily the yarn is undyed.

The warp and weft count or sett is given in inches and centimeters: epi and epc mean ends (warps) per inch and centimeter; ppi and ppc mean picks (wefts) per inch and centimeter; gauge for knitted textiles is spi and spc, which mean stitches per inch and centimeter.

Fabrication refers to the method utilized to create the textile, including cut-and-sew tailoring if present; most *randas* are in buttonhole stitch unless otherwise indicated.

Iconography is included where appropriate.

Comments derive from field notes, personal communication, textile analysts, primary and secondary sources, and the initials of the contributor are placed within parentheses. Otherwise the voice is that of the author.

The flow of the catalogue section is from the north of Mexico to the south of Guatemala, following the provenience of the textiles (see map). Because the bulk of this collection dates from the last thirty years, references have been consulted that deal with textiles from a similar time frame.

Initials are as follows.

OAG	Olga Arriola Geng		**JP**	Jone Pasha
E&JD	Edward and Jane Dwyer		**RP**	Ron Podell
CWH	Carl W. Haffenreffer		**FS**	Fern Sandhouse
DH	Dwight Heath		**MS**	Margot Schevill
WFM	Walter F. Morris, Jr.		**C&BS**	Clare and Burges Smith
			JS	Joyce Smith
			P&ES	Polly and Erwin Strasmich
			WT	Mr. and Mrs. William Traver

COSTUME AS COMMUNICATION

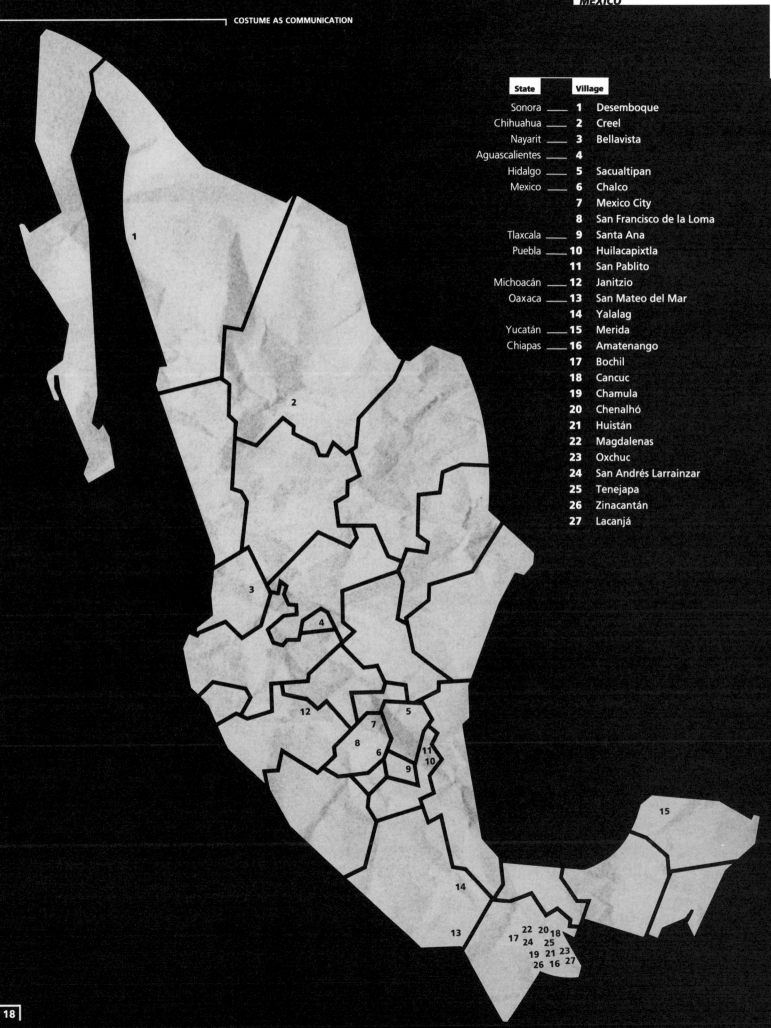

State		Village
Sonora	1	Desemboque
Chihuahua	2	Creel
Nayarit	3	Bellavista
Aguascalientes	4	
Hidalgo	5	Sacualtipan
Mexico	6	Chalco
	7	Mexico City
	8	San Francisco de la Loma
Tlaxcala	9	Santa Ana
Puebla	10	Huilacapixtla
	11	San Pablito
Michoacán	12	Janitzio
Oaxaca	13	San Mateo del Mar
	14	Yalalag
Yucatán	15	Merida
Chiapas	16	Amatenango
	17	Bochil
	18	Cancuc
	19	Chamula
	20	Chenalhó
	21	Huistán
	22	Magdalenas
	23	Oxchuc
	24	San Andrés Larrainzar
	25	Tenejapa
	26	Zinacantán
	27	Lacanjá

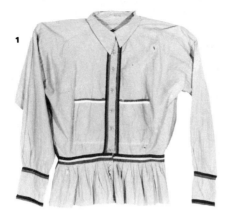

SONORA

Blouse

1

Sonora: Desemboque
Seri
Mrs. Mona Dayton   1970s   1973
21½" x 20"   (54.5cm x 51cm)
commercial cloth, rust
• *trims*: rickrack, tape hand-stitched, peplum at
waist.

**Semi-Victorian style, adopted at end of 19th
century, missionary influence.**

73–72
Johnston 1970
Sayer 1985:190
Cordry 1968:193–197
Fontana 1977:125–138

CHIHUAHUA

Blanket

2

Chihuahua: Creel
Tarahumara
CWH   1970s   1971
85½" x 64"   (217cm x 162cm)
• *warp*: wool, singles; brown, black; 7 epi (3 epc)
• *weft*: wool, singles; brown, yellow, orange,
white, red, green; 15 ppi (7 ppc)
Horizontal loom-woven; weft-faced plain weave;
tapestry-woven stars, weft stripes; braided fringe.

**Soft texture; worn around body Navajo-style
for warmth.**

71–5206

Blouse

3

Chihuahua: Creel
Tarahumara
CWH   1970s   1971
18¼" x 15"   (48cm x 39cm)
commercial cloth
Floral, green ribbon trim. Hand-stitched, set-in
sleeves, shoulder opening with buttons, ribbon
added on sleeve edges and cuffs.

See 1 for comments.

71–5206
See **9, 10**   Female Costume

Headband

4

Chihuahua: Creel
Tarahumara
CWH   1970s   1971
41¼" x ⅔"   (105cm x 1.5cm)
• *warp*: cotton, wool, 2-ply; red, yellow, blue,
white; 36 epi (16 epc)
• *weft*: cotton, 2-ply; white; 32 ppi (8 ppc)
Belt-loom woven; 2-color complementary warp-
faced plain weave; three 3-color braids.

**Similar techniques to *hakimas* of Central
Andes (see 421).**

71–5307
See **5**

Headband

5

Chihuahua: Creel
Tarahumara
CWH   1970s   1971
55" x 34"   (140cm x 2cm)
• *warp*: cotton, 2-ply, singles in pairs; red, white;
56 epi (20 epc)
• *weft*: cotton, 2-ply; multicolored; 14 ppi (5 ppc)
See **4** for fabrication.

**Iconography: geometric forms.
Worn by men and women with or without
head cloth.**

71–5211
See **4**

Sash, male

6

Chihuahua: Creel
Tarahumara
CWH   1970s   1971
104½" x 4½"   (265cm x 11cm)
• *warp*: wool, singles, handspun; brown, red, gold,
green, pink; 30 epi (12 epc)
• *weft*: wool, singles, handspun; dark brown;
10 ppi (4 ppc)
Horizontal belt-loomed; warp-faced plain weave;
2-color complementary pick-up; cut warp forms 8
braids of 4 strands with tassels, twined ends.

Iconography: geometric forms.

71–5305
Beardsley 1985:39–73
See **7**

Sash, male

7

Chihuahua: Creel
Tarahumara
CWH   1970s   1971
85" x 2½"   (24cm x 6cm)
• *warp*: wool, handspun singles; brown, white,
mustard, rust; 30 epi (12 epc)
• *weft*: wool, handspun singles; brown; 7 ppi
(3 ppc)
See **6** for fabrication; seven 2-color braids with 4
strands.

**Iconography: geometric forms.
Worn wrapped twice around the waist.**

71–5208
Beardsley 1985:39–73
See **6**

7

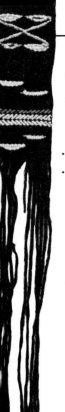

pascola

Sash, male

8

Chihuahua: Creel
Tarahumara
Gino Conti 1940–1950 1985
125½" x 3" (316cm x 7.5cm)
• *warp*: wool, handspun singles; black; 40 epi (16 epc)
• *weft*: wool, handspun singles; black, red, yellow; 25 ppi (10 ppc)
Horizontal belt-loomed; twill weave; cut warp forms thirteen 4-strand braids on each end; colored yarn creates weft geometric designs.

Worn for *Pascola* dances. *Pascola* dancers are individualists who perform as a result of dreamed visions (Fontana 1977:18).

85–788

Shawl

9

Chihuahua: Creel
Tamahumara
CHW 1970s 1971
73" x 64" (175cm x 161cm)
commercial cloth or *manta*, cotton; cotton embroidery thread, multicolored
A large white cloth sparsely embroidered with flowers and animals; some designs not completed.

To be worn around shoulders or as headdress (Fontana 1977:81). Embroidery personalizes bought cloth (Sayer 1985:154).

71–5205
See **3, 10** Female Costume

Skirt

10

Chihuahua: Creel
Tamahumara
CHW 1970s 1971
25" x 141" (63cm x 353cm)
commercial cotton cloth, plaid; yellow, blue, white
Hand-sewn; decorative tape on belt, hem, and skirt; gathered at waist.

71–5207
See **3, 9** Female Costume

NAYARIT

bolsa

Bag

11

Nayarit: Bellavista
Huichol
Museum Purchase 1980s 1983
7" x 6½" (17cm x 16.5cm)
• *straps*: 37" x ¾" (94cm x 2cm)
• *medallion*: 2½" x 2¼" (6.5cm x 6cm)
• *chain*: 23" x 1" (58cm x 2.5)
nylon thread, yellow and black beads, black and yellow wool; 25 ppi (10 ppc)
Lined with natural muslin; netted; strap woven on belt loom, six woolen pom-poms.

Iconography: double-headed eagle motifs surrounded with stars.
Agave, a vegetal fiber, was originally used for netting; bags take place of pockets; glass beads, called *chaquira*, replaced seeds and berries.

83–17
A,B,C,D,F (bracelet & ring included)
Sayer 1985:16,17,59,64,190,202,205
See **12**

bolsa

Bag

12

Nayarit: Bellavista
Huichol
DH 1950s 1961
8¾" x 8" (23.5cm x 20cm)
• *straps*: belt-loomed; 2 at 23½" x 1" (60cm x 2cm)
• *warp*: cotton, singles; white; 45 epi (18 epc)
• *weft*: same as warp; 55 ppi (22 ppc)
• *embroidery*: cotton, 2-ply; green, blue, yellow
• *straps*: wool; 2-ply; red, green, blue; plain-weave; cross-stitching, 2 wrapped tassels

Typical specimen, diagonal bands of cross-stitched Greek key motif, non-symbolic colors. Emphasis on overall design but disregard for uniformity in detail. Worn on one shoulder and crossing to opposite hip: used for carrying miscellaneous personal possessions, as many as eight may be worn at one time, the number serving as an index of wearer's socio-economic status. All costume items made by women (DH). Boys sometimes learn to cross-stitch (Sayer 1985:81).

61–2120
Sayer 1985:181
See **13, 14** Male Costume

sombrero

Hat

13

Nayarit: Bellavista
Huichol
DH 1950s 1961
4" x 14" (10cm x 35cm)
palm leaf, wool, glass beads, white commercial tape strap
Orange, yellow, green, red, violet, pink. Twill-plaited strips, single layer, stitched in spiral to form wide brim and short conical crown. Yarn pom-poms with glass beads on rim, yarn decoration.

Unmarried men often decorate crown of hat with playing cards (DH).

61–2119
See **12, 14** Male Costume

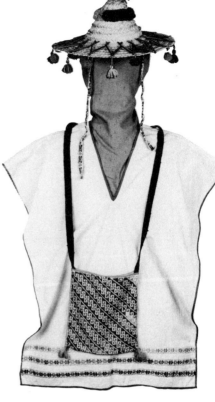

Male Costume 12–14

joronga

Shirt

14

Nayarit: Bellavista
Huichol
DH 1950s 1961
30" x 24" (76cm x 61cm)
commercial cotton, actually a sugar bag
Commercial tape, on outside edges and neck, three rows on front and back; side seams open.

A pre-Columbian dress form survival; a short tunic or *ehuatl*. Paucity of *manta* nowadays so use sugar sacks; printed inside "Vendido por U.S. P.A.S.A., Ingenio Bellavista, Santa Ana, Jal. Azucar granulado estandar blanco." Huichol created legend about *manta* "1930's, orders of their god, Sun Father, Mexicans cultivated cotton and North Americans started factories to make cloth" (Sayer 1985:154).

61–2116
See **12, 13** Male Costume & **88, 89, 90**

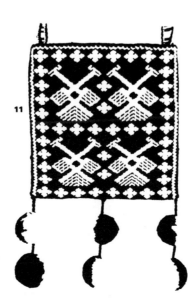

11

faja
Sash, female

17

Mexico: Chalco
Spanish/Mexica
DH   1950s   1961
88" x 6"   (224cm x 15cm)
• *warp*: cotton, 3 singles; blue, white; 64 epi
(28 epc)
• *weft*: cotton, multiple singles; blue; 8 ppi (4 ppc)
Belt-loomed, warp-faced plain weave; cut warps
create 5" fringe on each end.

**Wrapped tightly around skirt and ends
tucked in; a new style gaining popularity is
"tailored" – same cloth cut to approximate
waist length and fitted with hook-and-eye
closure (DH).**

61–2140
See **18, 19** Female Costume

Detail **15**

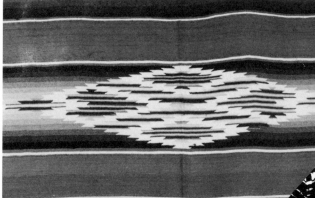

AGUASCALIENTES

sarape
Blanket

15

Aguascalientes: Aguascalientes type
Spanish
G. Bray   unknown   1975
88" x 40½"   (22cm x 103cm)
• *warp*: cotton, 2-ply; white; 36 epi, (12 epc)
• *weft*: wool, singles in pairs, 4-ply; multicolored;
30–45 ppi (12–18 ppc)
Treadle-loomed, weft-faced plain weave, tapestry
technique for motifs; delicate macramé fringe

Iconography: center diamond motif, weft-
striped patterning.
No opening for head, space-dyed yarns utilized.

72–263
Start 1948:83
Sayer 1985:102

HIDALGO

sombrero
Hat

16

Hidalgo: Sacualtipan
Huastec
DH   1950s   1961
5" x 18"   (13cm x 46cm)
palm fiber, cotton cord
Twill plaiting of strips, stitched in spiral to form
broad brim and high crown, usually thick. Cotton
cord running through rim, bow tie in back of rim.

**Is virtually the only handcraft product which
is distinctive of the Huastec, a member of the
Mayan linguistic family (DH).**

61–2114

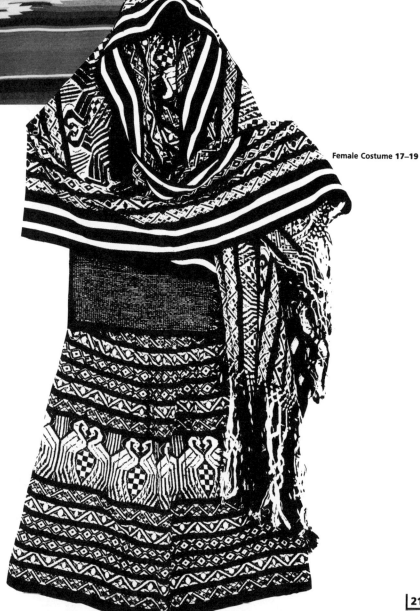

Female Costume 17–19

enagua

| Skirt |

18

Mexico: Chalco
Spanish/Mexica
DH 1950s 1961
25½" x 25" (65cm x 64cm)
• *warp*: cotton, singles in pairs, 2-ply; black, white;
40 epi (10 epc)
• *weft*: same as warp; 22 ppi (8 ppc)
• *supplementary weft*: same as warp, white
Treadle-loomed; warp-predominant plain weave;
machine-stitched, set in waist-band.

Iconography: band of stylized pairs of
birds.
Produced by *Ladinos*, for sale in markets;
"fancy" festive wear, workaday ones less ornate (DH).

61–2138
See **17, 19** Female Costume

rebozo

| Shawl |

19

Mexico: Chalco
Spanish/Mexica
DH 1950s 1961
65½" x 27½" (174cm x 70cm)
See **18** for cloth analysis.
Continuous warp creates 12" knotted fringe on
each end.
61–2139
See **17, 18** Female Costume

faja

| Sash, male |

20

Mexico: Chalco
Spanish/Mexica
DH 1950s 1961
84" x 3" (239cm x 7cm)
• *warp*: cotton, four singles; white, blue-black;
40 epi (16 epc)
• *weft*: cotton, fifty singles; white; 12 ppi (5 ppc)
Belt-loomed; warp-faced plain weave; narrow
blue-black stripes near selvedge; yarn may have
been stiffened with *atole*, a corn drink.

**Wrapped tightly around trousers and tucked
in; same new style appearing in men's sashes
as in women's (see 17) (DH).**

61–2141

blusa

| Blouse |

21

Mexico: Mexico City
Spanish
WT 1970s 1972
26¾" x 27" (68cm x 68cm)
commercial cotton cloth, *manta*, white
Tailored, machine-stitched, embroidered by hand,
satin stitch, multicolored silk, hem-stitched
edging; panels with gussets under arm; floral, eagle with snake in mouth, "Viva Mexico."

**National Costume of non-indigenous Mexico
until recent times; *mestizo* idea of femininity.
Indian maids from villages tried to replicate
dress of their mistresses; nowadays "fancy"
dress or for fiestas.**

72–2366 B
Sayer 1985:108–109
Pierce 1985:30
See **22, 23, 24** Female Costume, *China Poblana*

faja

| Sash |

22

Mexico: Mexico City
Spanish
WT 1970s 1972
58" x 3½" (147.5cm x 9cm)
• *warp*: silk, 2-ply; light green, rose, white; 150 epi
(60 epc)
• *weft*: same as warp; green; 25 ppi (10 ppc)
Belt-loomed; warp-faced plain weave; cut warps
create macramé fringe on both ends.

72–2366 C
See **21** for comments, references.
See **21, 23, 24** Female Costume, *China Poblana*

rebozo

| Shawl |

23

Mexico: Mexico City
Spanish
WT 1970s 1972
104" x 30" (264cm x 76cm)
• *warp*: cotton, singles; black; 60 epi (24 epc)
• *weft*: silk, untwisted; white, green, salmon;
45 ppi (18 ppc)
Treadle-loomed, warp-predominant plain weave
weft floats, two-faced brocading; warp ends tied
off, weft threads added to make macramé fringe.

Iconography: geometric forms.

72–2366 D
See **21** for comments, references.
See **21, 22, 24** Female Costume, *China Poblana*

enagua

| Skirt |

24

Mexico: Mexico City
Spanish
WT 1970s 1972
36" x 34" (91cm x 86cm)
Commercial cotton cloth; green, red, stamped
with patterns.

Iconography: image of an eagle holding a
serpent.
Gathered at waist, machine-stitched, decorated with sequins, glass beads.

72–2366 A
See **21** for comments, references.
See **21, 22, 23** Female Costume, *China Poblana*

rebozo

| Shawl |

25

Mexico: San Francisco de la Loma
Mazahua
Museum Purchase 1980s 1983
68¼" x 19" (173cm x 48cm)
• *warp*: wool, 2-ply; grey; 20 epi (8 epc)
• *weft*: same as warp; 20 ppi (8 ppc)
Backstrap-loomed, balanced plain weave, 4
loom-finished selvedges; white wool macramé
fringe added to both ends; surface decoration of
embroidery, cross-stitch in black, white 2-ply wool.

**Contemporary adaptation, made-for-sale, tra-
ditional cross-stitch technique of Mazahua; *rebozo* originated with *mestizos*, possibly derived from priests urging women to cover
heads when entering church, now used by all
classes.**

83–20
Sayer 1985:106
Goodman 1976:42

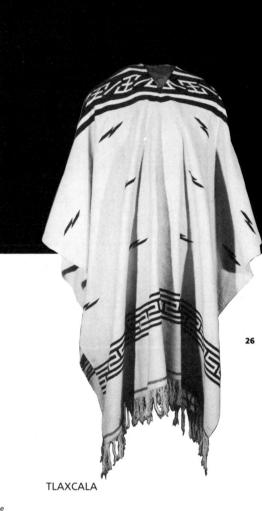

26

TLAXCALA

sarape

| Poncho |

26

Tlaxcala: Santa Ana
Otomi
DH 1960s 1961
44½" x 51" (118cm. x 130cm.)
• *warp*: wool, handspun singles; white; 13 epi 5
(epc)
• *weft*: wool, handspun singles; white, dark brown;
70 ppi (26 ppc)
Treadle-loomed; weft-faced plain weave; tapestry
inlay, warp fringes on both ends, head-hole created on loom.

Iconography: geometric motifs, weft bands,
diamond at neck.

This community is a center for extremely
varied weaving on a large-scale commercial
basis, involving several factories in which *Ladinos* employ as many as 15 Indian weavers;
this poncho produced for local use; design
distinctive of this community; relatively
affluent people of Santa Ana are virtually
only Otomi to use ponchos (DH).

61–2170

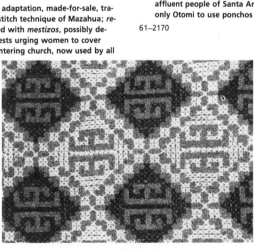

Detail 25

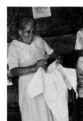

blusa, huipil
Blouse

29

Michoacán: Janitzio
Tarascan
DH   1950s   1961
22" x 25½"   (56cm x 65cm)
trade muslin
Tailored, set-in sleeves; white; 2-ply cotton, crochet neck and bodice; pink; drawn work on
sleeves; cuffs of sleeves embroidered.

> **Iconography: two goats eating at bush.**
> **Sleeve drawn-work accomplished by taking**
> **out individual threads from cloth, regrouping**
> **rest, edge bound, reinforced with decorative**
> **stitching; also known as needle weaving**
> **(Goodman 1976:74). Fine workmanship, worn**
> **on festive occasions; workaday blouse is simi-**
> **lar but embroidered without drawn-work**
> **(DH).**

61–2200
Goodman 1976:20, 74–75
Lechuga 1982:192–194
Sayer 1985:86
See **30**   Female Costume

falda
Skirt

30

Michoacán: Janitzio
Tarascan
DH   1950s
1961
75" x 35"   (190cm x 89cm)
• *warp*: wool, handspun singles; deep blue; 25 epi
(10 epc)
• *weft*: same as warp; 12 ppi (5ppc)
Backstrap-loomed, 4 selvedges, balanced plain
weave.

> **Woven by specialists. Worn tightly gathered**
> **around waist, supported with broad woolen**
> **sash (pink is in vogue); older women often**
> **wear this cloth as half-skirt with petticoat**
> **and white muslin apron (DH).**

61–2201
See **29**   Female Costume

OAXACA

faja
Sash

31

Oaxaca: unknown
Spanish
Museum education program
68½" x 3½"   (174cm x 9cm)
• *warp*: cotton, 2-ply, three singles; white, deep
blue, light brown; 30 epi (12 epc)
• *weft*: cotton, multiple groups of singles; white;
12 ppi (5 ppc)
• *supplementary warp*: cotton, 12 singles, slightly
twisted; light brown, deep blue; over 3–8 wefts
Belt-loomed, warp-faced plain weave, striped
boarders, warp floats create designs; cut warps
create four 3-color braids on both ends.

> **Atypical textile, probably created for sale to**
> **tourists, realistic male and female figures,**
> **carelessly woven, floats too long, loose ten-**
> **sion.**

74–75

27

PUEBLA

quechquémitl
Shoulder poncho

27

Puebla: Huilacapixtla
Nahua
Museum Purchase   unknown   1985
22" x 25"   (56cm x 64cm)
• *warp*: cotton, 2-ply; white; 30 epi (12 epc)
• *weft*: cotton, 2, 3, singles & single 2-ply; white;
35 ppi (14 ppc)
Backstrap-woven; gauze-weave bands alternating
with weft-faced plain weave bands giving seersucker effect; every 4th row 3 wefts are inserted
creating an undulating effect; 2 ends
loom-finished, 2 ends hand-sewn; 2 pieces joined
on the diagonal.

> **A pre-Columbian dress form survival, Type II**
> **(Cordry 1968:83).**

85–484
Cordry 1968:95
See **28, 140**

quechquémitl
Shoulder poncho

28

Puebla: San Pablito
Otomi
Museum Purchase   unknown   1985
26½" x 35"   (68cm x 89cm)
• *warp*: cotton, 2-ply; white; 80 epi (32 epc)
• *weft*: same as warp; 20 ppi (8 ppc); wool, singles; purple-orange, black; over 4 warps.
Two backstrap-woven pieces, warp-faced ground
cloth with weft-faced twill bands; loom-finished
and hemmed selvedges; rounded shape produced
on a loom.

> **A pre-Columbian dress form survival; curved**
> **weaving unknown outside of Americas, Type**
> **II (Cordry 1968:83). Cross-stitch decoration**
> **adorns more elaborate examples.**

85–485
Cordry 1968:94
Sayer 1985:146,178,165
See **27**

Ladina embroiderer doing drawn work. Aran-
za, Michoacán. 1973. Photo by Clare Brett
Smith. See **29**.

31

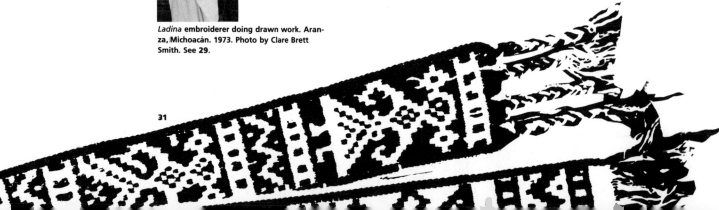

servilleta

Cloth, carrying

32

Oaxaca: San Mateo del Mar
Huave
DH   1960s   1961
37" x 30¼"   (94cm x 77cm)
• *warp*: cotton, singles in pairs; white; 32 epi
(13 epc)
• *weft*: same as warp; 20 ppi (8 ppc)
• *supplementary weft*: cotton, 6 singles; red; over
2–23 warps
Backstrap-loomed, warp-predominant plain
weave, single-faced supp. weft brocading, striped
borders, cut warps create fringe of twisted stiff
yarn.

Overall ornamentation includes repeated
small stylized deer, dog, bird, feline (*tigre*),
horned man (*diablo*), geometric motifs. Used
by women for carrying miscellaneous bur-
dens, especially food (DH). Pride of San
Mateo Huave weavers. Images appear in
white on reverse side of cloth.

61–2115
Cordry 1968:323–329

huipil

Long blouse

33

Oaxaca: Yalalag
Zapotec
C&BS   1970s   1985
37" x 33"   (94cm x 84cm)
• *warp*: cotton, pairs of 2-ply; white; 30 epi
(12 epc)
• *weft*: same as warp; 13 ppi (5 ppc)
Backstrap-loomed, warp-faced plain weave with
weft floats in shoulder area creating contrasting
texture; two pieces joined by wide *randas* of
multicolored rayon yarn, mutiple strands of 2 and
3-ply; rayon yarn braided with long fringes, sewn
onto front and back.

Neck decorated to protect cotton *huipiles*, removed when washed as rayon yarn colors
run (Sayer 1985:133). The neck decoration, a
"cross bar" and textural pattern in shoulder
area are present in a miniature *huipil* found
in a Mixteca Alta cave, in Oaxaca; possibly of
pre-Columbian origin (Johnson 1967:188).

85–174
Jopling 1975
Cordry 1968:260–265

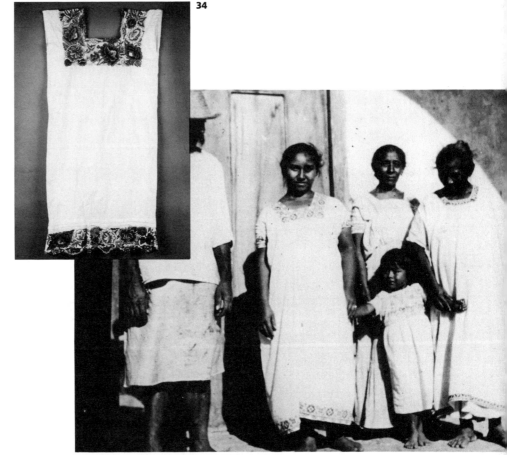

34

Group of Yucatec Maya, Yucatán. 1920–1930.
Herbert J. Spinden Photo Archives, Haffenreffer Museum of Anthropology.

YUCATÁN

huipil

Long blouse

34

Yucatán: unknown
Yucatec
JP   1970s   1985
88" x 20"   (96cm x 50cm)
commercial cloth, *manta*; white; one long piece
machine-stitched at sides; tucks above hem; head-
hole cut out; embroidered at neck and hem;
multicolored cotton, satin stitched.

Iconography: floral designs.
To be worn over long, white ruffled skirt.
Described as "de mestiza," worn on festive
occasions by non-Indians (Sayer 1985:156).

85–789
See **35, 36**

huipil

Long blouse

35

Yucatán: unknown
Yucatec
Museum education program   1985
36" x 29"   (91cm x 74cm)
See **34** for materials, fabrication.

Head-hole not cut out; floral designs drawn
on cloth with pen; not all embroidered.

85–790
See **34, 36**

huipil

Long blouse

36

Yucatán: Merida
Yucatec
MS   1983   1985
40" x 21½"   (102cm x 55cm)
commercial cloth, *manta*, light pink
One long piece, machine-stitched, with set-in
sleeves; band of gauze embroidered with multicolored cotton in satin stitch; sewn to neck, head-
hole cut out; multicolored cotton, gold and white
cotton crochet around band and on sleeves.

Iconography: geometric floral forms.

87–791
See **34, 35**

CHIAPAS

huipil

Blouse

37

Chiapas: Amatenango
Tzeltal
DH   1960s   1961
54" x 29"   (136cm x 74cm)
• *warp*: cotton, singles in pairs; white; 45 epi
(18 epc)
• *weft*: cotton, 3 singles; white; 33 ppi (13 ppc)
Backstrap-loomed; warp-predominant plain
weave; one piece; head-hole cut out; hemmed on
ends and sides; embroidered in satin stitch; *artisela*, artificial silk floss, and cotton in gold and red
decorate the neck area; long floats are fragile.

Iconography: rectangular blocks.
Women do not weave but embroider; are
acclaimed as fine potters (Sayer 1985:160).

61–2236
See **38**

37

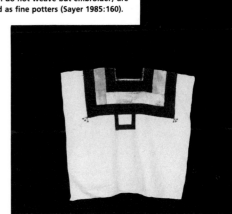

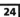

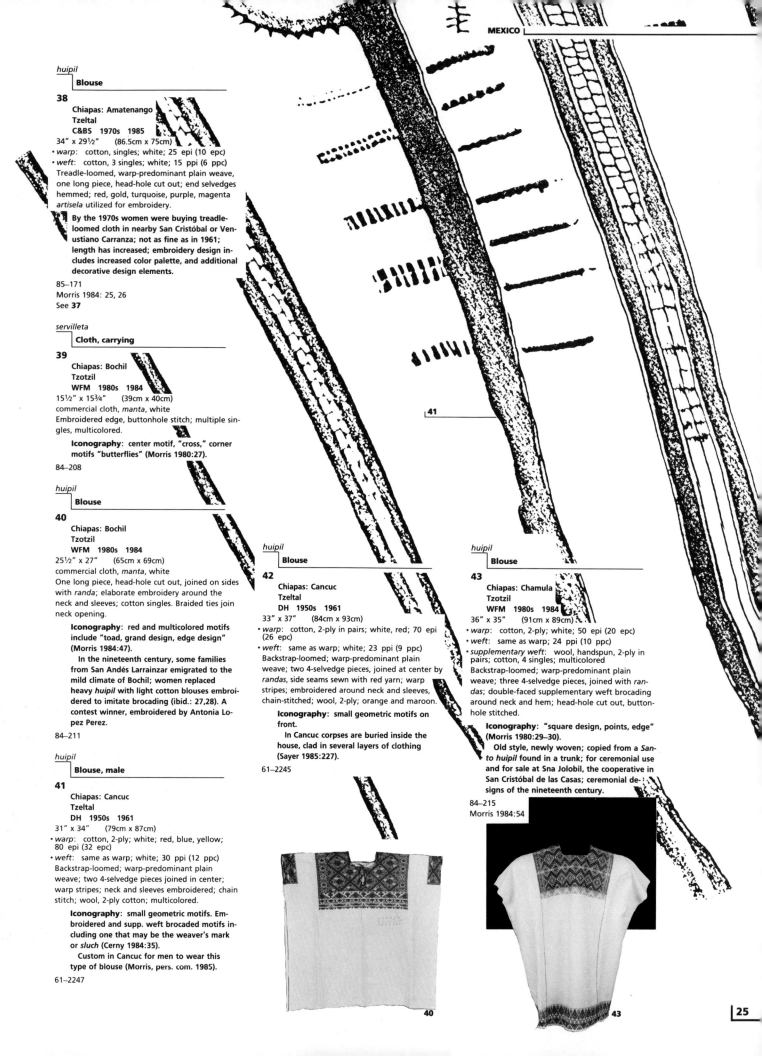

huipil

Blouse

38

**Chiapas: Amatenango
Tzeltal
C&BS 1970s 1985**
34" x 29½" (86.5cm x 75cm)
• *warp*: cotton, singles; white; 25 epi (10 epc)
• *weft*: cotton, 3 singles; white; 15 ppi (6 ppc)
Treadle-loomed, warp-predominant plain weave,
one long piece, head-hole cut out; end selvedges
hemmed; red, gold, turquoise, purple, magenta
artisela utilized for embroidery.

By the 1970s women were buying treadle-
loomed cloth in nearby San Cristóbal or Ven-
ustiano Carranza; not as fine as in 1961;
length has increased; embroidery design includes increased color palette, and additional
decorative design elements.

85–171
Morris 1984: 25, 26
See **37**

servilleta

Cloth, carrying

39

**Chiapas: Bochil
Tzotzil
WFM 1980s 1984**
15½" x 15¾" (39cm x 40cm)
commercial cloth, *manta*, white
Embroidered edge, buttonhole stitch; multiple singles, multicolored.

Iconography: center motif, "cross," corner
motifs "butterflies" (Morris 1980:27).

84–208

huipil

Blouse

40

**Chiapas: Bochil
Tzotzil
WFM 1980s 1984**
25½" x 27" (65cm x 69cm)
commercial cloth, *manta*, white
One long piece, head-hole cut out, joined on sides
with *randa*; elaborate embroidery around the
neck and sleeves; cotton singles. Braided ties join
neck opening.

Iconography: red and multicolored motifs
include "toad, grand design, edge design"
(Morris 1984:47).

In the nineteenth century, some families
from San Andés Larrainzar emigrated to the
mild climate of Bochil; women replaced
heavy *huipil* with light cotton blouses embroidered to imitate brocading (ibid.: 27,28). A
contest winner, embroidered by Antonia Lo-
pez Perez.

84–211

huipil

Blouse, male

41

**Chiapas: Cancuc
Tzeltal
DH 1950s 1961**
31" x 34" (79cm x 87cm)
• *warp*: cotton, 2-ply; white; red, blue, yellow;
80 epi (32 epc)
• *weft*: same as warp; white; 30 ppi (12 ppc)
Backstrap-loomed; warp-predominant plain
weave; two 4-selvedge pieces joined in center;
warp stripes; neck and sleeves embroidered; chain
stitch; wool, 2-ply cotton; multicolored.

Iconography: small geometric motifs. Embroidered and supp. weft brocaded motifs including one that may be the weaver's mark
or *sluch* (Cerny 1984:35).

Custom in Cancuc for men to wear this
type of blouse (Morris, pers. com. 1985).

61–2247

huipil

Blouse

42

**Chiapas: Cancuc
Tzeltal
DH 1950s 1961**
33" x 37" (84cm x 93cm)
• *warp*: cotton, 2-ply in pairs; white, red; 70 epi
(26 epc)
• *weft*: same as warp; white; 23 ppi (9 ppc)
Backstrap-loomed; warp-predominant plain
weave; two 4-selvedge pieces, joined at center by
randas, side seams sewn with red yarn; warp
stripes; embroidered around neck and sleeves,
chain-stitched; wool, 2-ply; orange and maroon.

Iconography: small geometric motifs on
front.

In Cancuc corpses are buried inside the
house, clad in several layers of clothing
(Sayer 1985:227).

61–2245

huipil

Blouse

43

**Chiapas: Chamula
Tzotzil
WFM 1980s 1984**
36" x 35" (91cm x 89cm)
• *warp*: cotton, 2-ply; white; 50 epi (20 epc)
• *weft*: same as warp; 24 ppi (10 ppc)
• *supplementary weft*: wool, handspun, 2-ply in
pairs; cotton, 4 singles; multicolored
Backstrap-loomed; warp-predominant plain
weave; three 4-selvedge pieces, joined with *randas*; double-faced supplementary weft brocading
around neck and hem; head-hole cut out, buttonhole stitched.

Iconography: "square design, points, edge"
(Morris 1980:29–30).

Old style, newly woven; copied from a *Santo huipil* found in a trunk; for ceremonial use
and for sale at Sna Jolobil, the cooperative in
San Cristóbal de las Casas; ceremonial designs of the nineteenth century.

84–215
Morris 1984:54

huipil

Blouse

44

Chiapas: Chamula
Tzotzil
WFM 1980s 1984
25" x 27"   (64cm x 68cm)
• *warp*: cotton, respun singles; white; 60 epi
(24 epc)
• *weft*: cotton, respun singles in pairs; white;
35 ppi (14 ppc)
One 4-selvedge backstrap-loomed piece; warp-predominant plain weave; hand-stitched at side
seams; head-hole cut out; embroidered with
multicolored 2-ply cotton at neck, bands along
shoulders and sleeves; satin stitch.

Iconography: floral, geometric motifs.
Worn by Christianized Chamulans who live
in low hot country, outside of municipality,
near Chenalo; could be worn under black
wool overblouse and is replacement for wool
huipil; won runner-up in embroidery contest
(Morris, pers. com. 1985).

84–216

blusa

Blouse

45

Chiapas: Chamula
Tzotzil
DH 1960s 1961
23" x 28"   (59cm x 71cm)
treadle-loomed, commercial cloth, white
Tailored, set-in sleeves, gussets under arm,
trimmed with commercial pink-white tape;
machine-stitched.

**Made in San Cristóbal de las Casas, worn as
underblouse; European-influenced design.**

61–2250
See **46, 51** Female Costume

Cloth, carrying

46

Chiapas: Chamula
Tzotzil
DH 1950s 1961
59½" x 22"   (151cm x 56cm)
• *warp*: wool, handspun, in pairs; black and white;
32 epi (epc)
• *weft*: same as warp; black; 10 ppi (4 ppc)
Backstrap-loomed; warp-faced plain weave; one
4-selvedge piece; warp stripes.

**Used by women for burden carrying, (DH)
and by Huistán men (Cordry 1968:346).**

61–2252
See **45, 51** Female Costume

sombrero

Hat

47

Chiapas: Chamula
Tzotzil
DH   1960s   1961
5" x 19"   (12.5cm x 48cm)
palm leaf fiber
Plaited strips sewn in continuous concentric
circles; multiple layers; braided hat band of 4
strands of pink and black fiber; black edging and
cord added.

**Palm hats woven by men in each community.
(Morris p.c.)**

61 • 2256

chamarro

Poncho

48

Chiapas: Chamula
Tzotzil
DH 1950s 1961
41" x 24½"   (104cm x 62cm)
• *warp*: wool, handspun, singles; cotton, singles;
white, red, green; 27 epi (11 epc)
• *weft*: same as warp; 10 ppi (4 ppc) Backstrap-loomed; warp-faced plain weave; one 4-selvedge
piece, neck opening created on loom; warp fringe
on both ends; neck binding machine-stitched on
commercial tape; open at sides.

**Shrunk, felted for warmth and water-proofing; neck machine-sewn in San Cristó-bal, made for sale and own use; Chamulans
trade wool for hoes and machetes with *Ladi-no* store keepers (Morris, pers. com. 1986).
Chamula female weavers provide these gar-ments to other villages in different styles; Zi-nacantán men wear a similar garment which
resembles costume of Spanish Knights of the
fifteenth century (Morris 1984:35). Like short
tunic, *ehuatl*, a pre-Columbian dress form sur-vival.**

61–2266
Blom in Harris and Sartor 1984:55,100
Morris 1984:35
Sayer 1985:169
See **49**

chamarro

Poncho

49

Chiapas: Chamula
Tzotzil
Museum Purchase   1970s   1983
39" x 25"   (100cm x 63cm)
• *warp*: wool, singles, handspun; white, some
brown; 30 epi (12 epc)
• *weft*: wool or goat, singles, handspun; tan;
12 ppi (5 ppc)
Backstrap-loomed; warp-faced plain weave; one
4-selvedge piece, head-hole not cut out.

Iconography: small geometric forms.
Embroidery pre-Columbian motifs (Morris
1984:45). Multicolored wool singles; 4 multi-colored wool tassels at each corner; consis-tency in dimensions, warp and weft counts
over ten-year period implies traditional gar-ment still in use.

83–25
See **48**

chamarro

Poncho

50

Chiapas: Chamula
Tzotzil
DM 1950s 1961
36" x 23½"   (92cm x 60cm)
• *warp*: wool, handspun, singles; black; 25 epi
(10 epc)
• *weft*: same as warp; 15 ppi (5 ppc)
Backstrap-loomed warp-predominant plain weave;
one 4-selvedge piece; head-hole cut out; side
seams unsewn.

Also worn in Tenejapa and by Chamula wo-men.

61–2257
See **48**

corte

Skirt

51

Chiapas: Chamula
Tzotzil
DH 1960s 1961
114" x 23"   (291cm x 59cm)
• *warp*: cotton, singles; deep blue; 52 epi (21 epc)
• *weft*: cotton, singles in pairs; deep blue and
white; 42 ppi (17 ppc)
Treadle-loomed; warp-predominant plain weave;
cut warp-ends, weft stripes.

**Produced by male weavers in Barrios Mexica-nos, outside of San Cristóbal de las Casas.
With introduction of the foot loom at the end
of colonial period, Aztecs who had settled
there began producing cloth for women's
skirts; fabric adopted by most Mayan high-land communities in Chiapas (Morris 1984:36).
Dark blue acheived by using indigo which is
soaked in lye, combined with *sacatinta* or
muicle, a native plant (Sayer 1985:136). Worn
wrapped around body, length becomes
width.**

61–2251
See **45, 46** Female Costume

morral

Bag, shoulder

52

Chiapas: Chenalhó
Tzotzil
WFM 1980s 1984
11½" x 9"   (29cm x 22cm)
• *cotton cord*: three 3-ply Z-spun yarns are S-spun
into cordage; white: 34 spi
Off-loom process, one set of elements, linking or
knotless netting; frame or stable parallel bars
used; woven band of green and red yarn; deer
skin strap (JS).

**A linked fabric is built up using a single
thread. Each new row of the fabric is formed
by whipping the thread around a previous
row (Drooker 1981:49).**

84–220

Cloth, shoulder or head

53

Chiapas: Huistán
Tzotzil
DH 1950s 1961
65" x 23½"   (164cm x 60cm)
• *warp*: cotton, 3 singles; white, deep blue; 28 epi
(11 epc)
• *weft*: same as warp; white
Backstrap-loomed, balanced plain weave, one
4-selvedge piece; dark blue borders, probably indi-go dye; light weight.

61–2286
Cordry 1968:347
See **55, 56, 57** Female Costume

Female Costume 45, 46, 51

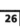

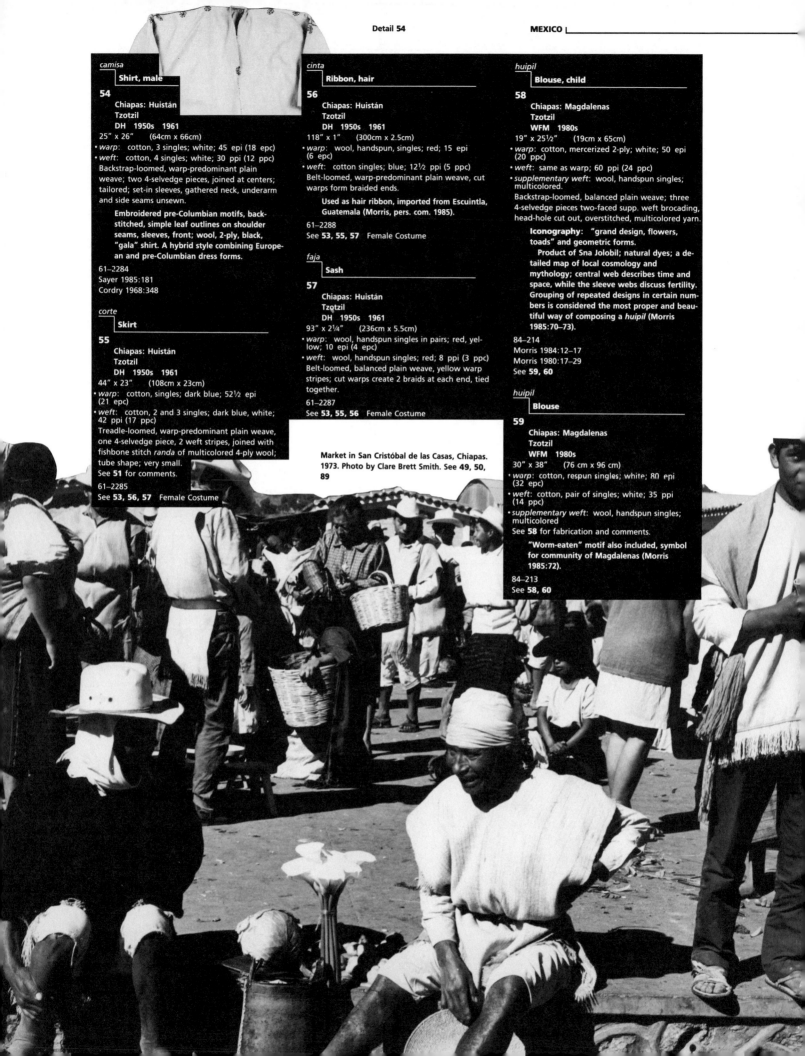

camisa

Shirt, male

54

Chiapas: Huistán
Tzotzil
DH 1950s 1961
25" x 26" (64cm x 66cm)
• *warp*: cotton, 3 singles; white; 45 epi (18 epc)
• *weft*: cotton, 4 singles; white; 30 ppi (12 ppc)
Backstrap-loomed, warp-predominant plain weave; two 4-selvedge pieces, joined at centers; tailored; set-in sleeves, gathered neck, underarm and side seams unsewn.

Embroidered pre-Columbian motifs, back-stitched, simple leaf outlines on shoulder seams, sleeves, front; wool, 2-ply, black, "gala" shirt. A hybrid style combining European- and pre-Columbian dress forms.

61–2284
Sayer 1985:181
Cordry 1968:348

corte

Skirt

55

Chiapas: Huistán
Tzotzil
DH 1950s 1961
44" x 23"   (108cm x 23cm)
• *warp*: cotton, singles; dark blue; 52½ epi (21 epc)
• *weft*: cotton, 2 and 3 singles; dark blue, white; 42 ppi (17 ppc)
Treadle-loomed, warp-predominant plain weave, one 4-selvedge piece, 2 weft stripes, joined with fishbone stitch *randa* of multicolored 4-ply wool; tube shape; very small.
See **51** for comments.

61–2285
See **53, 56, 57** Female Costume

cinta

Ribbon, hair

56

Chiapas: Huistán
Tzotzil
DH 1950s 1961
118" x 1"   (300cm x 2.5cm)
• *warp*: wool, handspun, singles; red; 15 epi (6 epc)
• *weft*: cotton singles; blue; 12½ ppi (5 ppc)
Belt-loomed, warp-predominant plain weave, cut warps form braided ends.

Used as hair ribbon, imported from Escuintla, Guatemala (Morris, pers. com. 1985).

61–2288
See **53, 55, 57** Female Costume

faja

Sash

57

Chiapas: Huistán
Tzotzil
DH 1950s 1961
93" x 2¼"   (236cm x 5.5cm)
• *warp*: wool, handspun singles in pairs; red, yellow; 10 epi (4 epc)
• *weft*: wool, handspun singles; red; 8 ppi (3 ppc)
Belt-loomed, balanced plain weave, yellow warp stripes; cut warps create 2 braids at each end, tied together.

61–2287
See **53, 55, 56** Female Costume

Market in San Cristóbal de las Casas, Chiapas. 1973. Photo by Clare Brett Smith. See 49, 50, 89

huipil

Blouse, child

58

Chiapas: Magdalenas
Tzotzil
WFM 1980s
19" x 25½"   (19cm x 65cm)
• *warp*: cotton, mercerized 2-ply; white; 50 epi (20 ppc)
• *weft*: same as warp; 60 ppi (24 ppc)
• *supplementary weft*: wool, handspun singles; multicolored.
Backstrap-loomed, balanced plain weave; three 4-selvedge pieces two-faced supp. weft brocading, head-hole cut out, overstitched, multicolored yarn.

Iconography: "grand design, flowers, toads" and geometric forms.
Product of Sna Jolobil; natural dyes; a detailed map of local cosmology and mythology; central web describes time and space, while the sleeve webs discuss fertility. Grouping of repeated designs in certain numbers is considered the most proper and beautiful way of composing a *huipil* (Morris 1985:70–73).

84–214
Morris 1984:12–17
Morris 1980:17–29
See **59, 60**

huipil

Blouse

59

Chiapas: Magdalenas
Tzotzil
WFM 1980s
30" x 38"   (76 cm x 96 cm)
• *warp*: cotton, respun singles; white; 80 epi (32 epc)
• *weft*: cotton, pair of singles; white; 35 ppi (14 ppc)
• *supplementary weft*: wool, handspun singles; multicolored
See **58** for fabrication and comments.

"Worm-eaten" motif also included, symbol for community of Magdalenas (Morris 1985:72).

84–213
See **58, 60**

huipil

Blouse

60

Chiapas: Magdalenas
Tzotzil
RP 1980s 1986
28" x 36"   (71.5cm x 91.5cm)
• *warp*: cotton, 2-ply; white; 50 epi (20 epc)
• *weft*: same as warp; 30 ppi (12 ppc)
• *supplementary weft*: wool, handspun singles;
multicolored
See **58** for fabrication and comments.

> "Saints and toad" along base, "grand design,
> flowers" above it; pretty good example (Morris, pers. com. 1986).

86–5
See **58, 59**

telar de palitos

Loom, backstrap

61

Chiapas: Magdalenas
Tzotzil
DH 1960s 1961
20½" x 18½"   (20.5cm x 47cm)
• *warp*: cotton, singles; white; 25 epi (10 epc)
• *weft*: cotton, pair of singles; white; 25 ppi
(10 ppc)
• *supplementary weft*: wool, handspun singles;
multicolored; over two warps

> One-fourth of web completed cloth; balanced
> plain weave; supp. weft two-faced
> brocading; shed sticks placed in web; motifs,
> "grand design, path of snake, stars" (Morris
> 1980:17–18).

61–2240

falda

Skirt

62

Chiapas: Magdalenas
Tzotzil
WFM 1980s 1984
91" x 35"   (232cm x 89cm)
• *warp*: cotton, pair of singles; indigo-*sacatina*;
60 epi (32 epc)
• *weft*: same as warp; also white; 24 ppi (9 ppc)
Backstrap-woven; warp-predominant plain weave;
two 4-selvedge pieces; weft stripes; two lengths
hand-sewn together, *randas*.

> Worn by women throughout Chiapas highlands; girls love to embroider large decorative *randas* attracting attention to their figures (Casagrande, pers. com. 1984). *Sacatina* or *muicle* "Jacobinia spicigera," an ingredient in indigo dyeing; left to rot for 3 days in vat of sugared water; then combined with indigo and lye; dipped frequently; hung to dry so dye can oxidize; color deepens (Sayer 1985:136).

84–212

morral, bolsa

Bag

63

Chiapas: Oxchuc
Tzeltal
DH 1960s 1961
22" x 7½"   (56cm x 19cm), not under tension
agave or ixtle, vegetal fiber; deer skin strap; knotless netting; top edge made by looping (JS).
See **52** for fabrication.

> Purchased in Zinacantán where it is also used; male burden carrying; highland men roll agave fibers on their legs with palm of their hands; as novices they suffer from leg hairs being caught and pulled out by the twisting of fiber; eventually have bald patches on legs; a pleasant social activity; a wooden frame small enough to rest on knees is used to support netting; held in place by nails (Sayer 1985:124).

61–2273

faja

Sash, female

64

Chiapas, Oxchuc
Txeltal
DH 1960s 1961
93" x 3¼"   (236cm x 8cm)
• *warp*: wool, handspun 2-ply; white, brown, red;
5 epi (2 epc)
• *weft*: same as warp but only white; same count
Belt-loomed; warp-faced warp stripes; one end
loom-finished; other cut warps, two braids.

> Purchased in Cancuc, more typical of Oxchuc
> (Morris, pers. com. 1985).

61–2246

Woman's purse

65

Chiapas: San Andrés Larrainzar
Tzotzil
DH 1960s 1961
4½" x 4½"   (11.5cm x 11.5cm)
• *warp*: cotton, pair of singles; white; 45 epi
(18 epc)
• *weft*: same as warp; white; 25 ppi (10 ppc)
• *supplementary weft*: wool, singles; red, orange,
and green; over 2–3 warps
Backstrap-loomed, warp-predominant plain
weave, one 4-selvedge piece, two-faced supp.
weft brocade, hand-sewn seams.

> **Iconography**: design motifs include
> "monkey, and points" (Morris 1980:6–7).

61–2238

huipil

Blouse

66

Chiapas: San Andrés Larrainzar
Tzotzil
DH 1960s 1961
23" x 30½"   (59cm x 77cm)
• *warp*: cotton, pair of singles; white; 55 epi
(22 epc)
• *weft*: cotton, 3 singles; white; 25 ppi (10 ppc)
• *supplementary weft*: cotton and wool, 3–5 singles; red, indigo, and orange; over 3–7 warps
Backstrap-loomed, warp-predominant plain
weave, three 4-selvedge pieces, two-faced supp.
weft brocade, head-hole cut out; all hand-
stitched.

> **Iconography**: geometric forms. "Square butterfly" dominates the neck and shoulder areas; diamonds symbolize the earth and sky as a unity; undulating forms like snakes symbolize the fertile earth (Morris 1984:10).
> In 1960 when purchased was the everyday style.

61–2262
Morris 1985
Morris 1984
Morris 1980
See **67, 68, 69, 70**

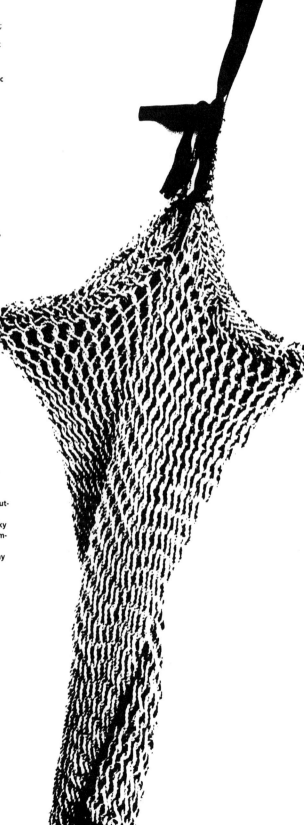

63

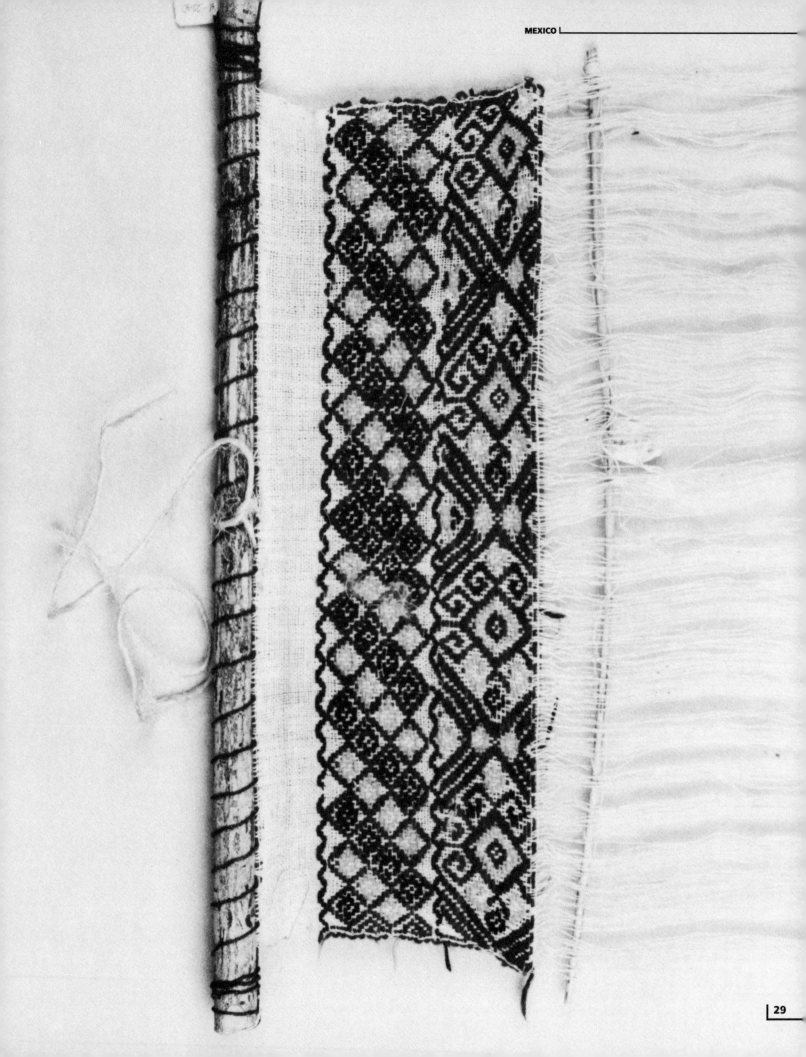

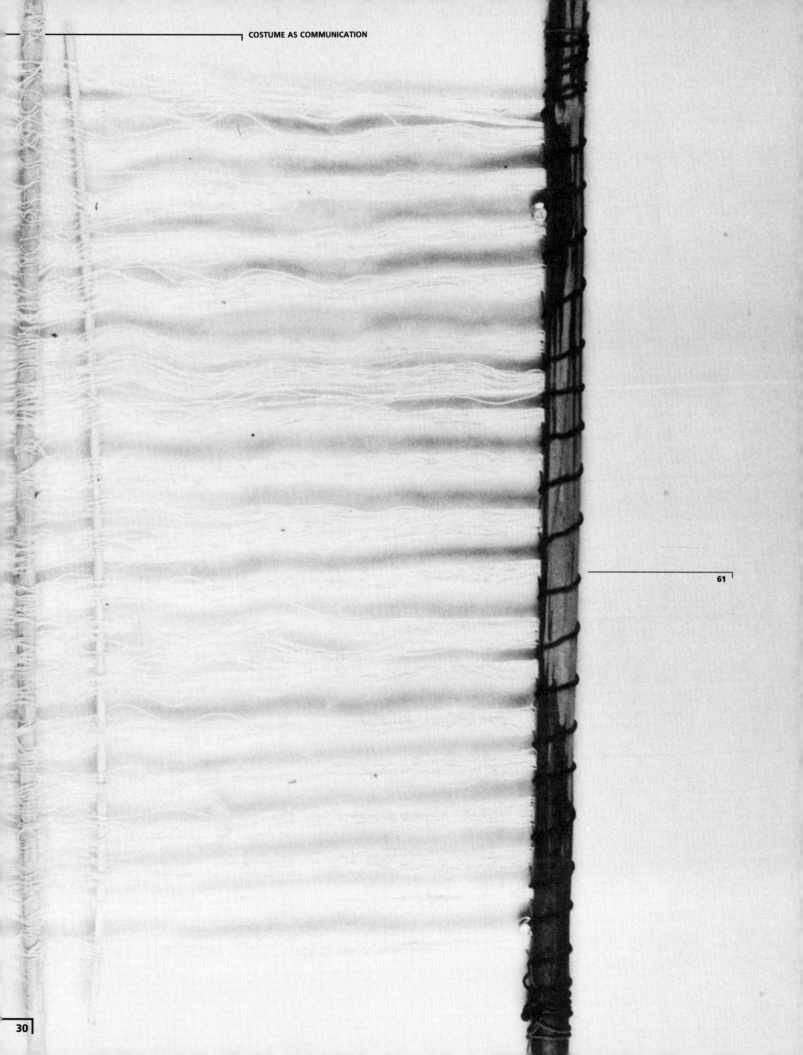

61

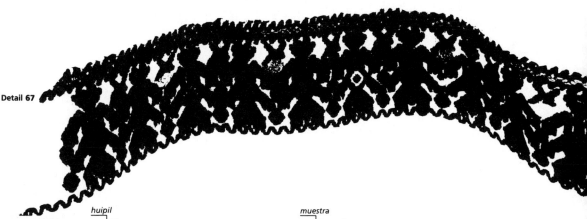

Detail 67

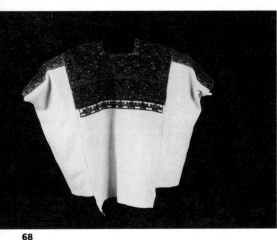

68

---

huipil
| **Blouse**

67

Chiapas: San Andrés Larrainzar
Tzotzil
WFM 1970s 1984
26½" x 37½"   (67cm x 95cm)
• *warp*: cotton, 2-ply; white; 60 epi (24 epc)
• *weft*: cotton, pair of 2-ply; white; 30 ppi (12 ppc)
• *supplementary weft*: cotton, 3–6 singles; red, indigo, and multicolored over 2–4 warps
See **66** for fabrication.

    Iconography: "saints, tarantella, feathered serpent" designs; feathered serpent is symbol of *cofradia* (religious organization) in Santa Rosario; weaver's mark present also (Morris, pers. com. 1985).
    Worn and woven by weaver for herself; purchased from Sna Jolobil.

84–207
See **66** for references.
See **66, 68, 69, 70**

---

huipil
| **Blouse**

68

Chiapas: San Andrés Larrainzar
Tzotzil
RP 1980s 1986
26" x 34"   (66cm x 86cm)
• *warp*: cotton, singles; white; 40 epi (16 epc)
• *weft*: cotton, 4 singles; white; 25 ppi (10 ppc)
• *supplementary weft*: cotton, singles; red, indigo, and multicolored; over 1–7 warps
See **66** for fabrication.

    Iconography: good saint figure along bottom of central panel; along one edge of sleeve "path of the snake or feathered serpent" designs (Morris, pers. com. 1986).
    From Sna Jolobil.

86–2
See **66** for references.
See **66, 67, 69, 70**

---

huipil
| **Blouse**

69

Chiapas: San Andrés Larrainzar
Tzotzil
RP 1970s 1986
24½" x 30½"   (62.5cm x 77.5cm)
• *warp*: cotton, pair of singles; white; 45 epi (18 epc)
• *weft*: cotton, 4 singles; white; 30 ppi (12 ppc)
• *supplementary weft*: cotton, wool, and rayon; red, indigo, and yellow; over 1–7 warps
See **66** for fabrication.

    Iconography: yellow diamonds called "wanderer" or "stars wandering across sky" (Morris, pers. com. 1986).
    Worn in late 1970s; simpler than **68**.

86–3
See **66** for references.
See **66, 67, 68, 70**

---

huipil
| **Blouse**

70

Chiapas: San Andrés Larrainzar
Tzotzil
RP 1970s 1986
22" x 32"   (56cm x 81cm)
• *warp*: cotton, 2-ply; white; 50 epi (20 epc)
• *weft*: cotton, pair of 2-ply; white; 35 ppi (10 ppc)
• *supplementary weft*: cotton and wool, singles; red, indigo, and multicolored; over 1–7 warps
See **66** for fabrication and comments.

86–4
See **66** for references.
See **66, 67, 68, 69**

---

muestra
| **Sampler**

71

Chiapas: San Andrés Larrainzar
Tzotzil
WFM 1980s 1984
51" x 21¼"   (130cm x 54cm)
• *warp*: cotton, 2-ply; white; 44 epi (19 epc)
• *weft*: cotton, pair of singles; white; 24 ppi (10 ppc)
• *supplementary weft*: cotton, singles; red and multicolored
Backstrap-loomed, warp-predominant plain weave, one 2-selvedge piece, two-faced supp. weft brocade, hand-sewn.

    All iconography in use included in **71**; Guatemalan style turkeys or peacocks in profile; unusual Chiapas designs – customarily woven straight on and spread out (Morris, pers. com. 1985).

84–210

---

faja
| **Sash, female**

72

Chiapas: San Andrés Larrainzar
Tzotzil
DH 1950s 1961
106" x 6"   (269cm x 15cm)
• *warp*: wool, handspun singles; red, black, and white; 35 epi (14 epc)
• *weft*: wool, singles; white; 10 ppi (4 ppc)
Belt-loomed, warp-faced plain weave, warp stripes, cut warps create 4 braids which are braided into 1 tie.

    Worn wrapped tightly around waist to hold up wraparound skirt. Women from San Andrés Larrainzar, Santiago, Magdalenas, and Santa Marta all use this belt (Morris, pers. com. 1986).

61–2242

---

faja
| **Sash, male**

73

Chiapas: San Andrés Larrainzar
Tzotzil
DH 1950s 1961
92" x 13"   (233cm x 33cm)
• *fringe*: 8" (20cm)
• *warp*: cotton, 2-ply; red, white, and indigo; 20 epi (8 epc)
• *weft*: cotton, pair of singles; white and red; 70 ppi (26 ppc)
Backstrap-loomed, weft-faced plain weave, one 2-selvedge piece, weft stripes, warp ends are twisted.

    Tightly beaten; no decorative end finish like **74**; weft-faced weavings unusual.

61–2265
See **74, 75** Male Costume

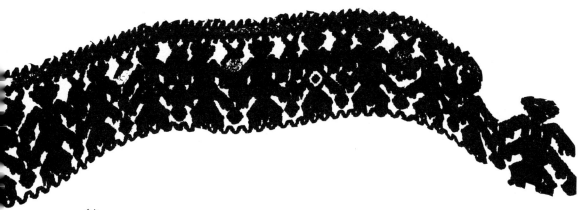

faja

Sash, male

74

Chiapas: San Andrés Larrainzar
Tzotzil
WFM 1960s 1986
93" x 10½"   (23.6cm x 27cm)
• *fringe*: 4½" (11.5cm)
• *warp*: cotton, 2-ply; red; 23 epi (9 epc)
• *weft*: wool and cotton, pair of singles; indigo, white, and red; 60 ppi (24 ppc)
• *supplementary weft*: wool, 3-ply; red, yellow, and green; 20 ppi (8 ppc)
See **73** for fabrication; supp. weft band at each end.

Old style; probably woven in the 1960s; purchased from Sna Jolobil; similar in dimensions and thread count to 73 with exception of wool used in the weft along with cotton.

84–209
See **73, 75**   Male Costume

Shirt

75

Chiapas: San Andrés Larrainzar
Tzotzil
DH 1950s 1961
23¼" x 23"   (59cm x 58cm)
• *warp*: cotton, 2-ply; white; 75 epi (30 epc)
• *weft*: same as warp; white; 25 ppi (10 ppc)
• *sleeves, warp*: cotton, pair of singles; red and black; 80 epi (32 epc)
• *sleeves, weft*: cotton, pair of singles; red and black; 40 ppi (16 ppc)
Backstrap-loomed, warp-predominant plain weave, two 4-selvedge pieces, hand-sewn center, head-hole cut out, sleeves set-in, narrow binding around neck.

European influenced hybrid-style shirt. Set-in sleeves of different cloth, unusual feature; similar to male and female shirt styles of Sololá, Guatemala (see 177, 186).

61–2263
See **73, 74**   Male Costume

Shawl, baby carrier

76

Chiapas: Santiago
Tzotzil
WFM 1980s 1984
56" x 34"   (136cm x 86.5cm)
• *warp*: cotton, 2-ply; natural dyed brown and white; 48 epi (28 epc)
• *weft*: same as warp; white; 19 ppi (8 ppc)
Backstrap-loomed, warp-faced plain weave, two 4-selvedge pieces, warp stripes, hand-joined.

Example of all-purpose cloth used for carrying babies, heavy loads of wood, food products; typical of the highlands; dye derived from elderbark and avocado pits.

84–219

Cap, baby

77

Chiapas: Tenejapa
Tzeltal
DH 1950s 1961
9" x 5½"   (22cm x 13.5cm)
• *warp*: cotton, pair of singles; white; 20 epi (8 epc)
• *weft*: cotton, singles; white, red, and indigo; 25 ppi (10 ppc)
• *supplementary weft*: wool, pair of singles; red, orange, and indigo; over 2–4 warps
Backstrap-loomed, balanced plain weave, one 4-selvedge piece, two-faced supp. weft brocade, weft stripes, one end hand-stitched, other end braided to form tie.

Iconography, materials, thread count are similar to 80, identified by Morris as old-style designs which might predate the 1960s.

61–2241
See **80**

sombrero

Hat, male

78

Chiapas: Tenejapa
Tzeltal
DH 1960s 1961
3" x 13¾"   (8cm x 35cm)
palm leaf
Twill plaiting, double layer, non-continuous strips, decorative cotton stitching, top and sides, ribbons on brim, twisted cotton, and horse hair tassel, extra construction of palm fronds to fill in opening of crown.

Palm hats are woven by men in each community; no significance to the colors used for ribbons although younger males wear brighter colors (Morris, pers. com. 1985).

61–2244

colera

Poncho

79

Chiapas: Tenejapa
Tzotzil
DH 1950s 1961
80" x 30"   (202cm x 76cm)
• *warp*: cotton and wool, singles and 2-ply; black and white; 36 epi (14 epc)
• *weft*: wool, 2-ply; white; 10 ppi (3 ppc)
Backstrap-loomed, warp-faced plain weave, one 4-selvedge piece, warp stripes.

Unfinished, no neck opening; some of the warp threads may have been dipped in *atole*, a corn drink, that is often used for stiffening warp yarns.

61–2243
Fisher 1986:21

faja

Sash, male

80

Chiapas: Tenejapa
Tzotzil
RP 1960s 1986
100" x 10½"   (254cm x 27cm)
• *warp*: cotton, singles; white; 25 epi (10 epc)
• *weft*: cotton, 1–4 singles; white; 75 ppi (30 ppc)
• *supplementary weft*: wool, singles and pairs of handspun singles; dark red, yellow, and orange; over 1–6 warps
Backstrap-loomed, weft-faced plain weave, one 4-selvedge piece, two-faced supp. weft brocading, weft stripes.

Iconography: female figures, geometric forms.
Ceremonial, religious official called "Capitan" in Tenejapa would wear it around his head, another draped around neck with ends hanging over his back and another as belt (Morris, pers. com. 1986).

86–1
See **73, 74, 77**

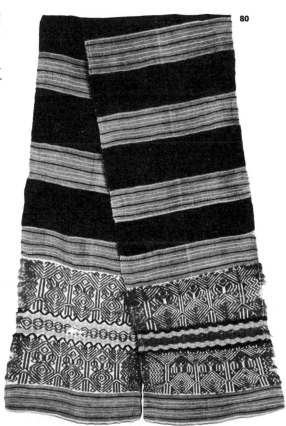

80

71. Teaching *Muestra* (sampler). Identifications by
Walter F. Morris, Jr.

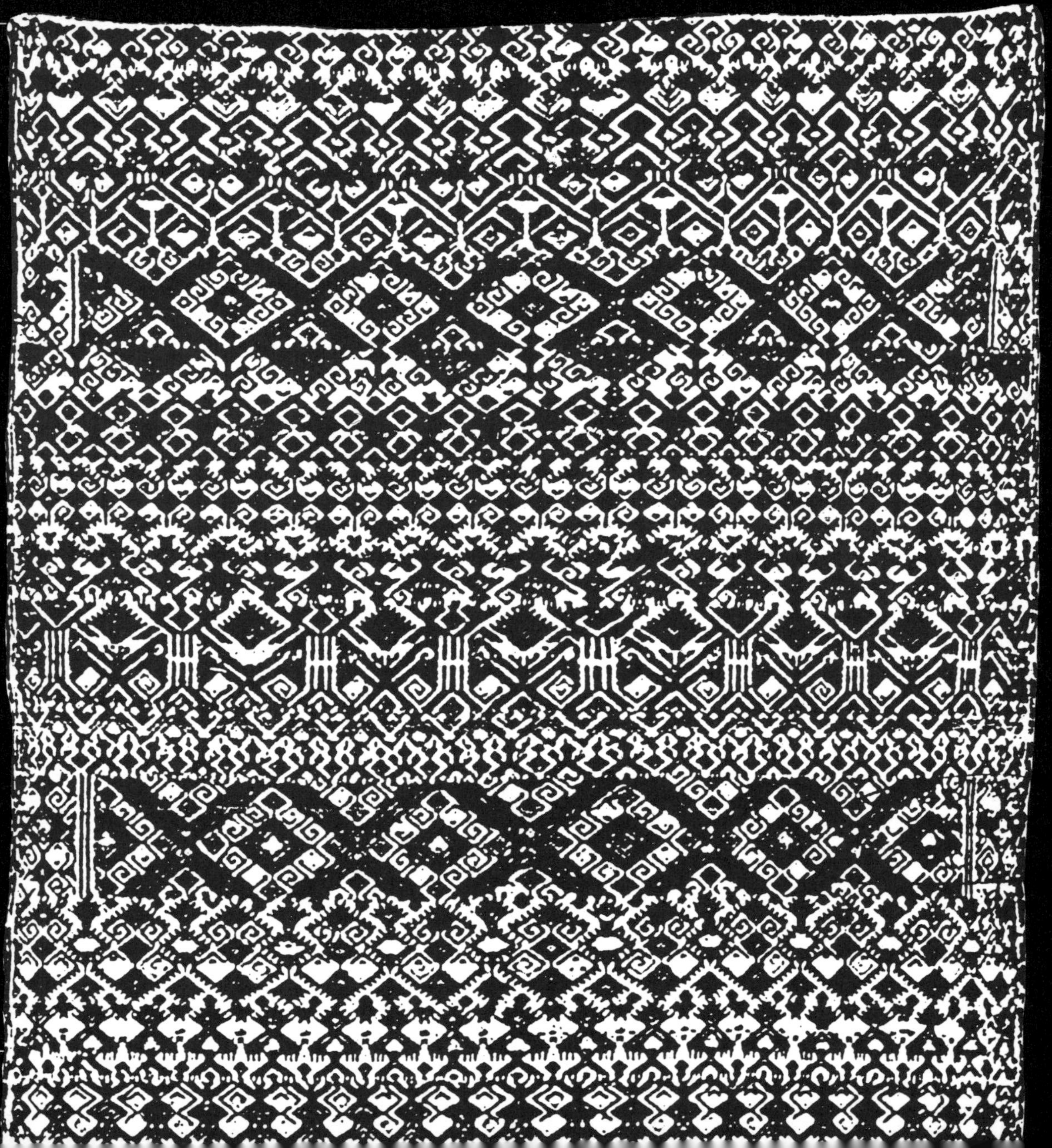

1 Saint without head
2 Saint
3 spider monkey
4 points
5 closure (where 2 woven sections meet)
6 Our Holy Mother
7 father and mother
8 toad
8a diamond design
9 hope
10 Saint
11 closure design

Designs from San Andrés Larrainzar

Designs fr

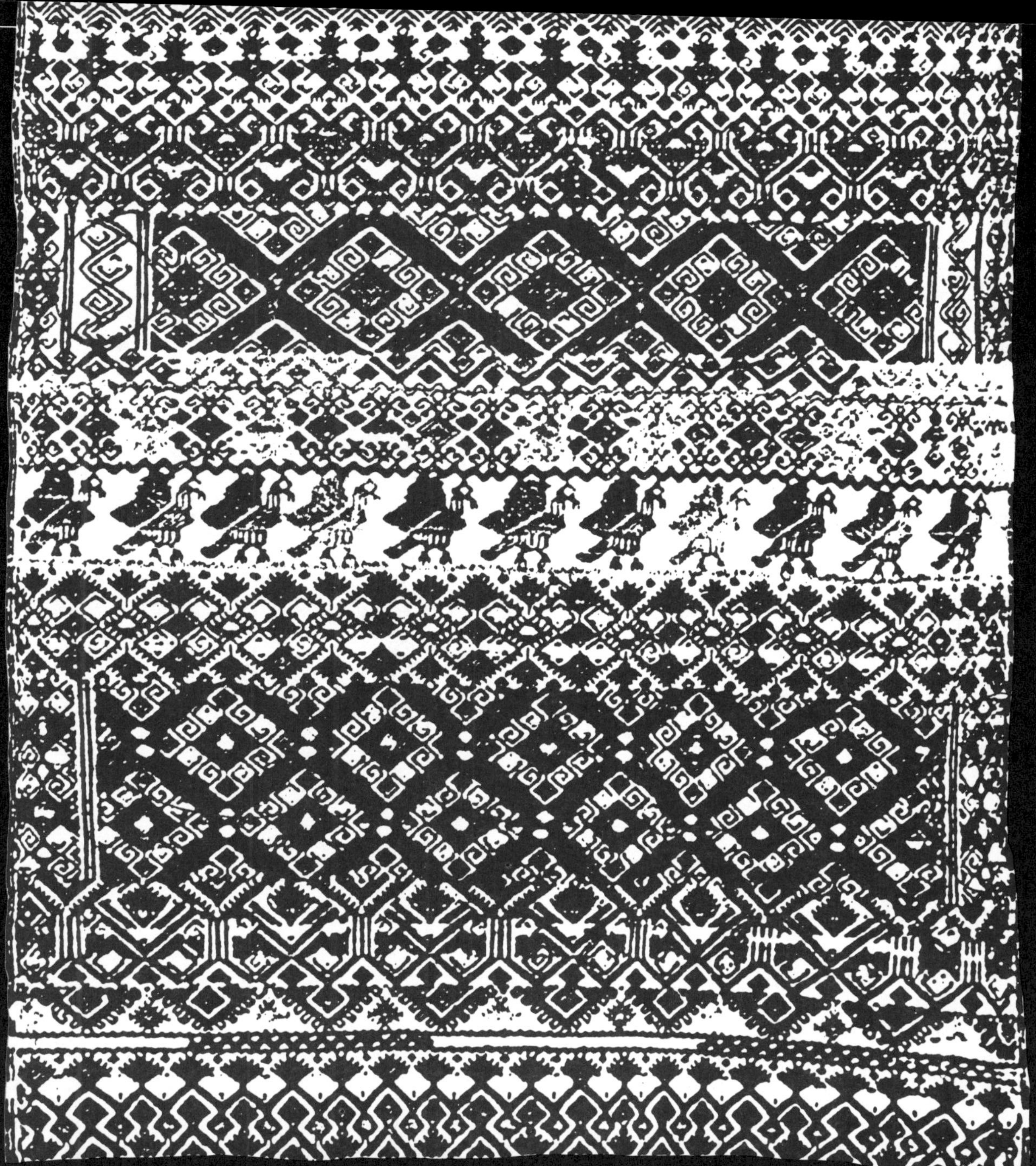

13 Saint

14 spider monkey

15 diamond design

15a Sideweaves

16 path of seeds

17 curl

18 bird (Guatemalan influence)

19 hope

20 refers to sunset

22 diamond design

24 Sideweave

23 Our Holy Mother

25 points

26 path of spines

27 Saint

Designs from Bochil

of Santa Rosario of Chamula

21 pineapple design

sombrero

Hat, male

81

Chiapas: Zinacantán
Tzotzil
DH 1960s 1961
2" x 15"   (5cm x 38cm)
palm leaf
Twill plaited stripes, sewn together in concentric circles, deer skin strap; black palm fiber edging; colored ribbons attached to brim; double layer of palm fronds fill in crown.
See **78** for comments.

61–2267
See **85, 86, 87, 88**   Male Costume

huipil

Blouse

82

Chiapas: Zinacantán
Tzotzil
WFM 1980s 1984
24½" x 25"   (62cm x 64cm)
• *warp*: cotton, pair of singles and 2-ply; white and multicolored; 60 epi (24 epc)
• *weft*: cotton, 3 singles; white; 25 ppi (10 ppc)
Backstrap-loomed, warp-faced plain weave, one 4-selvedge piece, warp stripes, head-hole cut out, buttonhole stitched at neck, sleeves, and adjacent to *randa* utilizing same colors as warp stripes.

Old style, newly made.

84–217

huipil

Wedding dress

83

Chiapas: Zinacantán
Tzotzil
C&BS 1970s 1985
41" x 35"   (105cm x 88cm)
• *warp*: cotton, 2 singles; white; 35 epi (14 epc)
• *weft*: cotton, 4 singles; white; 8 ppi (3 ppc)
• *supplementary weft*: wool and feathers, singles; multicolored, over 6 warps
Backstrap-loomed, warp-predominant plain weave, three 4-selvedge pieces, single-faced supp. weft brocading; head-hole cut out, folded over, and buttonhole stitched; decorative *randa* on center seams, side seams hand-sewn, feathers used as wefts; twisted and inserted.

A pre-Columbian survival resembling an Aztec-style garment.
The original technique involved spinning the feathers into the weft threads before weaving (Cordry 1968:344). The twined "cross bar" with long tassels survives on the feather-ornamented wedding *huipiles* of Zina-cantecos (Johnson 1967:188).

85–172
See **84**

huipil

Wedding dress

84

Chiapas: Zinacantán
Tzotzil
C&BS 1970s 1985
40" x 33"   (102cm x 86cm)
See **83** for thread makeup, count, fabrication, and comments.

85–173
See **83**

poc

Cloth, head

85

Chiapas: Zinacantán
Tzotzil
DH 1960s 1961
26" x 31"   (63 cm x 79 cm)
• *warp*: wool, singles; black and white; 30 epi (12 epc)
• *weft*: same as warp
Backstrap-loomed, balanced plain weave, one 4-selvedge piece, 4 large dark pink wool tassels attached at the corners.

Worn pirate-style, folded in half, wrapped around head or as a shoulder cape; can be worn with or without a hat (Sayer 1985:204).

61–2272
See **81, 86, 87**   Male Costume

poc

Cloth, head

86

Chiapas: Zinacantán
Tzotzil
Museum Purchase 1970s 1983
28¾" x 27"   (73 cm x 69 cm)
• *warp*: wool, singles; black and white; 30 epi (12 epc)
• *weft*: same as warp
See **85** for fabrication and comments. Blue and yellow ribbons attached at the 4 corners.

This example is made of treadle-woven cloth from San Cristóbal de las Casas.

83–24
See **81, 85, 87**   Male Costume

calzón

Pants

87

Chiapas: Zinacantán
Tzotzil
DH 1950s 1961
24" x 26"   (61cm x 66cm)
cotton; white
Treadle-loomed, commercially woven cloth, 2 pieces, hand-sewn together, cord at waist.

Shortest style pants worn in Chiapas; covered over by shirt; simplest construction of two rectangular pieces of cloth; a hybrid, non-fitted style (Fisher 1986:62).

61–2269
See **81, 85, 86**   Male Costume

colera

Poncho

88

Chiapas: Zinacantán
Tzotzil
DH 1960s 1961
28½" x 25½"   (72cm x 65cm)
• *warp*: cotton, 2–4 singles; white and red; 30 epi (12 epc)
• *weft*: cotton, 3 singles; white, red, and green; 30 ppi (12 ppc)
Backstrap-loomed, warp-predominant plain weave, two 4-selvedge pieces, warp stripes, ribbon trim at neck, braided warp fringe, open at side seams.

A pre-Columbian survival, a short tunic or *ehuatl*.
Similar to garment retained by Tarahumara, used by small boys and some men, a single open-sided width of cotton cloth worn over a shirt; may derive from *pita* garment found in local Basketmaker sites or later woolen garments likened by a Jesuit priest to a "dalmatic without sleeves" (Sayer 1985:200).

61–2270
See **81, 85, 86, 87**   Male Costume and **14, 89, 90**

Market in San Cristóbal de las Casas, Chiapas. 1973. Photo by Clare Brett Smith. See 81, 87, 89.

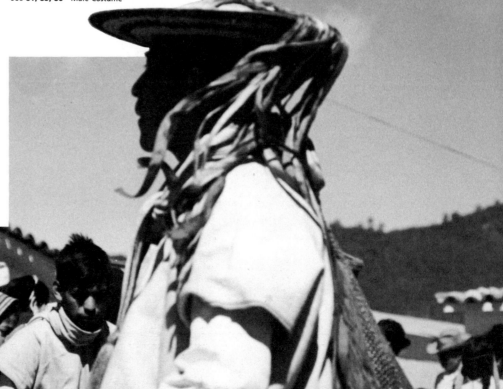

colera

| **Poncho** |

89

Chiapas: Zinacantán
Tzotzil
WFM 1980s 1984
28½" x 29"   (72cm x 74cm)
• *warp*: cotton, 2-ply; red and white; 70 epi
(28 epc)
• *weft*: cotton, pair of singles; white, purple, and
green; 35 ppi (10 ppc)
• *cords*: cotton and synthetic; multicolored
See **88** for fabrication and comments. Warp ends
twisted to make fringe.

84–218
See **14, 88, 90**

colera

| **Poncho, boy** |

90

Chiapas: Zinacantán
Tzotzil
DH 1960s 1961
13" x 13¾"   (33cm x 35cm)
• *warp*: cotton, pair of singles; white and red;
40 epi (16 epc)
• *weft*: cotton, 3 singles; white; 30 ppi (12 ppc)
• *supplementary weft*: cotton, 2-ply; green, and
magenta
Ties at sleeves and bottom, supp. weft borders on
bottom of front and back.
See **88** for fabrication and comments.

61–2271
See **14, 88, 89**

| **Shirt** |

91

Chiapas: Zinacantán
Tzotzil
DH 1960s 1961
21" x 24"   (53cm x 62cm)
• *warp*: cotton, 2 singles; white; 45 epi (18 epc)
• *weft*: cotton, 3 singles; white; 35 ppi (10 ppc)
Backstrap-loomed, warp-predominant plain
weave, two 4-selvedge pieces, hand-sewn center
seam, head-hole cut out, red neck binding, sleeves
set in.

A hybrid style.

61–2268
See **81, 85, 86, 87, 88**   Male Costume

huipil

| **Blouse** |

92

Chiapas: bought in Sacapulas, El Quiché, Guatemala
Lacandón
DH 1960s 1961
39½" x 27"   (100 cm x 78 cm)
• *warp*: cotton, 2 and 3 handspun singles and
2-ply; white, red, and blue; 35 epi (14 epc)
• *weft*: cotton, singles; white; 20 ppi (8 ppc)
Backstrap-loomed, warp-predominant plain
weave, one 4-selvedge piece, hand-sewn side
seams, head-hole cut out and bound, with whip
stitch; warp stripes.

**Made along Usumacinta River, Chiapas, Mexi-
co, worn loose, without belt, this is the sole
garment of both man and woman. This specimen is a fine old one; a growing trend is the
use of factory-made muslin (DH). Called *xikul*,
derives from *xicolli*, a pre-Columbian dress
form survival; before 1940s bark cloth was
utilized, now cotton (Sayer 1985:198, 192).
Uneven texture due to variation in make-up
of fibers.**

61–2125
Harris and Sartor, 1984
Perera and Bruce, 1982

92

State		Village
Huehuetenango	28	Colotenango
	29	San Mateo Ixtatán
	30	San Pedro Necta
	31	Todos Santos Cuchumatan
El Quiché	32	Chajul
	33	Chichicastenango
	34	Nebaj
Alta Verapaz	35	Cobán
	36	Tactic
	37	Tamahú
Totonicapán	38	Momostenango
	39	Totonicapán
Baja Verapaz	40	Rabinal

State		Village
Chimaltenango	47	Sololá
	48	Comalapa
	49	Patzún
	50	San Martin Jilotepeque
	51	Tecpán
	52	Parramos
Sacatepéquez	53	San Antonio Aguas Calientes
	54	Santiago Sacatepéquez
	55	Santo Domingo Xenacoj

State		Village
Quezaltenango	41	San Miguel Chicaj
	42	Quezaltenango
	43	San Martin Sacatepéquez, Chili Verde
Sololá	44	Nahualá
	45	San Lucas Tolimán
	46	Santiago Atitlán

State		Village
	56	Santa Maria de Jesús
	57	Sumpango
Guatemala	58	Chuarrancho
	59	San Juan Sacatepéquez
	60	San Pedro Sacatepéquez
Escuintla	61	Palin

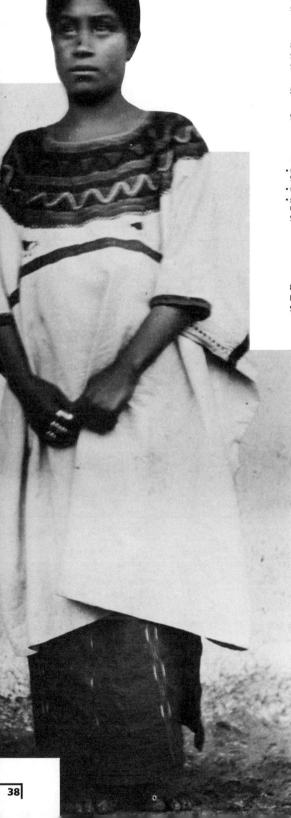

Mam woman, San Mateo Ixtatán. 1920–1930. Herbert J. Spinden Photo Archives, Haffenreffer Museum of Anthropology.

huipil

Blouse

93

Huehuetenango: Colotenango
Mam
C&BS 1970s 1985
23½" x 42"   (60cm x 110cm)
• *warp*: cotton, singles; white, red, and orange; 75 epi (30 epc)
• *weft*: same as warp; white; 25 ppi (10 ppc)
• *supplementary weft*: cotton, 3 singles; red, and multicolored; over 4–7 warps
Backstrap-loomed, warp-predominant plain weave, three 4-selvedge pieces, hand-sewn seams, head-hole cut out, bound stitch of 2 colors around neck and arm holes, dense single-faced brocading; solid squares of color on front, back, and sleeves.

　Iconography: geometric; contrast of square and lozenge shapes.

85–61
Sperlich and Sperlich 1980:147–150
See **94**

huipil

Blouse

94

Huehuetenango: Colotenango
Mam
C&BS 1970s 1985
19½" x 33"   (49cm x 84cm)
• *warp*: cotton, singles; red and multicolored; 90 epi (36 epc)
• *weft*: same as warp; white; 30 ppi (12 ppc)
• *supplementary weft*: cotton, 2 singles; red and multicolored; over 4–7 warps
See **93** for fabrication.

　Small single-faced brocaded geometric motifs against red/white striped background creates a very active impression; a ceremonial style that relates to an older design. Contrasts with 93.

85–162
Deuss 1981:34
See **93**

huipil

Blouse

95

Huehuetenango: San Mateo Ixtatán
Chuj
E&JD 1970s 1973
33½" x 31½"   (85cm x 80cm)
commercial cloth, *manta*, white; two pieces in two layers
• *embroidery*: cotton, 6 singles, three 2-ply; multi-colored, single-faced embroidery, false satin stitch, head-hole cut out, bound in whip stitch; side seams hand-sewn; additional motifs embroidered on bottom of front and back

　Iconography: overall geometric design; star and sun images.
　San Mateo is the only Chuj village with a costume that is documented; these colorful *huipiles* are popular with tourists and are sold as far away as San Cristóbal de las Casas, Chiapas.
　The female costume is a pre-Columbian dress form survival in design; a wraparound skirt, distinctive *huipil*, and unique hair ornament, but the basic material is commercially produced in an outside area (Anawalt 1984:17).

73–33
Rowe 1981:144–147
See **96**

huipil

Blouse

96

Huehuetenango: San Mateo Ixtatán
Chuj
RP 1970–1985 1986
29" x 41½"   (74cm x 105.5 cm)
commercial cloth, *manta*, two pieces in two layers
• *embroidery*: cotton, pearl cotton, and wool, singles and three 2-ply; multicolored
See **95** for fabrication; two-faced embroidery utilized.

　Iconography: birds, flowers, and butterflies; see 95.
　Earlier piece than **95**; sometimes worn with a ruffled collar, and rickrack is added to the decoration (Rowe 1981:147). A textural contrast is made by using threads that are twisted in an opposite manner.
　See **95** for further comments and references.

86–10
See **95**

94
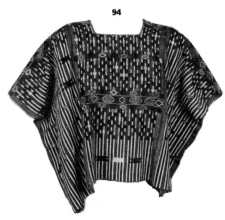

96
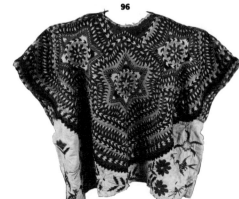

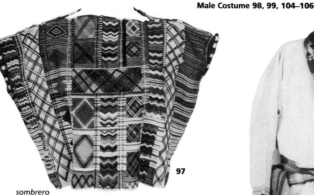

Male Costume 98, 99, 104–106

huipil

| **Blouse**

97

Huehuetenango: San Pedro Necta
Mam
FS 1970s 1978
17½" x 25"   (44cm x 63cm)
• *warp*: cotton, two 2-ply singles; white and multi-colored; 47 epi (18 epc)
• *weft*: cotton, 2 singles; white; 10 ppi (4 ppc)
• *supplementary weft*: cotton and wool, four 2-ply singles, and two 2-ply singles; multicolored; over 4–6 warps
Backstrap-loomed, warp-predominant plain weave, 4-selvedge piece, warp stripes, two-faced supp. weft brocade, head-hole cut out, folded back and wrapped, hand-sewn seams, satin stitch, from neck down to sleeves, buttonhole stitch also utilized.

Iconography: geometric.
Great color play; some of the patterns are made by weft-wrapping. A unique *huipil* style; only one piece of cloth utilized; seamed at the shoulders and sides; contrast between warp stripes and supp. weft designs; this example particularly ornate, per-haps ceremonial.

78–264
Anderson 1978:86–88
Bjerregaard 1977:82–84
Deuss 1981:56

morral

| **Bag**

98

Huehuetenango: Todos Santos Cuchumatán
Mam
MS 1970s 1979
10½" x 12½"   (27cm x 32cm)
crochet; cotton, 2-ply; white, and multicolored; 12 spi (5 spc)
• *strap*: cotton, 2-ply; multicolored; sprang

Iconography: zigzag, blocks.
Men crochet these bags.
Sprang is the process of constructing a fab-ric by manipulating a set of parallel yarns that are fixed at both ends or wound continu-ously around two poles (Kent 1983:298).

79–35
Deuss 1981:46
See **99, 103, 104, 105, 106** Male Costume

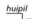
97

sombrero

| **Hat, male and female**

99

Huehuetenango: Todos Santos Cuchumatán
Mam
MS 1970s 1979
3" x 12½"   (8cm x 32cm)
twisted palm fiber
Twill plaiting, fine strips, layered, metal eyelets, leather hat band, reinforcement at rim and edge, sewn with cotton.

Made in Jacaltenango (Pancake, pers. com. 1978). Male and female identical hats are made on a sewing machine using plaited palm from Quiché (Anderson 1978:31). Eyelets might serve for ventilation.

79–36
See **98, 103, 104, 105, 106** Male Costume

huipil

| **Blouse**

100

Huehuetenango: Todos Santos Cuchumatán
Mam
RP 1940–1960 1986
24¾" x 30"   (63cm x 76cm)
• *warp*: cotton, handspun singles and pair of sin-gles; red, white, and multicolored; 80 epi (32 epc)
• *weft*: cotton, handspun singles; white; 25 ppi (10 ppc)
• *supplementary weft*: cotton, and wool, pair of singles; red and multicolored; over 2 warps
Backstrap-loomed, warp-predominant plain weave, three 4-selvedge pieces, single-faced supp. weft brocade, warp stripes, head-hole cut out, sep-arate neck piece added, gathered to fit neck, hand-sewn seams.

In outer panels, dense red supp. weft blocks create gathered effect of background cloth; center panel densely brocaded. The collar ex-emplifies European influence on native cos-tume.
Sometime between 1950–1965 Todos Santos women began adding designs other than simple rectangles to their huipils. The colored threads that form these designs are supplementary to the red wefts. Sometimes they are merely interlaced parallel to the red wefts, but linear designs (usually diagonals) are done by wrapping (Rowe 1981:122).

86–16
See **101, 102**

huipil

| **Blouse**

101

Huehuetenango: Todos Santos Cuchumatán
Mam
RP 1960–1975 1986
29½" x 35"   (75cm x 84cm)
• *warp*: cotton, handspun singles and pairs; red, white, and multicolored; 75 epi (30 epc)
• *weft*: cotton, handspun singles; white; 25 ppi (10 ppc)
• *supplementary weft*: cotton and wool, pair of sin-gles, and 2-ply; red and multicolored; over 2 warps
See **100** for fabrication and comments.

Underarm seams open; sleeve selvedges fold-ed over and hand-sewn; slightly different pat-terning of warp stripes in center and outside panels; badly worn at neck; geometric supp. weft designs only on center panel.

86–11
See **100, 102**

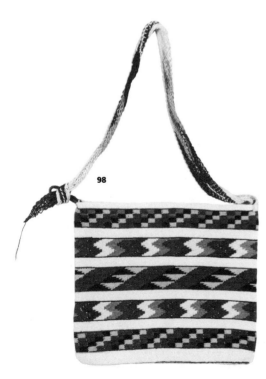
98

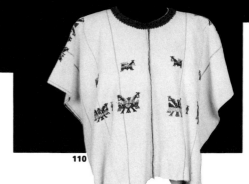

110

huipil

Blouse

102

Huehuetenango: Todos Santos Cuchumatán
Mam
RP 1980–1985 1986
29¼" x 32½" (74.5cm x 82.5cm)
- *warp* (center panel): cotton, 2 handspun singles; white, red, and multicolored; 75 epi (30 epc)
- *warp* (side panels): cotton, 2-ply; red; 120 epi (48 epc)
- *weft* (center panel): cotton, handspun singles, white; 25 ppi (10 ppc)
- *weft* (side panels): same as weft of center panel.
- *supplementary weft*: cotton, wool, and synthetic, pair of singles, and two 2-ply; red, yellow, and hot pink; over 1–3 warps.

More contemporary piece than **100**, **101**; brightly colored synthetic yarns, neck piece in good shape; finely woven cloth of side panels. Over a forty-year period warp and weft counts, colors, and iconography have remained consistent; by 1980s only the center panel is adorned with supp. weft brocading; neck piece is still present but in **102** rickrack has been added for decoration.

86–9
Arriola Geng n.d.
See **100, 101**

pantalón

Pants

103

Huehuetenango: Todos Santos Cuchumatán
Mam
MS 1970s 1979
40½" x 17½" (103cm x 44cm)
- *warp*: cotton, singles and 4-ply; red, white, orange, dark blue; 80 epi (32 epc)
- *weft*: cotton, pair of singles; white; 20 ppi (8 ppc)
Backstrap-woven; warp-predominant plain weave; two 2-selvedge pieces; warp stripes; cuffs and seams hand-sewn; gusset added to crotch.

A hybrid style; two rectangular pieces of cloth sewn together with the addition of a gusset; ankle length; a transition between fitted and nonfitted pants (Fisher 1986:62). No cording at waist to hold pants up.

79–32
Rowe 1981:125–127
See **98, 99, 104, 105, 106** Male Costume

sobre-pantalón

Overpants

104

Huehuetenango: Todos Santos Cuchumatán
Mam
MS 1950s 1979
27" x 16½" (68cm x 42cm)
treadle-loomed black twill wool
Material is felted before it is tailored, machine-stitched; buttons and buttonholes are placed on the front.

The tailoring is relatively elaborate, and not unlike that of the ceremonial overpants from other towns. In the late nineteenth century these overpants were the same length as the pants. Today they are only about knee height and lack the buttonholes on the legs found in older examples (Rowe 1981:127).

The French Navy visited Guatemala in the mid-nineteenth century and their costume included overpants worn over white, ruffled long pants. Somehow this style traveled to the mountains of Huehuetenango and there it was frozen in time (Bell, pers. com. 1978). Another example of European cut-and-sew technology.

79–34
See **98, 99, 103, 105, 106** Male Costume

faja

Sash, male

105

Huehuetenango: Todos Santos Cuchumatán
Mam
MS 1960s 1979
97" x 9" (246cm x 23cm)
- *warp*: cotton, pair of singles; red, white, blue, and yellow; 60 epi (24 epc)
- *weft*: same as warp; red, yellow, green, white, and blue; 35 ppi (14 ppc)
Backstrap-loomed, warp-predominant plain weave, 4-selvedge piece, warp and weft stripes create plaid; one end machine-stitched.

Sash is used to hold the pants up; sometimes it is visible and sometimes it is hidden by the overpants. Due to simplicity of patterning, **105** was probably woven before 1965.

79–33
Rowe 1981:125–127
See **98, 99, 103, 104, 106** Male Costume

camisa

Shirt, male

106

Huehuetenango: Todos Santos Cuchumatán
Mam
MS 1970s 1979
31½" x 26" (80cm x 68cm)
- *warp*: cotton, singles; white, red, blue, and orange; 30 epi (12 epc)
- *weft*: cotton, singles; white; 15 ppi (6 ppc)
- *supplementary weft* (collar and cuffs): cotton and wool, multiple strands; red and multicolored; 15 ppi (6 ppc)
- *shirt*: backstrap-loomed, warp-predominant plain weave, two 4-selvedge pieces, warp stripes, set-in sleeves
- *collar and cuffs*: backstrap-loomed, warp-predominant plain weave, three 4-selvedge pieces; single-faced supp. weft brocade; all seams hand-sewn; tie used for closing neck opening

Iconography: geometric, similar to motifs of the bag, **98**.
When collar and cuffs wear out, they are taken off, turned around and resewn to the shirt; contemporary examples have buttons down the front, and patch pockets have been added.

79–31
Rowe 1981:130
See **98, 99, 103, 104, 105** Male Costume and **107, 108**

camisa

Shirt, male

107

Huehuetenango: Todos Santos Cuchumatán
Mam
E&JD 1970s 1978
30" x 27" (76cm x 74cm)
See **106** for makeup of thread, count, and fabrication.

Warp stripes set farther apart; no neck tie.

78–202
See **106, 108**

camisa

Shirt, male

108

Huehuetenango: Todos Santos Cuchumatán
Mam
P&ES 1970s 1983
28" x 26" (71cm x 66cm)
See **106** for thread makeup, count, and fabrication.

Warp stripes are blue and green; cuffs of **107** and **108** narrower than **106**.

83–314
See **106, 107**

EL QUICHÉ

huipil

Blouse

109

El Quiché: Chajul
Ixil
FS 1970s 1978
23½" x 32" (60cm x 82cm)
- *warp*: cotton, pair of singles; red; 22 epi (9 epc)
- *weft*: same as warp; red; 10 ppi (4 ppc)
- *supplementary weft*: cotton, pearl cotton, and wool, three 2-ply; multicolored; over 6–16 warps
Backstrap-loomed, warp-predominant plain weave, two 4-selvedge pieces, two-faced supp. weft brocade, head-hole cut out, machine-stitched seams and at neck.

Iconography: birds and chevrons.
Notable for the simplicity of design layout, the paucity of motifs utilized. Weaving patterns of Nebaj, Chajul, and San Juan Cotzal, all Ixil speakers, are similar in techniques and pattern motifs (Hearne 1985). A variety of laced weft wrapping is practiced, and gives a dense, raised effect; sometimes simple weft wrapping is done in Chajul (Anderson 1978:93).

78–269
See **110**

huipil

Blouse

110

El Quiché: Chajul
Ixil
C&BS 1970s 1985
23½" x 35" (60cm x 90cm)
- *warp*: cotton, 3-singles; white and red; 45 epi (18 epc)
- *weft*: cotton, singles; white; 13 ppi (5 ppc)
- *supplementary weft*: cotton, 2-ply and 4-ply; multicolored; over 2–5 warps
Backstrap-loomed, warp-predominant plain weave, two selvedge pieces, two-faced supp. weft brocade; head-hole cut out, folded over and hand-sewn in purple silk with satin stitch; all seams are hand-sewn.

Iconography: 4-legged animals and double-headed eagle.
The eagle is a shared Mayan motif with both pre-Columbian and European significance (Schevill 1986:18–22).
See **109** for comments.

85–158
See **109**

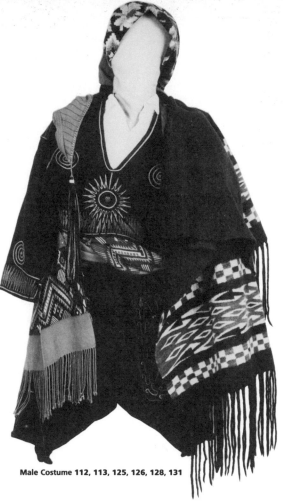

Male Costume 112, 113, 125, 126, 128, 131

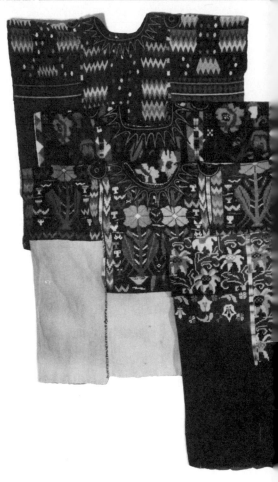

---

sarape

Blanket, shoulder

112

> El Quiché: Chichicastenango
> Quiché
> CWH 1960s 1967

78½" x 28½"   (198cm x 72cm)
- *warp*: wool, handspun singles; black and grey on borders; 15 epi (6 epc)
- *weft*: same as warp

Treadle-loomed, simple twill weave; cut warp creates twisted fringes.

> Different kinds of blankets are used by Chichicastenango men; some for carrying burdens, others for wrapping around the body, as protection from the rain; mixed colors in warp and weft give checkered effect.

67–10071
Anderson 1978:171–172
See **113, 125, 126, 128, 131** Male Costume

sarape

Blanket

113

> El Quiché: Chichicastenango
> Quiché
> CWH 1960s 1967

88½" x 30"   (228cm x 77cm)
- *warp*: wool, handspun singles; black and brown; 15 epi (6 epc)
- *weft*: same as warp
- *tapestry-woven bands, weft*: wool, finely spun singles; white, red, deep blue; 40 ppi (16 ppc)

Treadle-loomed, twill weave; one-over-three warps for center section; tapestry weave, weft-faced, both ends, cut warp ends for fringe, twisted.

> **Iconography**: geometric, blocks, arrows.
> Probably cochineal and indigo dyes for red and blue; made by specialists for sale to Chichicastenango men; first noted in the Guatemalan textile collection made by Gustavus Eisen in 1902 in the Lowie Museum of Anthropology, University of California, Berkeley; still worn by Chichicastenango men in 1978; when not in use, it is folded over the right shoulder.

67–10024
Anderson 1978:171–172
Rowe 1981:91–94
See **112, 125, 126, 128, 131** Male Costume

huipil

Blouse

114

> El Quiché: Chichicastenango
> Quiché
> CWH 1960s 1967

28½" x 32½"   (72cm x 83cm)
- *warp*: cotton, singles; white; 65 epi (26 epc)
- *weft*: cotton, pair of singles; white; 25 ppi (10 ppc)
- *supplementary weft*: wool, singles and 4-ply; purple and multicolored; over 3 warps

Backstrap-loomed, warp-predominant plain weave, three 4-selvedge pieces, two-faced supp. weft brocade, head-hole cut out, 2 black taffeta medallions sewn onto shoulders; black taffeta neck piece added; *randa* buttonhole stitch in design areas; other seams whip stitch; chain stitch around medallions.

> **Iconography**: some geometric; "new" floral designs originating in the 1940s.
> Symbolic layout of design field; medallions, representing four cardinal points positioned around the head-hole, the sun; chain-stitched neck piece can be seen as rays of the sun (Rodas, Rodas, and Hawkins 1940:124). *Huipil* is worn with extra fullness pulled around to the back, with right side folded over the left; held in place by the belt but not tucked into the skirt (Rowe 1981:90, Goodman 1976:5). Men embroider.

67–10009
See **123, 130, 132** Female Costume and **115–120**

---

faja

Sash, female

111

> El Quiché: Chajul
> Ixil
> FS 1970s 1978

118" x 11½"   (300cm x 29cm)
- *warp*: cotton, pair of singles; red; 84 epi (36 epc)
- *weft*: same as warp; red; 28 ppi (12 ppc)
- *supplementary weft*: cotton and pearl cotton, 3-ply and 2-ply; multicolored

Backstrap-loomed, warp-predominant plain weave, two-faced supp. weft brocade, macramé finish with pom-poms on ends.

> **Iconography**: lozenges and zigzags.
> Similar iconography appears on *huipiles*, outlining effective with color contrast. The traditional dress of a woman from Chajul includes a *huipil* like **109** or **110**, a red treadle-loomed skirt, a headband, and a sash which can be very impressive due to the supplementary weft brocading on each end. A small weaver's mark appears on the larger brocaded band of **111**.

78–272

---

huipil

Blouse

115

> El Quiché: Chichicastenango
> Quiché
> C&BS 1970s 1985

27" x 35½"   (68cm x 90cm)
- *warp*: cotton, singles; brown; 55 epi (22 epc)
- *weft*: cotton, pair of singles; brown; 25 ppi (10 ppc)
- *supplementary weft*: cotton, 5 singles or 2-ply; purple, multicolored; over 3 warps

Backstrap-loomed, warp-predominant plain weave, three 4-selvedge pieces, two-faced supp. weft brocade; 2 medallions on shoulders, black taffeta used in each medallion, and chain-stitched around; *randa*, sewn with multicolored and space-dyed yarn; head-hole cut out, embellished with black taffeta chain-stitched neck piece.

> **Iconography**: "new" floral style with some geometric motifs. Extra shed stick utilized to speed up weaving process, indicated by vertical ridges in supp. weft brocading; use of brown as background suggests a ceremonial *huipil*, since highly valued *ixcaco* or *cuyuscate* (natural brown cotton) was utilized in the past. See **114** for description of design layout.

85–144
Bjerregaard 1977:55–57
See **114, 116, 117, 118, 119, 120**

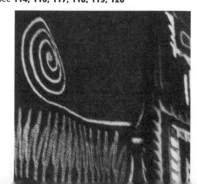

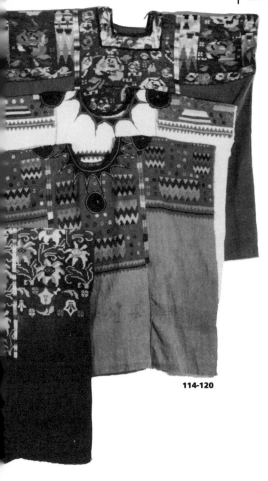

114-120

huipil

| Blouse |

116

El Quiché: Chichicastenango
Quiché
C&BS 1970s 1985
29½" x 32"   (75cm x 82cm)
- *warp*: cotton, singles; black, 70 epi (28 epc)
- *weft*: cotton, 4 singles; dark and light blue; 15 ppi (6 ppc)
- *supplementary weft*: wool, three 2-ply and singles; brown and multicolored; over 3 warps
See **115** for fabrication, neck treatment, surface embellishments, iconography, and technique.

85–145
See **114, 115, 117, 118, 119, 120**

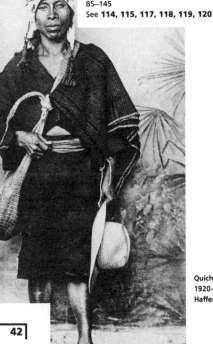

Quichean man from Chichicastenango, El Quiché.
1920-1930. Herbert J. Spinden Photo Archives,
Haffenreffer Museum of Anthropology.

huipil

| Blouse |

117

El Quiché: Chichicastenango
Quiché
C&BS 1970s 1985
29" x 33"   (74cm x 84cm)
- *warp*: cotton, singles; brown; 60 epi (24 epc)
- *weft*: cotton, pair of singles; brown; 20 ppi (8 ppc)
- *supplementary weft*: cotton and wool, four singles and 2-ply; red and multicolored; over 3 warps
See **115** for fabrication, neck treatment, surface embellishments, and use of color brown.

Iconography: abstracted double-headed eagle.

The use of the double-headed eagle in Chichicastenango male and female costume elements has persisted over a century; blocks of zigzag forms in **117** represent vestiges of wing and claw feather motifs seen in the bird image as it was woven into cloths from 1900–1940; might be interpreted as a *cofradia* or ceremonial style.

It would be worn loosely over the costume and not tucked in (Rowe 1981:90). The weaver is using the background or negative space to set off some of the design elements.

85–146
Schevill 1986: 29, 30; 40–48
See **114, 115, 116, 118, 119, 120**

huipil

| Blouse |

118

El Quiché: Chichicastenango
Quiché
C&BS 1970s 1985
28½" x 33"   (72cm x 84cm)
- *warp*: cotton, singles; white; 65 epi (26 epc)
- *weft*: cotton, 3 singles; white; 20 ppi (8 ppc)
- *supplementary weft*: cotton and synthetic, five 2-ply; red and multicolored; over 4 warps
See **115** for fabrication, neck treatment, medallions on shoulders.

Hand-sewn seams present a variation of buttonhole stitch but only in the upper part of the *huipil*; white was the traditional color for *huipiles* in the early part of the twentieth century; the separation of central design area from the neck and the use of geometric designs suggest an older style; this example was woven for sale; pick-up technique utilized; see **117** for use of negative space.

85–147
Goodman 1976: 55, 66
See **114, 115, 116, 117, 119, 120**

huipil

| Blouse |

119

El Quiché: Chichicastenango
Quiché
C&BS 1970s 1985
29½" x 30½"   (75cm x 78cm)
- *warp*: cotton, 3 singles; brown; 65 epi (26 epc)
- *weft*: cotton, 3 singles; brown; 15 ppi (6 ppc)
- *supplementary weft*: cotton and rayon, singles and 2-ply; purple and multicolored; over 3 warps
See **115** for fabrication, neck treatment, surface embellishments, use of color brown. See **117** for iconography.

Black velvet replaced taffeta for neck piece and medallions; rayon has taken the place of silk for supp. weft brocading giving a lustrous, rich impression; a recent example recalling older style iconography, materials, and techniques.

85–148
See **114, 115, 116, 117, 118, 120**

huipil

| Blouse |

120

El Quiché: Chichicastenango
Quiché
C&BS 1970s 1985
29½" x 35"   (75cm x 90cm)
- *warp*: cotton, singles; brown; 65 epi (26 epc)
- *weft*: cotton, 3 singles; brown and red; 25 ppi (10 ppc)
- *supplementary weft*: cotton and wool; 2–4 singles and four 2-ply; purple, space-dyed, and multicolored; over 3 warps
See **115** for fabrication, iconography, use of color brown. Neck treatment differs from other examples; an embroidered floral design piece outlined with black velvet was sewn to neck; **120** exhibits signs of wear, frequent washings until cloth has a soft, silky touch; extra shed stick was utilized for supp. weft patterning.

This group of seven *huipiles*, **114–120**, woven over a thirty-year period, exhibits a consistency in the use of single warps, dimensions, and fabrication. There is a wide range of variety in other categories for Chichicastenango weavers have always responded to outside as well as internal pressures. Innovations have been integrated into textile design more rapidly than in other, more conservative Mayan villages. The acceptance of an extra shed stick to speed up the process of weaving is an outstanding example. However, it is interesting to note that the use of pick-up technique, which can produce rounded forms, coexists with the new technique.

85–149
Schevill 1986: 61
Rowe 1981: 86–97
See **114, 115, 116, 117, 118, 119**

tzute

| Cloth, carrying |

121

El Quiché: Chichicastenango
Quiché
Museum Purchase   1920–1940   1983
20" x 25¼"   (50.5cm x 64cm)
- *warp*: cotton, a pair of handspun singles; white, red, and indigo; 80 epi (32 epc)
- *weft*: cotton, handspun singles; white; 30 ppi (12 ppc)
- *supplementary weft*: cotton and silk, singles; red, white, green, blue, and lavender
Backstrap-loomed, warp-predominant plain weave, one 4-selvedge piece cut in half; warp stripes; two-faced supp. weft brocade; 2 ends hand-sewn; silk used in *randa*.

Iconography: female figures, double-headed eagles, copulating animals, birds.

An old and valued piece; great care taken in patching worn edges, cloth with similar stripes from newer textiles used; relates to examples from the early twentieth century in the American Museum of Anthropology and the Lowie Museum of Anthropology.

Certain very interesting textiles used for ceremonial purposes, and not duplicated in other parts of the country, attract the interest and admiration of all visitors to Chichicastenango. These are called *tsibal kaperrah*, "pictured cloth" (Rodas, Rodas, and Hawkins 1940:134).

83–147
Rodas, Rodas, and Hawkins 1940:127–135
See **122, 123**

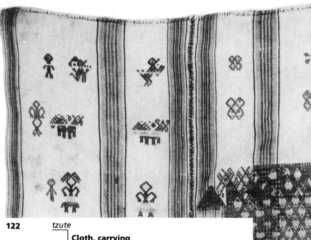

122

tzute

Cloth, carrying

122

El Quiché: Chichicastenango
Quiché
Museum Purchase   1920–1940   1983
25¼" x 20"   (64cm x 51cm)
• *warp*: cotton, handspun singles and pairs; white, brown (natural), red, and yellow; 70 epi (26 epc)
• *weft*: cotton, pair of singles; white; 25 ppi (10 ppc)
• *supplementary weft*: cotton, 6 singles; red, light green, and yellow
Backstrap-loomed, warp-predominant plain weave, one 4-selvedge piece cut in half; 2 ends hand-sewn; warp stripes, two-faced supp. weft brocade.
See **121** for comments and references.
Iconography: large double-headed eagles, male and female figures, birds, stars, and feathered serpents.

Ixcaco or *cuyuscate* is utilized for warp stripes, a sign of the ceremonial importance of this textile. Female *tzutes* are multifunctional, and therefore the weaver can be quite free in use of motifs, dimensions, and colors. No attempt has been made to match designs in the two pieces of cloth, woven as one web.

Some of these animals recall primitive totemic beliefs or legends regarding animals; others celebrate the hunt or care of domestic fowl. What one could take to be a horse is actually the *danta* or tapir, the largest animal known to the Guatemalan Indians before the arrival of the Spaniards (Rodas, Rodas, and Hawkins 1940:134).

83–149
See **121, 123**

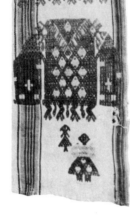

tzute

Cloth, carrying

123

El Quiché: Chichicastenango
Quiché
Museum Purchase   1940s   1983
31" x 30"   (79cm x 76cm)
• *warp*: cotton, pair of singles; red, blue, and white; 70 epi (28 epc)
• *weft*: same as warp; red; 25 ppi (19 ppc)
• *supplementary weft*: cotton, 12 singles; light and dark blues, white, touches of yellow, and rust; over 4–6 warps
Backstrap-loomed, warp-predominant plain weave, two 4-selvedge pieces, two-faced supp. weft brocade, warp stripes, one end hand-sewn, perhaps due to wear.

Iconography: female figures, stars, and one horse (see **122**).

The largest figures seen on the *tsibal kaperrah* are the horses (with their tails curved over their backs), the highly conventionalized double-headed eagles, and women with large triangular skirts and arms akimbo. These latter have been declared to represent Kiche princesses; but the Kiche who are well versed in their hereditary symbols say that these are *ishtan*, or domestic servants of royalty. We should hardly expect to find princesses surrounded by animals (Rodas, Rodas, and Hawkins 1940:135). The fine thread count and iconography are consistent in **121, 122,** and **123. 123** is considerably larger, with red as a dominant color, more typical of the 1930s or 1940s.

83–148
See **114, 130, 132**   Female Costume and **121, 122**

Hats, children

124

El Quiché: Chichicastenango
Quiché
JP   1970s   1978
15" x 23"   (38cm x 58.5cm) for both hats
cotton, singles and doubles; multicolored; 5–6 spi (2–3 spc)
Crochet; begun in center, worked outward, increasing in size.

Mayan women cover their children's head from birth until they are weaned and walking, around two years old. Some caps are very ornate and women take great care in weaving them on the backstrap loom. Others like **124** are crocheted rapidly by men.

78–239 A & B

tzute

Cloth, head

125

El Quiché: Chichicastenango
Quiché
CWH   1960s   1967
35" x 40½"   (89cm x 103cm)
• *warp*: cotton, 3 singles, red and black; 40 epi (16 epc)
• *weft*: cotton, 2 singles, red; 24 ppi (9 ppc)
• *supplementary weft*: silk floss; multicolored
Backstrap-loomed, warp-predominant plain weave, one 4-selvedge piece cut in half, two-faced supp. weft brocading; ends hand-sewn with red and black silk; *randa*, multicolored silk; four multicolored 2-ply silk tassels affixed to corners; extra purple silk wrapping on joining; silk knobs on each tassel.

Iconography: "new" floral designs, like **114**; some lozenge forms; narrow floral borders at top and bottom of supp. weft design area.

Rich use of color including space-dyed or *manchada* silk; two sides match well but within design areas, no attempt was made to weave identical motifs. Extra shed stick used for some of the brocading as well as a pick-up stick; yellow silk sewn stitches below left design area might be weaver's mark.

A pre-Columbian dress form, worn pirate-style wrapped around head with tassels hanging over shoulders.

67–10004
Schevill 1986: 55
See **112, 113, 126, 128, 131**   Male Costume

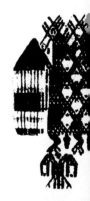

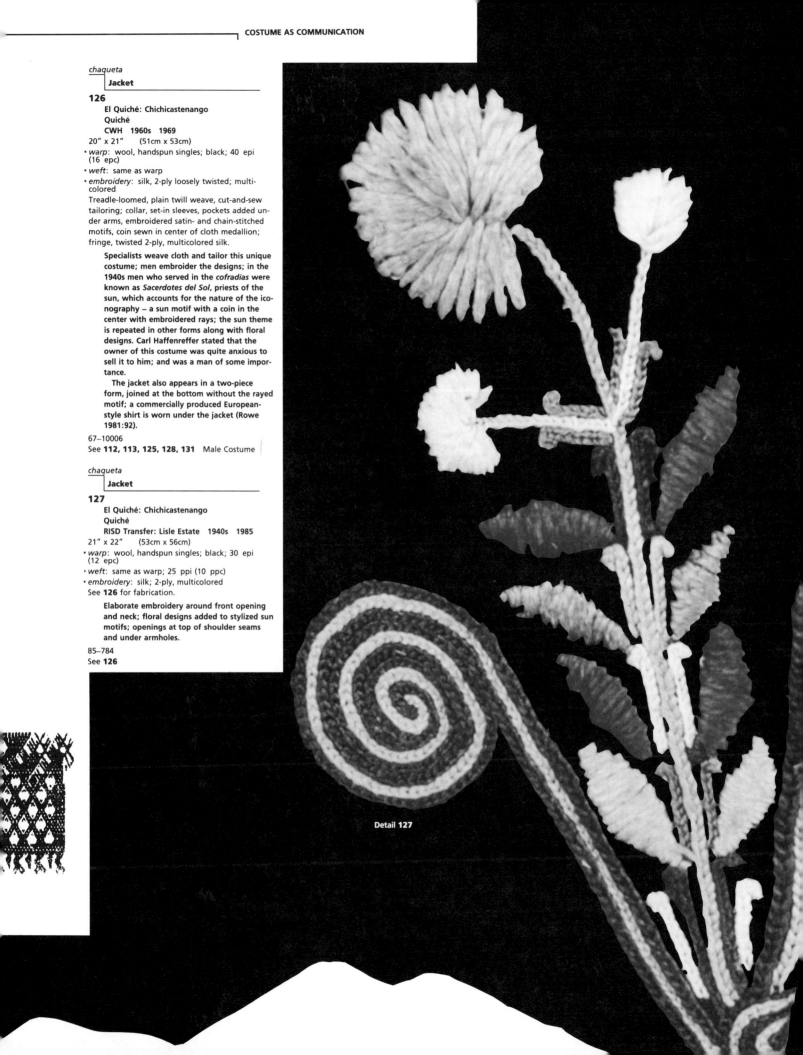

chaqueta

Jacket

126

El Quiché: Chichicastenango
Quiché
CWH   1960s   1969
20" x 21"   (51cm x 53cm)
- *warp*: wool, handspun singles; black; 40 epi (16 epc)
- *weft*: same as warp
- *embroidery*: silk, 2-ply loosely twisted; multi-colored

Treadle-loomed, plain twill weave, cut-and-sew tailoring; collar, set-in sleeves, pockets added under arms, embroidered satin- and chain-stitched motifs, coin sewn in center of cloth medallion; fringe, twisted 2-ply, multicolored silk.

Specialists weave cloth and tailor this unique costume; men embroider the designs; in the 1940s men who served in the *cofradias* were known as *Sacerdotes del Sol*, priests of the sun, which accounts for the nature of the iconography – a sun motif with a coin in the center with embroidered rays; the sun theme is repeated in other forms along with floral designs. Carl Haffenreffer stated that the owner of this costume was quite anxious to sell it to him; and was a man of some importance.

The jacket also appears in a two-piece form, joined at the bottom without the rayed motif; a commercially produced European-style shirt is worn under the jacket (Rowe 1981:92).

67–10006
See **112, 113, 125, 128, 131**   Male Costume

chaqueta

Jacket

127

El Quiché: Chichicastenango
Quiché
RISD Transfer: Lisle Estate   1940s   1985
21" x 22"   (53cm x 56cm)
- *warp*: wool, handspun singles; black; 30 epi (12 epc)
- *weft*: same as warp; 25 ppi (10 ppc)
- *embroidery*: silk; 2-ply, multicolored

See **126** for fabrication.

Elaborate embroidery around front opening and neck; floral designs added to stylized sun motifs; openings at top of shoulder seams and under armholes.

85–784
See **126**

Detail 127

pantalón

Pants

128

El Quiché: Chichicastenango
Quiché
CWH 1960s 1967
26¾" x 18½"   (68cm x 47cm)
- *warp*: wool, handspun singles; black; 40 epi (16 epc)
- *weft*: same as warp
- *embroidery*: silk, 2-ply; multicolored
Treadle-loomed, plain twill weave, cut-and-sew tailoring, hand-sewn seams, added pieces of cloth create flaps on back, pants open at bottom; chain-stitched embroidery.

> **Iconography**: the rayed-sun motif.
> Embroidered motifs on each flap, visible from the back of the garment; held in place by a wide sash.
> Perhaps the best-known of European-derived Guatemalan costumes is the famous black wool overtunic and short "eared" pants of Chichicastenango (Anawalt 1984:17). Formerly worn on a daily basis, now for *cofradía*, of European cut and form, but archaic – perhaps nineteenth century – in origin (Rowe 1981:91).
> Employees of the Mayan Inn in Chichicastenango were wearing this costume in 1977.

67–10008
See **112, 113, 125, 126, 131** Male Costume

Detail 141

faja

Sash

129

El Quiché: Village unknown
Linguistic group unknown
CWH 1960s 1967
54½" x 3½"   (138cm x 9cm)
- *warp*: cotton, 2 and 3 singles; multicolored; 35 epi (14 epc)
- *weft*: cotton, 3 singles; green; 20 ppi (8 ppc)
Backstrap-loomed, warp-faced plain weave, warp stripes, twisted fringe.

> Belts of this kind are popular with tourists and can be bought in many parts of Guatemala. **129** may have been woven in Santa Eulalia, Huehuetenango (Dieterich, Erickson, and Younger 1979:43).

67–10005

faja

Sash, female

130

El Quiché: Chichicastenango
Quiché
CWH 1960s 1967
97" x 2½"   (246 cm x 6 cm)
- *warp*: wool, 2-ply; white and brown; 55 epi (22 epc)
- *weft*: same as warp; brown; 15 ppi (6 ppc)
- *embroidery*: cotton and silk, 2-ply and 3-ply; maroon, space-dyed, and multicolored
Backstrap-loomed; warp-faced plain weave; warp stripes; embroidery: chain, satin, and fishbone stitches; cut warp make fringe.

> **Iconography**: flowers.
> Belts are woven by men, sold all over the highlands; each village has their own motifs (see **221**); wound around the waist several times so that patterning shows on outside of front (Rowe 1981:90).

67–10007
See **114, 123, 132** Female Costume

faja

Sash, male

131

El Quiché: Chichicastenango
Quiché
C&BS 1970s 1985
103" x 15½"   (262 cm x 40.5cm)
- *warp*: cotton, pair of singles; red; 37 epi (15 epc)
- *weft*: cotton, 4 singles; red; 12 ppi (5 ppc)
- *supplementary weft*: pearl cotton, eight 2-ply; multicolored; over 3–15 warps
Backstrap-loomed, warp-predominant plain weave, two-faced supp. weft brocade, warp twisted fringe on both ends.

> **Iconography**: zigzag or feathered serpent motifs.
> These motifs present in headdresses or *tzutes* of the 1960s and 1970s; zigzags may also be related to the double-headed eagle motif, a visual rendering of the wings, which has become abstracted over time. Plain red as well as supp. weft brocaded sashes are part of the man's costume.

85–150
See **112, 113, 125, 126, 128** Male Costume

corte

Skirt

132

El Quiché: Chichicastenango
Quiché
CWH 1960s 1967
92" x 33"   (234cm x 84cm)
- *warp*: cotton, singles; dark blue; 55 epi (22 epc)
- *weft*: cotton, singles and in pairs; white and blue; 55 ppi (22 ppc)
- *randa*: cotton, 5 singles; maroon, multicolored, and space-dyed
Treadle-loomed, balanced plain weave; 2 pieces, weft stripes, joined with *randa*, to make length, additional *randa* creates a tube.

> The skirt is wrapped smoothly around the body, the extra length passing around the back, ending on one side (Rowe 1981:90). The sash holds the skirt in place.

67–10001
See **114, 123, 130** Female Costume

huipil

Blouse

133

El Quiché: Nebaj
Ixil
C&BS 1960s 1985
29½" x 38½"   (75cm x 98cm)
- *warp*: cotton, pair of 2-ply; white; 50 epi (20 epc)
- *weft*: cotton, three 2-ply; white and multicolored; 10 ppi (4 ppc)
- *supplementary weft*: cotton, pair of 2-ply; multicolored; over 1–10 warps
Backstrap-loomed, warp-predominant plain weave, two 4-selvedge pieces, single-faced supp. weft brocade, weft stripes with supp. weft brocade added; all seams machine-stitched; neck cut out and an extra piece of cloth added, machine-stitched; hand embroidered designs.

> **Iconography**: birds, horses, female and male figures.
> Densely brocaded, not much negative space; almost entire *huipil* covered with supp. weft designs; embroidered neck treatment is related to **117**; gives effect of medallions, white background sets off designs effectively.
> Profile and frontal bird images shared by Ixil speakers (Deuss 1981:50).
> Narrow vertical and slanting lines are made by wrapping the pattern wefts around two warp threads (Bjerregaard 1977:84). Two panel *huipil* common in the 1960s, replaced by three panel style (**134**) in the 1970s (Rowe 1981:134).

85–151
See **135, 136, 138** Female Costume

huipil

Blouse

134

El Quiché: Nebaj
Ixil
C&BS 1970s 1985
27½" x 44"   70cm x 112cm
- *warp*: cotton, pair of 4-ply; white; 20 epi (8 epc)
- *weft*: cotton, 4 singles; white and multicolored; 10 ppi (4 ppc)
- *supplementary weft*: cotton, four 2-ply; multicolored, over 1–3 warps
See **133** for fabrication and neck treatment.

> **Iconography**: lozenges, half-lozenges, female plant and bird figures; on bottom, female and bird figures stand out against white background.
> One of the newer styles, which echoes those woven in the early twentieth century; images only appear on the center panel, back and front; center of sleeve openings has been stitched together; weft wrapping along with supp. weft brocading.
> On the older piece, figures are arranged more randomly, while on the newer one (**134**) horizontal bands of supp. weft brocaded stripes compartmentalize the patterns into layers (Anderson 1978:91).

85–152
Rowe 1981:132–134
Bjerregaard 1977:84–85
See **135, 136, 138** Female Costume

tzute

Cloth, carrying

Female Costume 134, 135, 137

135

El Quiché: Nebaj
Ixil
C&BS 1970s 1985
56" x 24"   (141cm x 61cm)
- *warp*: cotton, pair of 2-ply; multicolored; 25 epi (10 epc)
- *weft*: cotton, 5-singles; red and multicolored; 8 ppi (3 ppc)
- *supplementary weft*: cotton, four 2-ply and pair of 2-ply; multicolored; white; over 8–16 warps.
Backstrap-loomed, warp-predominant plain weave, one piece, warp and weft stripes, single-faced supp. weft brocade, uncut warp fringe.

> **Iconography**: geometric, corn-plant, and bird images.
> Supp. weft bands divide piece into sections.

85–153
See **134, 136, 138** Female Costume

tocoyal

Headdress

136

El Quiché: Nebaj
Ixil
Museum Purchase 1970s 1980
117" x 13"   (275cm x 34cm)
- *warp*: cotton and pearl cotton, pair of singles and four 2-ply; red, purple, green, brown, blue, and white; 80 epc (32 epc)
- *weft*: cotton of singles; red; 20 ppi (8 ppc)
Backstrap-loomed, warp-predominant plain weave, 4 selvedges; warp stripes; ends are folded back, machine-stitched to make point, 7 tassels added; 4 on one end, 3 on other; single joinings wrapped.

> A pre-Columbian dress form; **136** unusual in its lack of supp. weft brocaded motifs.
> The women of Nebaj weave a long, brightly striped piece of fabric fifteen inches wide which is twisted round the hair and head to form a spectacular turban (Deuss 1981:33).
> Hair is wound with the band itself. When the hair becomes thin, a cord is added to it so that the band can be wound beyond the length of the hair to make a roll of the desired length (Rowe 1981:140).

80–158
See **134, 135, 138** Female Costume

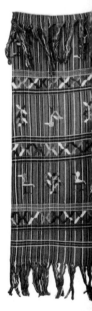

tocoyal

Headdress

137

El Quiché: Nebaj
Ixil
C&BS   1970s   1985
102" x 12½"   (269cm x 32.5cm)
• *warp*: cotton, two 2-ply; multicolored; 35 epi (14 epc)
• *weft*: cotton and pearl cotton, pair of singles and two 2-ply; red; 5 ppi (2 ppc)
• *supplementary weft*: pearl cotton, four 2-ply; multicolored; over 3–8 warps
See **136** for fabrication, comments, and references. Single-faced supp. weft brocade, 6 tassels added, 3 on each end; double wrapped joinings.

> **Iconography:** lozenges.
> Supp. weft stripes; supp. weft. brocading on one end only.

85–154

faja

Sash, female

138

El Quiché: Nebaj
Ixil
Museum Purchase   1970s   1980
99½" x 3¼"   (251cm x 8cm)
• *warp*: cotton, 2-ply; red, white, and black; 90 epi (40 epc)
• *weft*: cotton, 5 singles; red; 12 ppi (5 ppc)
• *supplementary weft*: pearl cotton, three 2-ply; multicolored.
Backstrap-loomed, warp-faced plain weave, single-faced supp. weft brocade, warp stripes; uncut warp ends create fringe on both ends; weft threads are increased and pulled tight on each end; sash becomes narrower.

> **Iconography:** geometric forms.
> Supp. weft brocaded section on one end only.
> The wraparound skirt, typical of Nebaj, is of treadle-loomed fabric, predominantly red with narrow weft stripes in yellow and ikat yarns at spaced intervals; the skirt is wrapped snugly with the end passing around the back, ending on the left side and held in place by a belt (Rowe 1981:135–137, 25).
> Cloth for skirts is woven in Huehuetenango and is also used by women from Chajul (Anderson 1978:158).

80–154
See **134, 135, 136**   Female Costume

ALTA VERAPAZ

huipil

Blouse

139

Alta Verapaz: Cobán
Kekchí
Museum Purchase   1970s   1983
15½" x 34½"   (40cm x 86cm)
• *warp*: cotton, single; white; 15 epi (6 epc)
• *weft*: same as warp
• *supplementary weft*: cotton, 4 singles; white; over 1–3 warps
Backstrap-loomed, three 4-selvedge pieces, widely spaced balanced plain weave, single-faced supp. weft brocade, head-hole cut out; embroidery at neck and sleeves, multicolored cotton yarn, all seams hand-sewn.

> **Iconography:** images of corn plants, deer, floral and geometric forms.
> Floral designs are embroidered around the neck and sleeves; a piece of cotton is used as facing for this process since the cloth is fragile; satin and chain stitches are employed.
> A year-round warm climate requires that clothing in the Cobán area be light; gauze-weave white-on-white cloth is a specialty; *huipiles* are short and not tucked into the gathered European-style ikat skirts (see **156**).

83–72
Anderson 1978:140–142
Dieseldorff 1984

huipil

Blouse, uncut

140

Alta Verapaz: Cobán
Kekchí
OAG   1970s   1984
31½" x 38"   (80cm x 98cm)
• *warp*: cotton, pair of singles; white; 20 epi (8 epc)
• *weft*: same as warp
• *supplementary weft*: cotton, 4 singles; white; over 1–4 warps
Backstrap-loomed, three 4-selvedge pieces, hand-sewn together; head-hole uncut; rows of gauze weave alternate with rows of two-faced supp. weft brocading on balanced plain weave.

> **Iconography:** animal and plant images.
> Warp threads stiffened with *atole*, a corn drink, to facilitate the weaving process.
> It is the custom to use the head-hole area for weaving experimentations; weavers cut these squares out and save them for future reference (Baizerman, pers. com. 1986).
> Gauze weave is one in which the odd-numbered warps are crossed over the even-numbered warps and held in the position by a passage of the weft, thus creating a line of openwork (Kent 1983:296).
> Gauze weave has been practiced by Mayan weavers over time; recent excavations at Rio Azul, A.D. 450–500, produced a gauze-woven shroud (Adams 1986:436).

82–203
Dieseldorff 1984
Pancake and Baizerman 1982:1–26
See **27, 141, 142, 143**

huipil

Blouse, uncut

141

Alta Verapaz: Cobán
Kekchí
OAG   1970s   1984
35" x 40"   (90cm x 101cm)
• *warp*: cotton, singles; white; 32 epi (13 epc)
• *weft*: same as warp; 27 ppi (11 ppc)
• *supplementary weft*: cotton, 4 singles; white; over 1–4 warps
Backstrap-woven, three 4-selvedge pieces, hand-sewn together; head-hole uncut; balanced plain widely spaced weave; two-faced supp. weft brocading.

> **Iconography:** rows of horses alternate with an abstracted representation of the spider.
> A Kekchí myth attributes the art of weaving to the spider, from whom the weavers learned their craft (Dieseldorff 1984:11).

84–204
See **140** for references.
See **140, 142, 143**

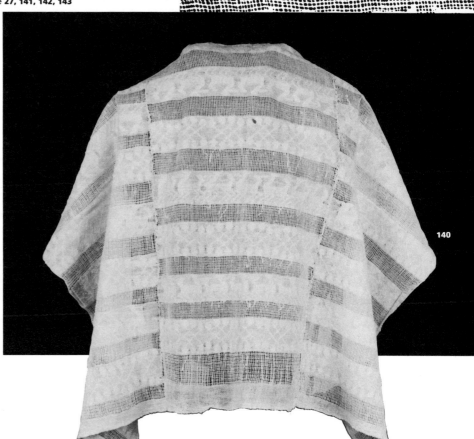

140

139

46

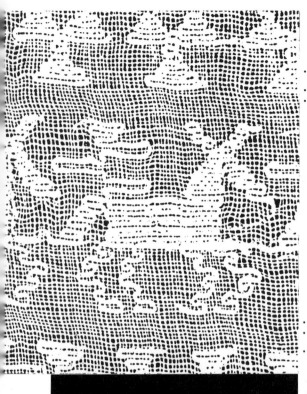

huipil

Blouse, uncut

143

    Alta Verapaz: Cobán
    Kekchí
    OAG 1970s 1984
43½" x 38"   (110.5cm x 90cm)
• *warp*: cotton, pair of singles; white; 50 epi (20 epc)
• *weft*: same as warp; white; 30 ppi (12 ppc)
• *supplementary weft*: cotton, 6-singles; white; over 3–10 warps
Backstrap-loomed, three 4-selvedge pieces; rows of single-faced supp. weft brocading alternate with rows of warp-predominant plain weave, pieces hand sewn together; head-hole uncut.

    Iconography: animals and geometric forms.
    A heavier piece of cloth than **140–142**; relates to designs of Tamahú, where multicolored supp. weft yarns are utilized.

84–206
See **140, 141, 142, 145**

huipil

Blouse

144

    Alta Verapaz: Tactic style
    Kekchí
    RP 1970s 1985
26½" x 37½"   (67.5cm x 95cm)
• *warp*: cotton, pair of 2-ply; red; 35 epi (14 epc)
• *weft*: cotton, singles and 2-ply; red; 25 ppi (10 ppc)
• *supplementary weft*: cotton and synthetic; multicolored, over 2–4 warps
Backstrap-loomed, balanced plain weave, three 4-selvedge pieces; commercial gray cloth machine-stitched to bottom for length; single-faced supp. weft brocade; head-hole and sleeves cut out and bound with blue velvet, all machine-stitched.

    A *huipil* with the designs of Tactic but made in Chimaltenango to be used in Quezaltenango and in other areas; the gray cloth is added so that the *huipil* can be tucked into the skirt whereas in Tactic it is worn loosely without addition of commercial cloth (Arriola Geng, pers. com. 1986).

86–6

huipil

Blouse, uncut

145

    Alta Verapaz: Tamahú
    Kekchí
    C&BS 1970s 1985
34½" x 41½"   (88cm x 106cm)
• *warp*: cotton, pair of singles; dark blue, 40 epi (16 epc)
• *weft*: same as warp; dark blue and green; 20 ppi (8 ppc)
• *supplementary weft*: cotton, 6 singles; red, green, blue, yellow, purple, over 2–6 warps
Backstrap-loomed, warp-predominant plain weave, three 4-selvedge pieces, single-faced supp. weft brocade, pieces hand-sewn together; head-hole uncut.

    Iconography: zigzags with diamonds and triangles; background used as a triangular design element; green bands on bottom of center panel.
    Tamahú weavers utilize single-faced supplementary weft weaving with a pick-up stick, similar to Tactic and San Antonio Aguas Calientes (see **202**); their weaving resembles that of neighboring villages except for color (Anderson 1978:95).
    The *huipil* is worn loose over a European-style gathered skirt; no belt is worn.

85–169
See **143**

huipil

Blouse, uncut

142

    Alta Verapaz: Cobán
    Kekchí
    OAG 1970s 1984
34" x 37"   (86cm x 94cm)
• *warp*: cotton, singles; white; 40 epi (16 epc)
• *weft*: singles and 3 singles; white; 30 ppi (12 ppc)
Backstrap-woven, three 4-selvedge pieces, hand-sewn together, head-hole uncut; seersucker weave.

    Seersucker or *tzot*; 3 weft singles are inserted every third or fourth shot for several rows alternating with bands of balanced plain weave, creating a sheer texture; multiple wefts are pulled tight making a wrinkled effect; formerly a common weave, now difficult to find.

84–205
Dieseldorff 1984:14
See **140, 141, 143**

Backstrap loom set up for gauze weave.
Drawing by Suzanne Baizerman.

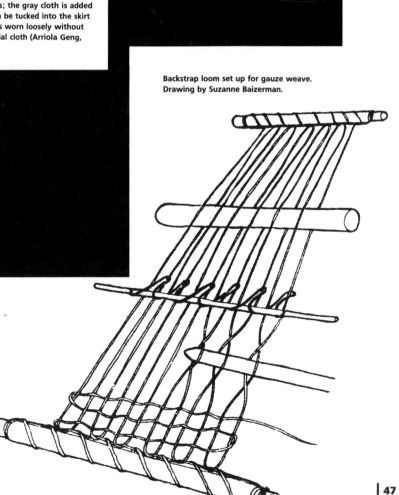

TOTONICAPÁN

Blanket

146

Totonicapán: Momostenango
Quiché
CWH   1960s   1967
85½" x 59"   (217cm x 150cm)
• *warp*: wool, handspun singles; dark blue; 15 epi (6 epc)
• *weft*: same as warp; 20 ppi (8 ppc)
• *supplementary weft*: white, red, and yellow; over 2–4 warps
Treadle-loomed, weft stripes, supp. weft double-faced patterning, brushed finish, twisted ends.

Iconography: rows of *quetzal* birds, the national symbol of Guatemala, boys and girls, rabbits, stylized zigzags on top and bottom.

The blankets are used by Indians and *Ladinos* alike; a family operation with each member having a special task from spinning, through dyeing and weaving, which is sometimes shared by two boys or men; one throws the ground weft, the other lays in the supp. weft; the loom is wide, so one throws the bobbin to the other who returns it for the next throw. Blankets are washed and trampled in nearby hot springs to shrink them; while still damp, brushed with teasals to give them their attractive finish (Anderson 1978:162–163).

Another type of tapestry-woven blanket is also produced in Momostenango.

67–10010

cinta
Belt

147

Totonicapán: Totonicapán
Quiché
FS   1960s   1978
71" x 1½"   (180cm x 3.5cm)
• *warp*: cotton, 4 singles; white; 20 epi (8 epc)
• *weft*: cotton and silk; singles; multicolored; 24 ppi (12 ppc), 60 ppi (23 ppc) for the silk
Treadle-loomed, weft-faced plain weave; eccentric tapestry technique; cored corn cobs used as base for black fuzzy tassels (Pancake, pers. com. 1978); cobs covered with cloth, warps pulled through hollow cobs; extra fringe of silk added.

Iconography: abstract, geometric forms, plain bands.

Woven on a four harness counterbalance treadle loom that uses the weaver's body as the primary warp tensioning device; woven warp is wrapped over a small rod which the weaver has attached to her apron or belt; the warp is tensioned when the weaver adjusts her belt and body to a suitable position (McEldowney 1982:26). Two types of *cintas* are being produced by Totonicapán weavers: traditional-functional (**147**) and tourist; there are special characteristics or combination of characteristics of tapestry *cintas* that are capable of distinguishing town or municipio-specific identity (ibid.: 3).

78–274
McEldowney 1982

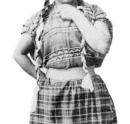

147

BAJA VERAPAZ

huipil
Blouse

148

Baja Verapaz: Rabinal
Quiché
FS   1970s   1978
22½" x 26"   (57cm x 66cm)
• *warp*: cottons, two 2-ply; pink; 35 epi (14 epc)
• *weft*: cotton, three 2-ply; pink; 20 ppi (8 ppc)
• *supplementary weft*: cotton and wool, four 2-ply; multicolored; over 1–10 warps
Backstrap-loomed, warp-predominant plain weave, one 4-selvedge piece, single-faced supp. weft brocade; cut out neck, buttonhole stitched, also at arm holes; hand-sewn side seams.

Iconography: zigzags with geometric border on the bottom of design area; one square icon on the front, may be the weaver's mark.

148 resembles the neighboring San Miguel Chicaj style; unusual for *huipil* to be made out of one 4-selvedge piece of cloth; worn with a wraparound weft ikat skirt woven in Rabinal on treadle loom; a *cinta* or hair ribbon woven in Totonicapán (see **147** for comments), and a belt.

78–265
Deuss 1981:32
Bunch and Bunch 1977:25

corte
Skirt

149

Baja Verapaz: San Miguel Chicaj
Quiché
Museum Puchase   1980s   1985
4' 30" x 35"   (444cm x 89cm)
• *warp*: cotton, singles; multicolored and ikat; 50 epi (20 epc)
• *weft*: same as warp; multicolored and ikat; 40 ppi (14 ppc)
Treadle-loomed, balanced plain weave, ends machine-stitched together to make tube.

Produced by male weavers in Salcajá, Quezaltenango, in workshops; sometimes six or more motifs are used in both warp and weft, giving an effect of undulating colors and shapes without clearly delineated motifs; vendors sell these *cortes* all over the highlands and can be heard calling "cortes" in the streets when festival time is near.

85–486
Anderson 1978:157–158
Deuss 1981:58
Dieterich, Erickson, and Younger 1979:86

QUEZALTENANGO

faja
Belt, child's

150

Quezaltenango: Quezaltenango
Quiché
DH   1960s   1961
48" x 1"   (122cm x 2.5cm)
• *warp*: cotton, 2-ply; white and red-orange; 90 epi (36 epc)
• *weft*: cotton, 4 singles; light brown; 20 ppi (8 ppc)
Warp-faced plain weave; warp stripes, warp fringe.

61–2197
See **153, 156**   Child's Costume

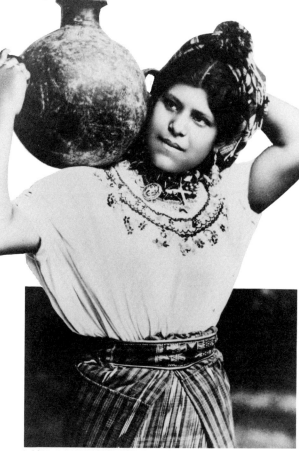

Quichean woman, San Cristóbal, Totonicapán. 1920–1930. Herbert J. Spinden Photo Archives, Haffenreffer Museum of Anthropology. See **147**.

149

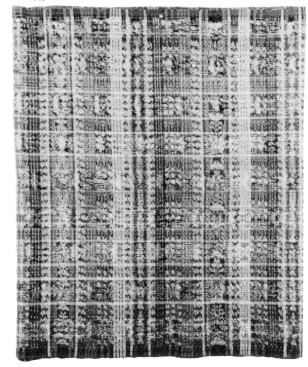

Quichean woman, Totonicapán. 1920–1930. Herbert J. Spinden Photo Archives, Haffenreffer Museum of Anthropology.

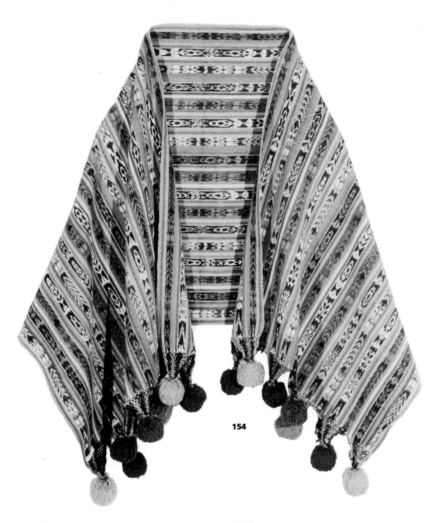

154

huipil
Blouse, child

153

Quezaltenango: Quezaltenango
Quiché
DH   1960s   1961
19" x 15"   (49cm x 38cm)
• *warp*: cotton, pair of singles; black; 45 epi
(18 epc)
• *weft*: same as warp; black and white; 41 ppi
(14 ppc)
• *supplementary weft*: pearl cotton, 2-ply; green,
white, purple, and blue; over 2–6 warps
Treadle-loomed, balanced plain weave; one piece,
two-faced supp. weft brocade, cut-out neck; embroidered piece added at neck, hand-sewn sides.

> **Iconography: geometric designs.**
> Handwoven by specialists; neck opening
> decorated with 2 in. band embroidered over-
> all with flowers; stitched up both sides
> except small arm hole at top; this specimen
> typical except for being hemmed at bottom
> (DH).

61–2195
See **150, 156**   Child's Costume

perraje
Shawl

154

Quezaltenango: Quezaltenango
Quiché
Museum Purchase   1980s   1982
71½" x 27½"   (200cm x 69cm)
• *warp*: cotton, two 2-ply; multicolored, metallic,
and ikat; 55 epi (22 epc)
• *weft*: cotton, three 2-ply; white; 15 ppi (6 ppc)
Treadle-loomed, warp-predominant plain weave,
warp stripes; cut warp ends are finished with macramé; 6 pom-poms on each end.

> **Iconography: plant and geometric images in
> ikat stripes.**
> A popular textile worn by *Ladinas* as well
> as traditional Mayan women of Santo Domin-
> go Xenacoj, Sacatepéquez, and San Pedro Sa-
> catepéquez, Guatemala (Barrios 1983: cover,
> 45).
> The knotting of the fringe into triangular
> points is typical (Rowe 1981:109,113).

82–70
Deuss 1981: 57
See **155**

perraje
Shawl

155

Quezaltenango: Quezaltenango
Quiché
Museum Puchase   1980s   1982
See **154** for complete description.

82–71

huipil
Blouse, uncut

151

Quezaltenango: Quezaltenango
Quiché
RISD Transfer: Lisle Estate   1950s   1985
156" x 15"   (396cm x 39 cm)
• *warp*: cotton, singles; white; 40 epi (16 epc)
• *weft*: cotton, pair of singles; multicolored and
ikat; 30 ppi (12 ppc)
• *supplementary weft*: cotton, 2–6 singles; yellow
and purple; over 2–4 warps
Treadle-loomed, warp-predominant plain weave,
double-faced supp. weft brocade, cut ends.

> **Iconography: geometrics, chevrons.**
> Woven in Totonicapán on a draw loom
> called a *falseria* in Guatemala; which is said
> to have originated in the department of San
> Marcos in 1865; weavers who use these
> looms use pattern harnesses attached to a
> regular treadle loom to raise the warps for in-
> sertion of supp. wefts; a draw boy selects the
> cords of the pattern harnesses; endless possi-
> bilities for patterning (Anderson
> 1978:163–167). To make a *huipil* three
> treadle-woven pieces are joined by *randas*;
> head-hole cut out and embroidered neck
> piece added.

85–787
Rowe 1981:106–108

huipil
Blouse, uncut

152

Quezaltenango: Quezaltenango
Quiché
DH   1960s   1961
67" x 35"   (170cm x 89cm)
• *warp*: cotton, pair of singles; white; 40 epi
(16 epc)
• *weft*: cotton, 2–3 singles; white; 34 ppi (14 ppc)
• *supplementary weft*: cotton, three singles and
2-ply; multicolored; over 1–10 warps
Treadle-loomed, balanced plain weave; two-faced
supp. weft brocade, cut at both ends.

> **Iconography: stylized *quetzal* birds, plants,
> flowers.**
> Woven on foot looms and embroidered by
> Quiché women who are specialists; blouses
> are normally sold unfinished; all that remains
> to be done to prepare for wear is to cut 8 in.
> slit across center and sew 1 in. ribbon (any
> color) around it; or insert a more elaborate
> trim (see **153**); designed for pullover fit, with-
> out sleeves – about half of the women put a
> few stitches in each side to prevent it from
> being entirely open; worn tucked into skirt,
> which is held up by tightly wrapped sash; for
> workaday or festive wear (DH).

61–2192
Bunch and Bunch 1977:72
See **157, 158**   Female Costume

falda
Skirt, child

156

Quezaltenango: Quezaltenango
Quiché
DH   1960s   1961
17½" x 14"   (45cm x 36cm)
• *warp*: cotton, pair of singles; green, black, and
white ikat; 45 epi (18 epc)
• *weft*: cotton, singles; same as warp; 40 ppi
(16 ppc)
Treadle-loomed, balanced plain weave, wide *randa* in front, gathered at waist with woolen
thread, cut warp ends hand hemmed.

> Cloth is machine-made locally by *Ladinos* for
> this sole purpose – sold in market by
> standard length for skirts only; short full skirt
> of this area constrasts with long tight skirt of
> most Quiché people, although cloth is similar
> (DH). A similarly styled skirt is worn in Cobán,
> Alta Verapaz.

61–2186
See **150, 153**   Child's costume

nagua

Skirt

157

Quezaltenango: Quezaltenango
Quiché
DH 1960s 1961
58" x 38"   (147.5cm x 96cm)
• *warp*: cotton, pair of singles; white, green, and black; 57 epi (23 epc)
• *weft*: same as warp; 52 ppi (21 ppc)
Treadle-loomed, balanced plain weave; double ikat, cut ends.

Same material as 156.

A simple rectangle that is wrapped around waist and legs very tightly and held in place with sash; for workaday or festive wear; typical of Quezaltenango and surrounding area, also much of the department of San Marcos (DH). Similar to **210**, old-style skirt of San Antonio Aguas Calientes, Sacatepéquez; worn in many other highland villages.

61–2193
See **152, 158** Female Costume

perraje

Shawl

158

Quezaltenango: Quezaltenango
Quiché
DH 1960s 1961
45" x 20½"   (114cm x 52cm)
• *warp*: wool, 2-ply; blue, green, and purple; 30 epi (16 epc)
• *weft*: wool, pair of singles; black; 20 ppi (8 ppc)
Backstrap or treadle-loomed, warp-predominant plain weave, warp stripes; cut warps create fringe; 10 tassels on each end.

A popular tourist item, still for sale in 1978.

61–2194
See **152, 157** Female Costume

capixay

Cape

159

Quezaltenango: San Martín Sacatepéquez,
Chili Verde
Mam
MS 1970s 1979
107½" x 36"   (273cm x 92cm)
• *warp*: wool, handspun singles; black; 15 epi (6 epc)
• *weft*: same as warp; 20 ppi (8 ppc)
Treadle-loomed, twill weave, 1 long piece, head-hole cut out; tailored; pieces added for sleeves, under arm seams open but stitched at wrist; fringe on one end; adds to garment length on one end.

The man's costume is one of the most spectacular in Guatemala; the *capixay* shows 16th-century European influence on a pre-Columbian dress form survival, the long tunic; the cassock of the Catholic priests and the Spanish riding coat are two sources for this unusual costume element; sleeves are purely ornamental; a fringe at the joining of the sleeves shows only when the wearer throws the sleeves onto his back.

79–24
Rowe 1981:119–121
Anderson 1978:118–123
See **160, 161, 162, 163** Male Costume

159

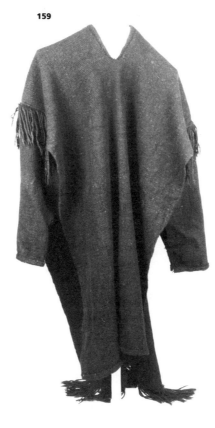

tzute

Cloth, head

160

Quezaltenango: San Martín Sacatepéquez,
Chili Verde
Mam
MS 1970s 1979
49½" x 47"   (126cm x 119cm)
• *warp*: cotton, three singles; red, yellow, orange; 35 epi (14 epc)
• *weft*: same as warp; red; 25 ppi (10 ppc)
Backstrap-loomed, warp-predominant plain weave, twill weave; one 4-selvedge piece cut in half, warp stripes; one end cut warps create fringe, the 2 pieces joined with orange stitching.

Worn pirate-fashion, folded in half, tied around the head, with extra cloth hanging down the back.

79–24
See **159** for references.
See **159, 161, 162, 163** Male Costume

pantalón

Pants

161

Quezaltenango: San Martín Sacatepéquez,
Chili Verde
Mam
MS 1970s 1979
34" x 25"   (85.5cm x 64cm)
• *warp*: cotton, pair of singles and 3 singles; white and red; 25 epi (10 epc)
• *weft*: cotton, 3-singles; white; 25 ppi (10 ppc)
• *supplementary weft*: cotton and pearl cotton, 3-singles and 2-ply; blue and multicolored; over 1–4 warps
Backstrap-loomed, warp-predominant plain weave, 2 pieces, single-faced supp. weft brocade on cuffs of pants; hand-sewn seams, 2 loom finished and 2 hemmed ends.

Iconography: geometric diamond motifs.
An example of European cut-and-sew process; a hybrid style; gusset is added to the crotch, and drawstring at the waist; very short in length, sometimes not visible under long tunic shirt.

79–21
See **159** for references.
See **159, 160, 162, 163** Male Costume

faja

Sash, male

162

Quezaltenango: San Martín Sacatepéquez,
Chili Verde
Mam
MS 1970s 1979
62" x 11½"   (314cm x 29cm)
• *warp*: cotton, 3-ply; red; 30 epi (12 epc)
• *weft*: same as warp
• *supplementary weft*: cotton and pearl cotton, 3-ply and 4-ply; blue, yellow, green, magenta, space-dyed blue; over 1–4 warps
Backstrap-loomed, warp-predominant plain weave, 1 piece, single-faced supp. weft brocade, warp fringe twisted.

Iconography: lozenges, horizontal bands.
The sash is worn wrapped around the waist twice, starting with the center in back, and finishing with the ends in back, where they are tied; the ends hang down; the sash is worn in this same way either over the *capixay*, or over the shirt if a *capixay* is not worn (Rowe 1981:120).

79–22
See **159** for references.
See **159, 160, 161, 163** Male Costume

camisa

Shirt

163

Quezaltenango: San Martín Sacatepéquez,
Chili Verde
Mam
MS 1970s 1979
48" x 25"   (123cm x 63cm)
• *warp*: cotton, 4-ply; white and red; 30 epi (12 epc)
• *weft*: cotton, 3-ply; white; 25 ppi (10 ppc)
• *supplementary weft*: cotton, pearl cotton, 3-ply; red, multicolored; space-dyed; over 2–10 warps
Backstrap-loomed, warp-predominant plain weave, 2 pieces hand-sewn together with opening for neck; double-faced supp. weft brocade on sleeves, 1 loom finished end, the other warp fringe.

Iconography: long-necked birds, small birds, geometric forms.
Weavers utilize both single- and two-faced supp. weft brocading; **163** represents another hybrid style; a combination of a long tunic, a pre-Columbian dress form, with set-in sleeves and cuffs, European tailoring devices.

79–23
See **159** for references.
See **159, 160, 161, 162** Male Costume

SOLOLÁ

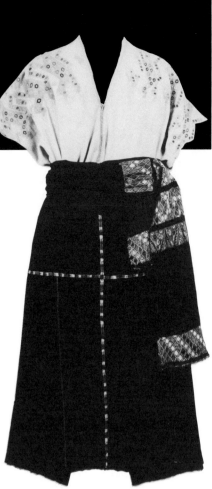

huipil
Blouse

164
Sololá: Nahualá
Quiché
MS 1960s 1979
29" x 32"   (74cm x 82cm)
- *warp*: cotton, pair of singles; white; 60 epi (24 epc)
- *weft*: same as warp; 36 ppi (12 ppc)
- *supplementary weft*: cotton, 4-singles; purple, orange, and multicolored; over 4 warps
Backstrap-loomed, warp-predominant plain weave, two 4-selvedge pieces, two-faced supp. weft brocade; only on shoulder area; *randa*, center seam left open for head.

> **Iconography**: 4-legged animals standing on their hind legs, birds, geometric fillers.
> These animals have been identified as lions (Morales Hidalgo 1982:67–68).
> There is much cerise in the everyday (164) and ceremonial blouses; it runs and stains each time it is washed, but the wearer likes the softened effect this gives (Pettersen 1976:98). Colors are almost indiscernible in this example due to excessive washing. Foundation cloth looks pink, due to running of purple dye.

79–28
Rowe 1981:74–78
See **165, 168** Female Costume

faja
Sash, female

165
Sololá: Nahualá
Quiché
MS 1970s 1979
99" x 9"   (252cm x 23cm)
- *warp*: cotton, pair of singles; indigo, lavender; 72 epi (28 epc)
- *weft*: same as warp; indigo; 18 ppi (7 ppc)
- *supplementary weft*: cotton, pair of 2-ply and 3-singles; multicolored; over 8–18 warps
Backstrap-loomed, warp-faced plain weave, two-faced supp. weft brocade, warp stripes, ends stitched with multicolored thread.

> **Iconography**: lozenges and zigzags; bands on bottom and lower third of sash; middle undecorated; bright colors of supp. weft brocading stand out against dark background.
> The woman steps into the skirt, places top of skirt above waist level, holds fabric to one side, makes skirt fit tightly on opposite hip; still holding fabric out, she pinches skirt together at hip, folding the rest flat; *huipil* is tucked in, belt wrapped around the body once, tied in a half-hitch; longer end wrapped around the waist; two brocaded ends secured in a square knot (Rowe 1981:81).

78–30
See **164, 168** Female Costume

Shirt, child

166
Sololá: Nahualá
Quiché
FS 1970s 1970
11½" x 14"   (30cm x 35.5cm)
- *warp*: cotton, pair of singles; black and rose; 40 epc (16 epc)
- *weft*: same as warp; black; 25 ppi (10 ppc)
- *supplementary weft*: see **165** for makeup, count, technique, iconography
Three kinds of cloth; 1 treadle-loomed; 2 backstrap-loomed; two-faced supp. weft brocade and warp ikat striped cloth; set-in sleeves which are pieced; machine-stitched throughout; neck is bound.

> **Made for sale to tourists; elements newly produced and typical of Nahualá except for warp ikat striped cloth; could be the product of a cooperative that supplies importers.**

78–237
See **167**

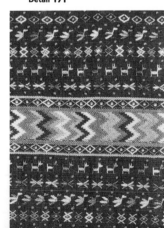

166

Female Costume 164, 165, 168

Shirt

167
Sololá: Nahualá
Quiché
FS 1970s 1978
16" x 22"   (41cm x 56cm)
- *warp*: cotton, pair of singles; indigo and white; 40 epi (16 epc)
- *weft*: same as warp; indigo
- *supplementary weft*: see **165** for makeup, count, technique, and iconography

> Ikat stripes differ from **166**; added colors and metallic thread; center backstrap-woven yoke is worn; body is very soft and somewhat faded indicating it is used fabric.

78–238
See **166**

corte
Skirt

168
Sololá: Nahualá
Quiché
MS 1970s 1979
44½" x 89"   (113cm x 226cm)
- *warp*: cotton, 2-ply; indigo; 40 epi (16 epc)
- *weft*: same as warp; indigo and white
Treadle-loomed; balanced plain weave; weft stripes; pieces are joined with *randas* of multicolored cotton yarn.

> Woven on treadle looms in Sololá; length used is seven *varas*, one *vara* equals approximately 33"; length cut in two and two lengths are sewn together side to side, then into a tube with a narrow *randa* (Rowe 1981:79).
> See **165** for manner of putting on the skirt.

79–29
See **164, 165** Female Costume

huipil
Blouse

169
Sololá: San Lucas Tolimán
Cakchiquel
FS 1970s 1978
25½" x 25"   (65cm x 63.5cm)
- *warp*: cotton, pair of singles; white; 40 epi (16 epc)
- *weft*: same as warp; 28 ppi (11 ppc)
- *supplementary weft*: cotton, 3 singles; blue and multicolored; over 4–6 warps
Backstrap-loomed, warp-predominant plain weave, one 4-selvedge piece, cut in half, single-faced supp. weft brocade, dark red velvet ribbon added at neck and sleeves, machine-stitched seams.

> **Iconography**: geometric with band of zig-zags over the chest area.
> A treadle-loomed double ikat wraparound skirt and a belt complete this costume; weavers use a pattern shed to lay in supp. weft yarn; simple weft wrapping or soumak for spots of weft or zigzags; foundation cloth colors vary.

78–270
Anderson 1978:102–106
See **170, 171**

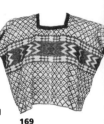
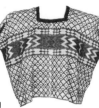

169

172

huipil
Blouse

170
Sololá: San Lucas Tolimán
Cakchiquel
FS 1970s 1978
21½" x 26"   (54cm x 66cm)
- *warp*: cotton, pair of singles; maroon; 70 epi (26 epc)
- *weft*: same as warp; 28 ppi (11 ppc)
- *supplementary weft*: cotton, 3-singles; green and multicolored; over 4–6 warps
See **169** for fabrication, comments, and references.

78–271
See **169, 171**

huipil
Blouse, uncut

171
Sololá: San Lucas Tolimán
Cakchiquel
Museum Purchase 1970s 1980
50½" x 27½"   (128cm x 71cm)
- *warp*: cotton, 2-ply; purple; 75 epi (28 epc)
- *weft*: cotton, 4-singles; purple, 25 ppi (10 ppc)
- *supplementary weft*: cotton, three 2-ply; multicolored; over 2–18 warps
Backstrap-loomed, warp-predominant plain weave, one 4-selvedge piece, cut in half, hand-sewn center seam; one end cut warps; head-hole uncut.

> **Iconography**: animals, geometric forms.
> See **169** for comments and references.

80–156
See **169, 170**

Detail 171

pantalón
Pants

172

Sololá: Santiago Atitlán
Tzutujil
E&JD 1970s 1978
38½" x 27"   (98cm x 68cm)
- *warp*: cotton, pair of singles; purple and white; 75 epi (30 ppc)
- *weft*: same as warp; white; 25 ppi (10 ppc)
- *embroidery*: cotton and synthetic, 2-ply; multi-colored

Backstrap-loomed, warp-predominant plain weave, 2 pieces, machine-stitched seams and cuffs, warp stripes, satin-stitched embroidery.

Iconography: birds with long tail feathers.

Powerful visual effect of embroidery done by women on warp-striped background; a hybrid style; costume is completed with a white or striped shirt, a wide wraparound belt which holds the pants up, and a head cloth or *tzute*, pants are ankle-length; men still wear traditional costume in the villages that border Lake Atitlán.

78–312

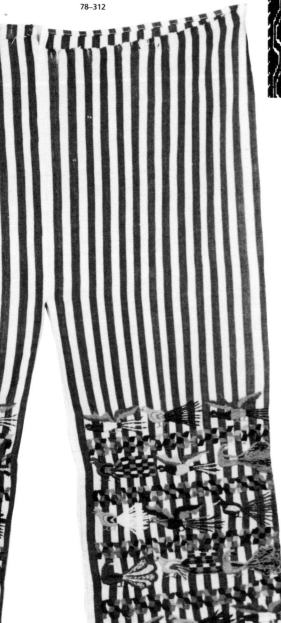

corte
Skirt

173

Sololá: Santiago Atitlán
Tzutujil
FS 1960s 1978
126" x 40"   (320cm x 102cm)
- *warp*: cotton, singles; white and deep blue; 42 epi (16 epc)
- *weft*: same as warp; red, white, deep blue, and white ikat

Treadle-loomed, weft ikat, balanced plain weave, narrow warp stripes, seams hand-sewn; length becomes width.

Iconography: animals, human figures, and plants in ikat patterns.

By the mid-seventies some women no longer were wearing the red skirt (**173**) but instead one with polychrome weft stripes alternating with ikat stripes; this type of fabric is not specific to Santiago Atitlán as the red skirt was, but is also worn in other villages (Rowe 1981:66).

Wraparound skirt cloth is woven in Santiago Atitlán; several different patterns are produced but red is the predominant color. Weavers in a cooperative had assembled a thick sample book of all kinds they could weave on order (Anderson 1978:158).

78–273
See **174**

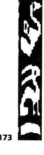

Detail **173**

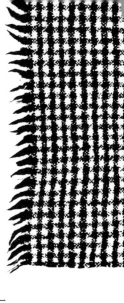

corte
Skirt

174

Sololá: Santiago Atitlán
Tzutujil
Museum Purchase 1970s 1980
83" x 64¾"   (210cm x 167cm)
- *warp*: cotton, 2-ply; red and white; 60 epi (24 epc)
- *weft*: cotton and metallic; singles; red, black, and white ikat; 35 ppi (14 ppc)

Treadle-loomed, balanced plain weave; weft ikat, two pieces machine-stitched together; length becomes width.

See **173** for comments.

80–155
See **173**

Detail **173** (vertical, left margin)

bolsa
Bag

175

Sololá: Sololá
Cakchiquel
DH 1950s 1961
12" x 12½"   (31cm x 32cm)
- *bag*: wool, singles; brown and white; 10 spi (4 spc)
- *strap, warp*: wool, singles; brown and white; 10 epi (4 ppc)
- *strap, weft*: same as warp; brown; 7 ppi (3 ppc)

Knitted bag; backstrap belt-loomed strap, warp stripes, crochet edging on top; strap handsewn to bag.

Knitted on two metal needles by men; a double knit stitch is used which gives the bag a strong moisture resistant texture.

Worn hung from left shoulder, used for carrying miscellaneous personal possessions; some men who work part-time as porters keep an extra cloth folded over top of this bag to be used as carrying pad (DH).

61–2112
Anderson 1978:188
See **179–182, 185, 187**   Male Costume

huipil
Blouse, child

176

Sololá: Sololá
Cakchiquel
MS 1980s 1986
15" x 12½"   (38cm x 32cm)
- *warp*: cotton, pair of singles; red and multicolored ikat; 100 epi (44 epc)
- *weft*: cotton, 2-singles; red; 25 ppi (10 ppc)
- *sleeves, warp*: cotton, 2-singles; multicolored and ikat; 50 epi (20 epc)
- *sleeves, weft*: same as warp; red; 25 ppi (10 ppc)

Backstrap-loomed, warp-predominant plain weave, warp stripes, one 4-selvedge piece, cut in half, one end hand-sewn, head-hole cut out.

Mayan children wear the same costume as their parents; see **150, 153, 156**; the cut-and-sew European influence is reflected in many aspects of Sololá clothing; sleeves are set-in, extra fabric around the neck is gathered into a small band, sometimes cuffs and pockets are added.

86–19

huipil
Blouse

177

Sololá: Sololá
Cakchiquel
DH 1950s 1961
31" x 18"   (94cm x 46cm)
- *warp*: cotton, pair of singles; red, multicolored, indigo and white ikat; 80 epi (32 epc)
- *weft*: same as warp; 3 singles; red; 25 ppi (10 ppc)
- *sleeves, warp*: cotton, pair of singles; red, multicolored, and ikat; 50 epi (20 epc)
- *sleeves, weft*: same as warp; red; 25 ppi (10 ppc)

Backstrap-loomed, warp-predominant plain weave, pieces of cloth hand-stitched together; set-in sleeves, warp stripes, fringe on front and cuffs of sleeves; *randa* on shoulders, joins front and back pieces.

See **176** for comments. Chevron-shaped *randa* is decorative and functional.

Worn tucked into skirt, this style is typical for both workaday and festive wear. Note similarity to man's shirt, **187** (DH). There is a ceremonial *huipil* reserved for those who serve in the *cofradía*, worn over the skirt.

61–2101
See **178, 184, 188**   Female Costume

Detail **173**

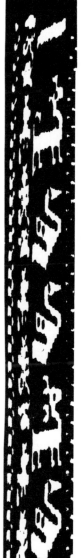

180

tzute
Cloth, carrying

178

Sololá: Sololá
Cakchiquel
DH 1950s 1961
40½" x 35½"   (103cm x 90cm)
- *warp*: cotton, pair of singles; red, multicolored, and ikat; 60 epi (26 epc)
- *weft*: cotton, 3 singles; red; 20 ppi (8 ppc)
Backstrap-loomed, warp-predominant plain weave, 2 pieces, joined by a multicolored *randa*, warp stripes, 3 hemmed ends.

Used by women for carrying baby and/or miscellaneous bundles, slung over shoulder to the back and tied in front. Sometimes rolled as padding for basket carried on head. When not in use, folded and carried on head (DH).

61–2104
See **177, 184, 188**   Female Costume

gabán
Cloth, shoulder

179

Sololá: Sololá
Cakchiquel
DH 1950s 1961
84" x 54½"   (210cm x 131cm)
- *warp*: wool, handspun singles; black and white; 20 epi (8 epc)
- *weft*: same as warp; 18 ppi (7 ppc)
Backstrap-loomed, checked pattern, balanced plain weave, warp and weft stripes, 2 identical pieces, hand-sewn together, warp fringe.

Usually folded to about 12" width and draped around back of neck and over shoulders. Used as poncho, and as blanket when sleeping. Not used on festive occasions when replaced by jacket, **181** (DH).

61–2110
See **175, 180, 181, 182, 185, 187**   Male Costume

rodillera
Cloth, hip

180

Sololá: Sololá
Cakchiquel
DH 1950s 1961
34" x 19"   (86cm x 49cm)
- *warp*: wool, handspun singles; brown and white; 15 epi (6 epc)
- *weft*: same as warp
Backstrap-loomed, balanced plain weave, warp and weft stripes; warp fringe, twisted; checkered pattern.

A pre-Columbian dress form survival.
Usually wrapped around waist to hang like a skirt, over trousers; sometimes unwrapped and used as pad for cushioning loads carried on back by tump strap (DH).

61–2109
See **175, 179, 181, 182, 185, 187**   Male Costume

chaqueta
Jacket

181

Sololá: Sololá
Cakchiquel
DH 1950s 1961
24" x 18½"   (61cm x 47cm)
- *warp*: wool, handspun singles; black and white; 25 epi (10 epc)
- *weft*: wool, pair of singles; white; 20 ppi (8 ppc)
Treadle-loomed, balanced plain weave, extra piece of cloth added at sleeve and front joining, lined with sturdy cloth, 4 pockets machine-stitched, black cloth for collar, black commercial tape for trim on back, sleeves, and lapels.

Iconography: black tape forms abstracted image of a bat on back.
During the time of the conquest, the ruling house of the Cakchiquel tribe was the clan of the bat. Of this, the Spanish chronicler Ximenez explains, "Another tribe or group stole the fire from the smoke and these were from the House of the Bats; their idol was called *Chamalcan* and belonged to the Cakchiquel, and it had wings like a bat" (Rugg 1974:63).
Worn open (there is no provision for closure) or, in hot weather, hung over one shoulder. Reserved for festive occasions (DH). Stable design of jacket since early twentieth century; made for tourist trade and export as well. Example of European-influenced dress form; pockets and fitted shape.

61–2111
See **175, 179, 180, 182, 185, 187**   Male Costume

pantalón
Pants

182

Sololá: Sololá
Cakchiquel
DH 1950s 1961
30" x 20½"   (77cm x 52cm)
- *warp*: cotton, pair of singles; red, white, blue, green, and ikat; 75 epi (30 epc)
- *weft*: same as warp; white; 25 ppi (10 ppc)
Backstrap-loomed, warp-predominant plain weave, narrow warp stripes; hand-stitched seams, hemmed, large opening for fly.

A hybrid style; no drawstring at waist. Short inseam and mode of wearing trousers very high at waist makes these knee-length. Held in place at waist by tightly wound sash, **184**; typical for both workaday and festive wear (DH).

61–2107
See **175, 179–181, 185, 187**   Male Costume

faja
Sash, male or female

183

Sololá: Sololá
Cakchiquel
CWH 1960s 1967
90" x 6¼"   (230cm x 16cm)
- *warp*: cotton, pair of singles; red-orange; 32 epi (12 epc)
- *weft*: same as warp; 16 ppi (6 ppc)
Backstrap-loomed, warp-predominant plain weave, cut warp fringe.

A common sash worn all over the highlands by men and women; small embroidered purple rectangle may be the weaver's mark.

67–10002
See **185**

faja
Sash, female

184

Sololá: Sololá
Cakchiquel
DH 1960s 1961
104" x 7½"   (264cm x 19cm)
- *warp*: cotton, pair of singles; red, multicolored, and ikat; 96 epi (36 epc)
- *weft*: same as warp; red; 24 ppi (10 ppc)
Backstrap-loomed, warp-predominant plain weave, warp stripes, fringe of warp ends.

Cloth similar to **177**; wound around waist several times, with end tucked in (DH).

61–2103
See **177, 178, 188**   Female Costume

faja
Sash, male

185

Sololá: Sololá
Cakchiquel
DH 1950s 1961
116" x 9"   (216cm x 24.5cm)
- *warp*: cotton, pair of singles; red; 30 epi (12 epc)
- *weft*: same as warp; 15 ppi (6 ppc)
Backstrap-loomed, warp-predominant plain weave, twisted fringe of cut warps, knotted ends.

Wound around waist several times, and end tucked in (DH).

61–2108
See **175, 179–182, 187**   Male Costume

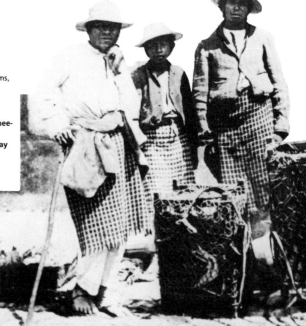

Carriers, Sololá. Herbert J. Spinden Photo Archives, Haffenreffer Museum of Anthropology. See **180, 181**.

camisa
Shirt

186
> Sololá: Sololá
> Cakchiquel
> E&JD 1970s 1978
> 28" x 25" (72cm x 63cm)

• *warp*: cotton, pair of singles; blue, yellow, and multicolored ikat; 55 epi (22 epc)
• *weft*: same as warp; blue; 25 ppi (10 ppc)
Backstrap-loomed cloth, warp-predominant plain weave; warp stripes, machine-stitched, set-in sleeves, collar, cuffs.

> **European cut-and-sew tailoring, western style; made for sale to tourists, for export, and also to be worn by Mayan men.**

78–313

camisa
Shirt

187
> Sololá: Sololá
> Cakchiquel
> DH 1950s 1961
> 21½" x 33½" (54cm x 85cm)

• *warp*: cotton, pair of singles; multicolored and ikat; 55 epi (22 epc)
• *weft*: same as warp; white; 25 ppi (10 ppc)
• *sleeves, warp*: cotton, pair of singles; multicolored and ikat; 55 epi (22 epc)
• *sleeves, weft*: same as warp; red; 25 ppi (10 ppc)
Backstrap-loomed, warp-predominant plain weave, one 4-selvedge piece cut in half, warp fringe front ends; warp stripes, set-in sleeves, collar and sleeves smocked with hand-stitched tab, hand-stitched seams.

> **See 177 for comments; cuffs remain unfastened; worn tucked into trousers (DH).**

61–2106
See **175, 179–182, 185** Male Costume

corte
Skirt

188
> Sololá: Sololá
> Cakchiquel
> DH 1960s 1961
> 92" x 37" (234cm x 94cm)

• *warp*: cotton, pair of singles; indigo; 60 epi (24 epc)
• *weft*: same as warp; dark blue and white; 40 ppi (16 epc)
• *embroidery*: cotton, 2-ply; multicolored
Treadle-loomed; balanced plain weave; weft stripes; *randa* joins 2 widths and 2 ends to make a tube; width becomes length.

> **Cloth is woven on foot-looms for this purpose by *Ladinos* in Sololá; sold in lengths at the market; worn wrapped tightly around waist and held by sash 185; typical for workaday and festive wear (DH).**
> **Male and female costume appeared to be much the same in 1978 as in 1961 when Dwight Heath collected the Sololá material.**

61–2102
See **177, 178, 184** Female Costume

huipil
Blouse

189
> Chimaltenango: Comalapa
> Cakchiquel
> RP 1950–1960 1986
> 23½" x 30" (60cm x 76.5cm)

• *warp*: cotton, singles and 2-ply; white; 40 epi (16 epc)
• *weft*: (lower ⅓) cotton, 3 singles; white, yellow, green, lavender; 30 ppi (12 ppc); (upper ⅔) cotton, singles and 2-ply; multicolored and orange; 130 ppi (56 ppc)
• *supplementary weft*: cotton, three 2-ply; multicolored; over 1–20 warps
Backstrap-loomed, warp-predominant plain weave, 2 pieces, cut warps, machine-stitched ends, two-faced supp. weft brocade and weft-faced striped banding; velvet strips on neck and sleeves removed; hand-sewn center and side seams.

> **Iconography: floral, birds, and geometric.**
> Bands of orange on shoulder formerly woven with a European red yarn called *crea*; now those bands are called *creya*; orange has badly faded; older style of neck treatment; not cut out; center seam left open for headhole; finely woven weft striping; to be worn tucked in and held in place with a belt; there is another style of *huipil* called a *sobre-huipil* that is worn over one like **189**, and covered with supp. weft brocading.
> Like those from San Jose Poaquil but has more red in horizontal lines (Arriola Geng, pers. com. 1986). Weft-faced cloth results from Comalapa weavers' practice of "compacting" the weft very tightly together to cover the warps; weft-faced plain weave and regular plain weaving on which supp. weft brocading is done are combined on a single panel (Anderson 1978:78).

86–13
Barrios 1985
See **190, 191**

huipil
Blouse

190
> Chimaltenango: Comalapa
> Cakchiquel
> FS 1970s 1978
> 24½" x 28½" (66cm x 72cm)

• *warp*: cotton, 2-ply; black; 55 epi (22 epc)
• *weft*: same as warp; light, dark blue; 22 ppi (9 ppc); pair of singles; red; 60 ppi (24 ppc)
• *supplementary weft*: cotton, metallic, and pearl cotton, 3 singles; multicolored; over 2–20 warps
Backstrap-loomed, warp-predominant plain weave, weft-faced banding; single- and two-faced supp. weft brocade, head-hole cut out; black velvet ribbon added to neck and sleeves, side and back seams machine-sewn.

> **Iconography: vase with flowers, geometric and floral bands; *creya* (see 189 comments) on shoulder.**
> A style that is still being produced in the 1980s combines new and old features including the square neckline, black color of ground, widening of central band, *creya* and combination of old and modern figures (Barrios 1985:34). Designs taken from magazines were introduced to Comalapa around the 1930s (ibid.: 76). An extra shed rod is used for supp. weft brocading that enables the weaver to lift alternate groups of four wefts at a time, attached by string heddles to the rod (Anderson 1978:78).

78–268
Barrios 1985
See **189, 191**

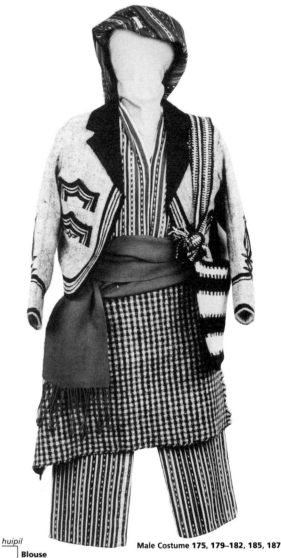
huipil
Blouse

191
> Chimaltenango: Comalapa
> Cakchiquel
> RP 1980s 1986
> 22¾" x 31½" (58cm x 80cm)

• *warp*: cotton, 2-ply; red; 40 epi (16 epc)
• *weft*: cotton, two and three 2-ply; red and multicolored; 35 ppi (14 ppc)
• *supplementary weft*: cotton, 3 singles; multicolored, over 2–10 warps
Treadle-loomed, balanced plain weave, 2 pieces, cut ends, machine-stitched side seams; two-faced supp. weft brocade, head-hole cut out, black velvet band added to neck and sleeves.

> **Iconography: flowers, horned animal, geometric forms.**
> Horizontal supp. weft bands separate design bands; see **190** comments; tucks in the front to make the *huipil* fit better, a European influence, have been let out; no *creya*.
> Woven by a male weaver; workshops exist in Comalapa owned by men that create *huipiles* for Comalapa, San Martín Jilotepeque and other neighboring municipalities; the family is involved, each with special tasks, also male and female employees; innovation is accepted in response to the tastes of the clientele; marketing efforts extend beyond the village; reproducing supp. weft patterns on the treadle or draw loom involves making drawings on graph paper indicating the required harnesses. Said one such weaver, "Night is an excellent time to draw when nothing bothers you, you see, because there's no noise from the looms" (Barrios 1985:61–63).

86–12
Barrios 1985
See **189, 190**

Male Costume 175, 179–182, 185, 187

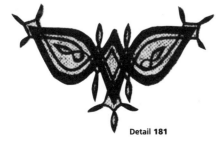

Detail 181

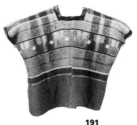

191

huipil
| **Blouse**

192

Chimaltenango: Patzún
Cakchiquel
RP 1975–1985 1986
23½" x 25"   (60cm x 63.5cm)
• *warp*: cotton, 2-ply; red and multicolored; 60 epi (24 epc)
• *weft*: cotton, pair of singles; red; 20 ppi (8 ppc)
Backstrap-loomed; warp-predominant plain weave; 4-selvedges, warp stripes, head-hole cut out, black velvet band added to neck and sleeves; ribbon facing; all seams machine-stitched; many tucks for close fitting.

    Iconography: appliqued flowers of commercial cloth applied on chest and shoulder areas with zigzag stitch.
    One of the most popular *huipiles*, and is sold in other villages; embroidery has been substituted by appliqued flowers sewn on with a sewing machine (Arriola Geng, pers. com. 1986).

86–15
See **193, 194**

huipil
| **Blouse**

193

Chimaltenango: Patzún
Cakchiquel
C&BS 1970s 1985
25½" x 29"   (65cm x 74cm)
• *warp*: cotton, 2-ply; red and multicolored; 80 epi (32 epc)
• *weft*: cotton, 8 singles; red; 20 ppi (8 ppc)
• *embroidery*: cotton, three 2-ply; multicolored
Backstrap-loomed; warp-predominant plain weave; two 4-selvedge pieces, warp stripes, center joined by *randa*, sides hand-sewn, embroidery around neck, pieces of blue cloth added for front and back medallions.

    Iconography: flowers, chevrons, leaf forms; only around neck.
    The decoration on the blouse shows it was once made bright with feathers for the feather shapes are now embroidered (Pettersen 1976:180). Ceremonial *huipil* has similar neck iconography but is embroidered in silk thread (Deuss 1981:25). **193** was woven for sale in the 1970s but is of an older style. Embroidered by women.

85–155
See **192, 194**

huipil
| **Blouse**

194

Chimaltenango: Patzún
Cakchiquel
RP 1980–1986 1986
21" x 29½"   (53cm x 75cm)
• *warp*: cotton, pair of 2-ply; red and multicolored; 50 epi (20 epc)
• *weft*: cotton, 6 singles; red; 15 ppi (6 ppc)
• *embroidery*: cotton, 2-ply; multicolored and space-dyed
Backstrap-loomed; warp-predominant plain weave; two 4-selvedge pieces, warp stripes, *randa* center, machine-stitched side seams, head-hole cut out, neck facing machine-stitched, black tape around neck and sleeves; satin stitch used for embroidery, smocking from shoulder to waist on front and back; fitted and flares out on bottom.

    Iconography: flowers, *quetzal* birds.
    Embroidery covers chest and shoulder areas; also on sleeve edges; smocking done in yellow yarn, creates another design element.
    The designs are of recent years, a substitute for the classical forms of the past (Arriola Geng, pers. com. 1986).

86–14
See **192, 193**

huipil
| **Blouse**

195

Chimaltenango: San Martín Jilotepeque
Cakchiquel
FS 1970s 1978
21" x 31½"   54cm x 80cm)
• *warp*: cotton, pair of singles; indigo; 45 epi (18 epc)
• *weft*: cotton, 4 singles; indigo; 13 ppi (5 ppc)
• *supplementary weft*: cotton, silk, and synthetic, four 2-ply and six 2-ply; multicolored; over 4–18 warps.
Backstrap-loomed; warp-predominant plain weave; two 3-selvedge pieces, single- and double-faced supp. weft brocade, large cut out head-hole, *randas* on front and sides, neck and sleeves folded back and whip-stitched, hand-sewn and loom-finished hems.

    Iconography: geometric motifs.
    San Antonio Aguas Calientes designs are quite similar (see **200**); in particular the double-faced supp. weft arch pattern across the chest area; **195** is a ceremonial style; everyday *huipil* can be treadle-loomed in Comalapa (see **191**).
    Double-faced supp. weft brocading called marker (*marcador*) is a direct or indirect introduction from San Antonio Aguas Calientes; the influence of the modern-style *huipil* of this community on Comalapa's *huipiles* can be appreciated in three aspects: marker technique; flowers, fruits, or birds such as parrots or macaws as designs; placement of these designs across the chest (Barrios 1985:77–78). San Martín designs have influenced Comalapa *huipiles*; one style is called the *sanmartineco huipil* (ibid.: 31).

78–263
Pettersen 1976:198

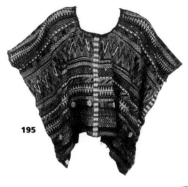

195

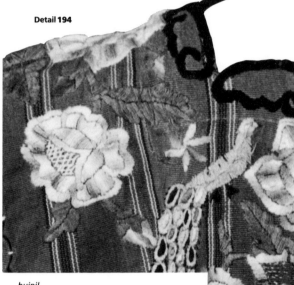

Detail **194**

huipil
| **Blouse**

196

Chimaltenango: Tecpán
Cakchiquel
FS 1970s 1978
24" x 25½"   (61cm x 65cm)
• *warp*: cotton, pair of singles; blue; 37 epi (15 epc)
• *weft*: same as warp; 13 ppi (5 ppc)
• *supplementary weft*: cotton, two 2-ply; multicolored; over 8 warps
Backstrap-loomed; warp-predominant plain weave; 2 pieces; single-faced supp. weft brocading, head-hole cut out, black velvet and white tape added at neck and edges, machine-stitched at hems.

    Iconography: geometric motifs.
    Organization of motifs in horizontal bands similar to San Antonio Aguas Calientes (see **200**); separated by several rows of floating wefts over 4 warps; an extra shed stick is utilized and the pattern is called *pepenado*: large tucks are placed next to the neck, extending down the front; **196** is the everyday style; the ceremonial *huipil* is woven with brown cotton and is worn over the everyday one, a *sobre-huipil*.

78–266
Deuss 1981:18

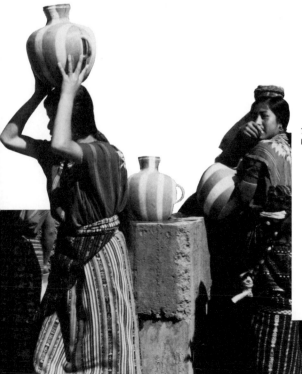

Cakchiquel young women at the fountain.
1976. Patzún. Photo by Clare Brett Smith. See 194.

SACATEPÉQUEZ

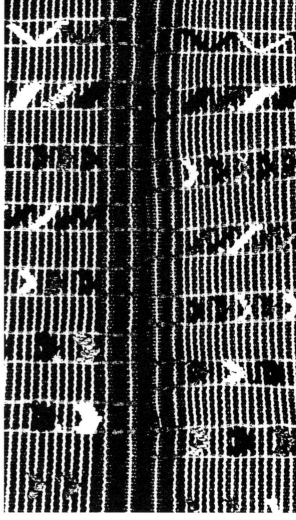

delantal

Apron

198

Sacatepéquez: San Antonio Aguas Calientes
Cakchiquel
MS 1980s 1983
30" x 36"   (76cm x 91cm)
- *warp*: cotton, 2-ply; dark brown; 25 epi (10 epc)
- *weft*: wool, cotton, synthetic, singles; multi-colored; 90 ppi (36 ppc)

Treadle-loomed; weft-faced plain weave, weft stripes; rickrack trim and facing for belt and pocket, and sash machine-stitched.

Small patterns in weft created by alternating colors; ikat yarn is also utilized for weft striping but not in 198; a European dress form that was adopted in most highland villages; cut-and-sew technology; when the Haffenreffer Museum wanted to acquire a complete wedding costume, this item was added to the new-style female costume, see 199, 202, 205, 211, 212, along with 213, earrings, a wedding ring, necklace, hair ribbon, and sandals. In 1978 in Santa María de Jesús, the bride wore a new towel over her head instead of a veil; commercial bath towels are highly valued and quite expensive.

83–364
See **213**

faja

Belt

199

Sacatepéquez: San Antonio Aguas Calientes
Cakchiquel
MS 1970s 1979
104" x 2"   (269cm x 5cm)
- *warp*: cotton, singles and 2-ply; multicolored; 50 epi (20 epc)
- *weft*: same as warp; 2-ply pink and blue; 20 ppi (8 ppc)
- *supplementary weft*: cotton; 4 singles and 2-ply; multicolored; over 2–4 warps

Backstrap belt-loomed; single-faced supp. weft brocading; warp floats; 1 large braid on each end; uncut ends, twisted first.

Iconography: flowers, animal, diamonds, and circular forms; woven into nine different pattern areas.

"We observed Totonicapán-style belts being woven in the town of San Antonio Aguas Calientes, where weavers have learned to copy textiles from many places. The belts look exactly like the ones from Totonicapán, but it is possible that Totonicapán weavers use a different loom setup...Weavers from San Antonio do *not* use extra heddles for weaving the belts" (Sperlich and Sperlich 1980:163). These belts are probably woven by specialists; when asked to demonstrate the technique on **206**, the weaver experienced difficulty in remembering how to proceed, although she assured me that she knew the process but hadn't woven one recently; worn by all the young women, for it can be pulled tightly around the wraparound skirt and shows off the waist and figure; adapted in the 1960s.

79–8
Sperlich and Sperlich 1980:163–166
Schevill 1980:15
See **202, 205, 211, 212**   New-style Female Costume 1960s–1980s and **206**

huipil

Blouse, uncut

197

Chimaltenango: Parramos
Cakchiquel
C&BS 1970s 1985
26¼" x 33½"   (67cm x 85cm)
- *warp*: cotton, singles; red and multicolored; 70 epi (28 epc)
- *weft*: same as warp; red; 20 ppi (8 ppc)
- *supplementary weft*: cotton, 4 singles; multicolored; over 6–10 warps

Backstrap-loomed; warp-predominant plain weave; two 4-selvedge pieces; single-faced supp. weft brocading; warp stripes; hand-sewn center seam; head-hole uncut.

Iconography: small geometric forms in single horizantal bands; widely spaced at bottom of *huipil*.
Woven for sale.

85–168

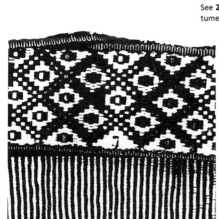

Detail 199

huipil   **Detail 197**

Blouse

200

Sacatepéquez: San Antonio Aguas Calientes
Cakchiquel
MS 1950s 1979
22½" x 26"   (57cm x 65.5cm)
- *warp*: cotton, 2-ply; black; 60 epi (24 epc)
- *weft*: cotton, 3-ply; black; 30 ppi (12 ppc)
- *supplementary weft*: cotton, pearl cotton, 2-ply and 3-ply; multicolored; over 2–4 warps

Backstrap-loomed; warp-predominant plain weave; two 4-selvedge pieces; single-faced supp. weft brocading; head-hole created by opening in center seam; dark green velvet bands sewn to neck and arm holes; side seams hand-sewn.

Iconography: geometric forms in horizontal bands, divided by 8 rows of *pepenado*, see **196**.

San Antonio weavers have names for each one of their designs such as *tijeras* (scissors), *jaspe* (ikat), *arco* (arch), *mosquito* (mosquito), *pie de chucho* (foot of the dog), *marimba* (marimba), and *pepita* (zigzags). **200** contains no double-faced supp. weft weaving which didn't become fashionable until the 1960s.

79–13
Schevill 1987
See **204, 209, 210**   Old-style Female Costume

huipil

Blouse

201

Sacatepéquez: San Antonio Aguas Calientes
Cakchiquel
FS   1970s   1978
26" and 22" x 25"   (66cm and 56cm x 64cm)
- *warp*: cotton, 2-ply; maroon; 60 epi (24 epc)
- *weft*: cotton, three 2-ply; maroon; 20 ppi (8 ppc)
- *supplementary weft*: cotton, three 2-ply; multi-colored; over 2–4 warps

Backstrap-loomed; warp-predominant plain weave; two 4-selvedge pieces of uneven lengths; single- and double-faced supp. weft brocading; head-hole created by opening in center seam; blue velvet ribbon hand-sewn on to neck and sleeves; side seams hand-sewn.

Iconography: floral and geometric motifs.
Floral band on shoulders done in double-faced weave; motifs adapted from cross-stitch pattern books imported from Mexico, Europe, and the U.S.; San Antonio weavers try to match horizontal design bands, so occasionally one length is longer than the other; since the *huipil* is worn tucked into the wraparound skirt and held in place with a belt, this unevenness is not noticeable; opening in front center seam facilitates nursing one's baby; sometimes a zipper is added.

78–267
Bjerregaard 1977:60–71, 90–92
Lathbury 1974
See **200, 202**

huipil

Blouse

202

Sacatepéquez: San Antonio Aguas Calientes
Cakchiquel
MS   1978   1979
24½" x 30"   (62.5cm x 76cm)
- *warp*: cotton, 3-ply; white; 28 epi (11 epc)
- *weft*: cotton, 2-ply; white; 28 ppi (11 ppc)
- *supplementary weft*: cotton and pearl cotton, 2-ply and 3-ply; multicolored; over 2–4 warps

Backstrap-loomed; warp-predominant plain weave; two 3-selvedge pieces; single- and double-faced supp. weft brocading; blue rayon added at neck and sleeves; 2 ends hand-sewn, 2 loom-finished; side seams hand-sewn.

Iconography: floral and geometric motifs.
Double-faced supp. weft brocading at shoulder called *flores y hojas* (flowers and leaves); a specialty of the fifteen-year-old male weaver who produced **202** as a commission for the Haffenreffer Museum; no particular meaning for the use of white as a background; in 1978 red and maroon were the popular choices; colors in the supp. weft brocading are contingent on what is available in the small shops in the village, otherwise a trip to nearby Antigua market must be made; 572 hours were required to complete **202** including the warping and finishing process done by the weaver's mother, sister, and grandmother; sometimes *huipiles* are produced by several members of a family, each one weaving his or her specialty; the use of double-faced supp. weft brocaded bands on San Antonio *huipiles* has increased in recent times; in the 1980s some are woven entirely with this technique; these *huipiles* are ablaze with brightly colored flowers, leaves, and fruits.

79–15
See **199, 205, 211, 212**   New-style Female Costume 1960s–1980s

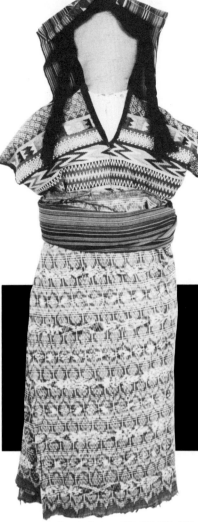

Female Costume 200, 204, 209, 210

tzute

Cloth, carrying

203

Sacatepéquez: San Antonio Aguas Calientes
Cakchiquel
RISD Transfer: Lisle Estate   1930s   1985
35" x 29"   (89cm x 74cm)
- *warp*: cotton, pair of singles; indigo, lavender, and multicolored; 70 epi (26 epc)
- *weft*: same as warp; indigo; 35 ppi (14 ppc)
- *supplementary weft*: silk and cotton, pair of singles; white, lavender, and red.

Backstrap-loomed; warp-predominant plain weave; two 4-selvedge pieces; double-faced supp. weft brocading; warp stripes; hand-sewn seams.

Iconography: stars, flowers, animals; yellow weft stripes at top and bottoms may be the weaver's mark.
Double-faced brocading was known to San Antonio weavers since the early twentieth century, but it was utilized only for small motifs as seen in **203**; in 1936 Lila M. O'Neale spent three months in the Guatemalan highlands documenting Mayan costume and weaving technology, among other subjects; she wrote about the weaving of San Antonio: "work like that done on huipiles exemplifies finest, most expertly developed craftsmanship in highlands" (O'Neale 1945:252). **203** resembles fig. 106a in O'Neale publication.

85–786
See **204**

tzute

Cloth, carrying

204

Sacatepéquez: San Antonio Aguas Calientes
Cakchiquel
MS   1950s   1978
39" x 30"   (97cm x 76cm)
- *warp*: cotton, singles; blue and multicolored; 56 epi (22 epc)
- *weft*: same as warp; blue; 30 ppi (12 ppc)
- *supplementary weft*: cotton and pearl cotton, singles and 2-ply; multicolored

Backstrap-loomed; warp-predominant plain weave; two 4-selvedge pieces; double-faced supp. weft brocading; warp stripes; hand-sewn seams.

Iconography: birds and floral.
Compared to **203**, motifs are much larger but still occupy the solid background areas of dark blue; old-style *tzutes* were hard to find in 1978; so much work is involved that women don't like to part with them; a sixty-year-old weaver had one that was given to her by her niece but she didn't want to sell it; **204** was made by a weaver who was eighty years old in 1978 and was said to have been fifteen years old when she wove it. Warp and weft count is not as fine as in **203**.

79–11
See **203** and **200, 209, 210**   Old-style Female Costume

tzute

Cloth, carrying

205

Sacatepéquez: San Antonio Aguas Calientes
Cakchiquel
MS   1970s   1979
38" x 33½"   (97cm x 85cm)
- *warp*: cotton, 2-ply; multicolored; 75 epi (28 epc)
- *weft*: cotton, three 2-ply; black, red, brown, and orange; 15 ppi (6 ppc)

Backstrap-loomed; warp-predominant plain weave; two 4-selvedge pieces; warp stripes; hand-sewn center seam.

Creative color warping gives variety in warp striping; **205** represents the everyday style of carrying cloth that evolved in the 1970s; similar patterning in a cloth for carying large loads, a *cargador*, and also used for a wide female sash; the double-faced supp. weft brocaded style, **203, 204**, is still being produced in the 1980s; supp. weft brocaded motifs cover solid colored background areas entirely.

79–10
See **203, 204** and **199, 202, 211, 212**   New-style Female Costume 1960s–1980s

telar de cinta

Loom, backstrap-belt

206

Sacatepéquez: San Antonio Aguas Calientes
Cakchiquel
MS   1970s   1979
96" x 3¼"   (243cm x 8cm)
- *warp*: cotton and pearl cotton, 2-ply and 3-ply; red, white and maroon; 35 epi (14 epc)
- *weft*: cotton, four 2-ply; red; 30 ppi (12 ppc)
- *supplementary weft*: cotton and pearl cotton, four 2-ply; multicolored; 13 ppi (5 ppc); single-faced supp. weft brocading; warp floats, over 2–4 warps

See **199** for fabrication, comments, references.

Rope is attached to the warp beam, then tied to a strap of leather or jute that goes around the weaver's waist or hips.

79–4
Schevill 1980: 7–10
See **199**

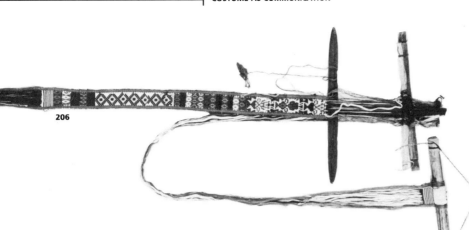

206

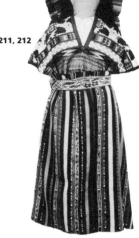

Female Costume 199, 202, 205, 211, 212

telar de palitos

Loom, backstrap

207

Sacatepéquez: San Antonio Aguas Calientes Cakchiquel
MS   1970s   1979
36¼" x 16¼"   (92cm x 41.5cm)
• *warp*: cotton, 3-ply; red and yellow; 25 epi (10 epc)
• *weft*: cotton, 3-ply; red; 25 ppi (10 ppc)
• *supplementary weft*:   cotton and pearl cotton, 3 singles; over 2–4 warps
Backstrap-loomed; warp-predominant plain weave; single-faced supp. weft brocading; warp stripes

Iconography: geometric forms, see **200**.
Woven to be sold as a wall hanging, without weaving tools; partially woven looms provide a constant source of income for San Antonio weavers; men participate in the marketing of these items, sometimes taking them to shops or to the textile market in Guatemala City for sale; **207** is not as fine a weave as **200, 201, 202** since it was not meant to be a *huipil*; a leather strap, a well-worn hardwood sword or batten, bamboo shuttles, and heddle rods out of softwood constitute the required weaving equipment.

79–5
Schevill 1980:67–69
See **206**

faja

Sash

208

Sacatepéquez: San Antonio Aguas Calientes Cakchiquel
MS   1930s   1979
128" x 9½"   (320cm x 24.5cm)
• *warp*: cotton, 2-ply; green, red, white, and blue; 100 epi (40 epc)
• *weft*: same as warp; 3-ply; blue; 20 ppi (8 ppc)
Backstrap-loomed; warp-faced plain weave; warp stripes; cut warp ends make fringe.

An old-style sash, well worn; mauve color has faded badly; woven by an older Mayan woman; she had to weave a new one before she would sell **208** which corresponds to the description of the male belt by O'Neale (1945:252).

79–9
See **209**

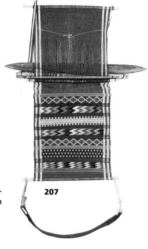

207

faja

Sash

209

Sacatepéquez: San Antonio Aguas Calientes Cakchiquel
MS   1960s   1979
127" x 9½"   (322cm x 24cm)
• *warp*: cotton, singles; multicolored; 100 epi (40 epc)
• *weft*: cotton, pair of singles; black; 25 ppi (10 ppc)
Backstrap-loomed; warp-faced plain weave; warp stripes; cut warp ends make fringe.

The old-style sash was worn by men and women; in 1978 the sash was the only costume element still used by some men in San Antonio and it was red; some women still prefer the old style.

79–14
Dieterich, Erickson, and Younger 1979:87
See **208** and **200, 204, 210**   Old-style Female Costume

falda

Skirt

210

Sacatepéquez: San Antonio Aguas Calientes Cakchiquel
MS   1950s   1979
174" x 36"   (442cm x 91cm)
• *warp*: cotton, 2-ply; white, blue, green, purple ikat; 45 epi (18 epc)
• *weft*: same as warp
Treadle-loomed; double ikat; balanced plain weave; cut warp ends and hand-sewn to make a tube.
See **157** for fabrication and comments.

79–16
See **200, 204, 209**   Old-style Female Costume

falda

Skirt

211

Sacatepéquez: San Antonio Aguas Calientes Cakchiquel
MS   1970s   1978
192" x 34½"   (448cm x 88cm)
• *warp*: cotton, pair of singles; red and black; 30 epi (12 epc)
• *weft*: cotton and wool, 2-ply; black and white ikat, multicolored; cotton: 60 ppi (24 ppc); wool: 100 ppi (40 ppc)
Treadle-loomed; weft-faced plain weave; weft stripes; cut warp ends.

Iconography: weft ikat stripes contain plant, floral, and geometric forms.
Woven in workshops in Salcajá, Quezaltenango; in 1978 very few women were wearing the old-style double ikat skirts, see **210**; **211** is much warmer and thicker and provides a nice cushion when kneeling on the ground backstrap weaving; vendors sell these in the streets; at fiesta time all the women try to buy new skirts, and weave or buy new *huipiles*.

78–253
See **199, 202, 205, 212**   New-style Female Costume 1960s–1980s

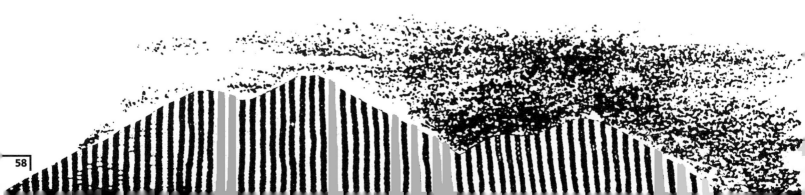

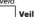

cotón
| **Underblouse**

212
> Sacatepéquez: San Antonio Aguas Calientes
> Cakchiquel
> MS 1970s 1979

25½" x 14"   (65cm x 36cm)
commercial cloth; tailored, machine-sewn, set-in sleeves; smocking in back; decorative tape at neck with buttons

> Unique to San Antonio, sewn by specialists; a European dress form, it resembles the undergarment of the nuns and is visible from the back and the front; it was said that women in San Antonio have been wearing *cotónes* for the past fifty years; it was also said that women didn't wear *huipiles* when cooking, only the *cotón*; this was the case with an older Mayan woman who had household responsibilities including care of the animals; when she was weaving she wore her *huipil*.

79–12
See **199, 202, 205, 211** New-style Female Costume 1960s–1980s

velo
| **Veil**

213
> Sacatepéquez: San Antonio Aguas Calientes
> Cakchiquel
> MS 1970s 1983

49½" x 39"   (126cm x 99cm)
machine-made cotton lace cloth; 2 pieces joined in center; decorative border

> **Iconography:** birds, crowns, crosses.
> An item that is probably shared by the extended family; a European dress form accepted by the predominantly Catholic Maya; see **198** for comments.

83–365
See **198**

huipil
| **Blouse**

214
> Sacatepéquez: Santiago Sacatepéquez
> Cakchiquel
> RP 1975–1985 1986

26" x 30"   (66cm x 76.5cm)
• *warp*: cotton, 3 singles; red and white; 60 epi (24 epc)
• *weft*: cotton, 6 singles; red and white; 20 ppi (8 ppc)
• *supplementary weft*: cotton and pearl cotton, 9 singles; multicolored; over 1–7 warps
Backstrap-loomed, warp-predominant plain weave; two 4-selvedge pieces, two-faced supp. weft brocading; warp stripes; hand-stitched side seams; *randa* at neck and sleeves

> **Iconography:** warp and weft stripes create a plaid effect; animal, geometric, and plant motifs utilized.
> Head opening might have been bound like **215**; well worn; binding removed because of wear.

86–7
See **215, 216**

huipil
| **Blouse**

215
> Sacatepéquez: Santiago Sacatepéquez
> Cakchiquel
> RP 1975–1985 1986

22" x 26"   (56cm x 66cm)
• *warp*: cotton, 3 singles; red and white; 45 epi (18 epc)
• *weft*: cotton, 6 singles; red and white; 20 ppi (8 ppc)
• *supplementary weft*: cotton, singles; multicolored; over 1–6 warps
Backstrap-loomed; warp-predominant plain weave; two 4-selvedge pieces; single- and two-faced supp. weft brocading; small *randa*; blue velvet binding at neck; hand-stitched side seams.

> **Iconography:** geometric blocks, five-pointed stars; plaid effect.

86–8
See **214, 216**

huipil
| **Blouse**

216
> Sacatepéquez: Santiago Sacatepéquez
> Cakchiquel
> C&BS 1970s 1985

26½" x 35"   (67cm x 90cm)
• *warp*: cotton, pair of singles; white and red; 55 epi (22 epc)
• *weft*: cotton, 3 singles; white; 20 ppi (8 ppc)
• *supplementary weft*: cotton and pearl cotton; 10 singles; multicolored; over 2–6 warps
Backstrap-loomed, warp-predominant plain weave, two 4-selvedge pieces; single-faced supp. weft brocading; warp stripes; not joined at sides; *randa* at center.

> **Iconography:** geometric blocks and five-pointed stars as in **215**.
> Satin stitch of *randa* decorates neck opening. Resembles description of *huipil* worn in the 1930s (O'Neale 1945:298); made-for-sale; an attempt to recreate older style; larger in dimensions than **214, 215**; warp count in three examples varies but weft count is consistent as is use of red warp stripes; plaid effect of recent popularity.

85–163
See **214, 215**

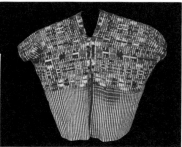
214

huipil
| **Blouse**

217
> Sacatepéquez: Santo Domingo Xenacoj
> Cakchiquel
> MS 1970s 1979

26" x 36"   (66cm x 90.5cm)
• *warp*: cotton and pearl cotton, 4-ply and 2-ply; red, blue, orange, and brown; 35 epi (14 epc)
• *weft*: cotton, singles; red; 18 ppi (7 ppc)
• *supplementary weft*: silk, cotton, and pearl cotton, singles; multicolored space-dyed; over 3 warps
Backstrap-loomed, warp-predominant plain weave, two 4-selvedge pieces; two-faced supp. weft brocading; warp stripes; not joined at sides; *randa*; head-hole cut out.

> **Iconography:** feathered serpent or worm along shoulder area along with diamond shapes.
> Xenacoj weavers use a particular technique of supp. weft brocading which creates a bubble effect; supp. weft is loosely laid in, then tightly beaten; the result is similar to a looped pile; center warp stripes are highlighted by the unusual *randa* which varies from hourglass shapes to lozenges; two flowers are embroidered on back; bought from weaver who traveled some distance each day to demonstrate weaving and to sell textiles; **217** was the everyday style of the 1970s; the weaver's mother was the acknowledged expert on the history of Xenacoj weaving; she claimed to have invented the use of large, animal designs on the front of Xenacoj weavings which then caught on in other highland villages, see **218**; sometimes an undergarment is worn too; **217** has a soft, silky feeling due to repeated washings; use of silk makes this a special example, but not ceremonial, see **219**.

79–20
See **220, 221, 222** Female Costume

Cakchiquel woman. San Antonio Aguas Calientes. 1978. Photo by Margot Schevill. See **200**.

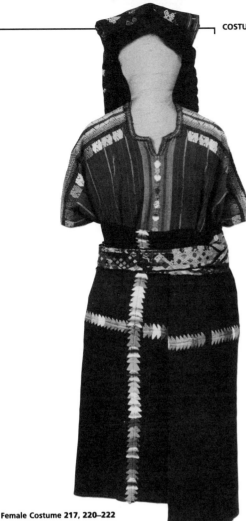

Female Costume 217, 220–222

huipil

Blouse

218

Sacatepéquez: Santo Domingo Xenacoj
Cakchiquel
C&BS   1970s   1985
28½" x 43"   (72cm x 110cm)
• *warp*: cotton, 2-ply and pair of singles; red, white, blue, pink, and light blue; 25 epi (10 epc)
• *weft*: cotton, 6 singles; red; 8 ppi (3 ppc)
• *supplementary weft*: cotton and silk, seven 2-ply; multicolored; over 1–21 warps
Backstrap-loomed, warp-predominant plain weave; two 4-selvedge pieces; two-faced supp. weft brocading; warp stripes; not joined at sides; *randa*; head-hole cut out

Iconography: feathered serpent or worm and stylized tree-of-life on shoulder area (see **217**), large lions across chest area.
　Elements in **217** have been expanded in this *huipil* made-for-sale; wide warp stripes contrast with those in **217**; similar shoulder treatment but large images on chest area, a recent innovation; same technique for supp. weft brocading and *randa* employed. Xenacoj weavers are very inventive and have been commissioned to weave *huipiles* for other villages on occasion; in 1976 after the earthquake, in which Xenacoj was badly damaged, weavers sold their work at a stand on the Pan American highway, as well as demonstrating backstrap weaving, it provided a good, additional income for many women in the village including *Ladinas* who were also fine weavers.

85–159
Morales Hidalgo 1982:17
See **217, 219**

huipil

Blouse

219

Sacatepéquez: Santo Domingo Xenacoj
Cakchiquel
C&BS   1970s   1985
29½" x 37"   (75cm x 94cm)
• *warp*: cotton, 3-ply; white, green, purple, and blue; 35 epi (14 epc)
• *weft*: cotton, 5 singles; white; 10 ppi (4 ppc)
• *supplementary weft*: cotton and synthetic, 5 singles; purple and multicolored; over 2–17 warps
Backstrap-loomed, warp-predominant plain weave; two 4-selvedge pieces; two-faced supp. weft brocading; green warp stripes on side selvedges; not joined at sides; *randa*; head-hole cut out.

Iconography: a rich visual repertoire of animal images including peacocks, worms, horses, lions, ducks, and hummingbirds; geometric fillers.
　An elaborately brocaded ceremonial huipil for *cofradia*; similar to the ceremonial huipiles of San Pedro Sacatepéquez, **237, 238**, Chuarrancho, **229, 230**; use of purple on white background suggests ceremonial use; lower area is less densely brocaded; white background sets off individual two-legged animals and motifs that look like letters of the alphabet.

85–160
Morales Hidalgo 1982:57, 67, 71
See **217, 218**

tzute

Cloth, carrying

220

Sacatepéquez: Santo Domingo Xenacoj
Cakchiquel
MS   1970s   1979
24½" x 23½"   (62cm x 60cm)
• *warp*: cotton, 3 singles; blue; 35 epi (14 epc)
• *weft*: cotton, 4 singles; blue; 32 ppi (9 ppc)
• *supplementary weft*: cotton, silk, and fine embroidery yarn; 4 and 6 singles; multicolored; over 2–4 warps
Backstrap-loomed, warp-predominant plain weave, one 4-selvedge piece; two-faced supp. weft brocading; warp stripes on sides.

Iconography: large and small animal repertoire, see **219**; feathered serpent or worm images create top and bottom borders; small bird in red cotton may be weaver's mark.
　Xenacoj weavers offered names for their motifs but when the weaver of this ceremonial *tzute* was asked about a small bird with what appeared to be a broken neck, she laughed, calling it a *chompipe muerto* (dead little bird); a similar image is woven into San Pedro Sacatepéquez, Guatemala, *huipiles*; called "a little bird scratching itself" (Barrios 1983:59). The sharing of a design repertoire among these Cakchiquel speakers reinforces aspects of Hearne's research (1985). It also suggests the way innovation, in respect to the use of new motifs, techniques, and materials, is integrated rapidly by Mayan weavers (see comments for **217**). **220** was praised by other Xenacoj weavers as a fine, older piece of weaving. Larger *tzutes* are in use for everyday.

79–17
See **217, 221, 222**   Female Costume

faja

Sash

221

Sacatepéquez: Santo Domingo Xenacoj
Cakchiquel
MS   1970s   1979
115" x 3"   (292cm x 6.8cm)
• *warp*: cotton, 2-ply; black and white; 30 epi (12 epc)
• *weft*: same as warp; 3-ply; black and white; 20 ppi (8 ppc)
• *embroidery*: wool and cotton, 3 singles; multicolored
Backstrap belt-loomed; warp-predominant plain weave; warp stripes; added fringe.

Iconography: ducks and four-legged animals, flowers, and small geometric motifs.
　Sashes are imported from Chichicastenango, see **130**; Xenacoj women embroider them using same iconography as on other textiles; stitches resemble two-faced supp. weft brocading but images are elongated. Men do not wear traditional costume in Xenacoj; many work in Guatemala City, but when in the village, participate in the buying and selling of textiles; one weaver wove under contract to a store owner in the capitol; her husband delivered the textiles; she would not sell to anyone else. Sash is tied tightly around the wraparound skirt with *huipil* tucked inside.

79–18
See **217, 220, 222**   Female Costume

corte or *morga*

Skirt

222

Sacatepéquez: Santo Domingo Xenacoj
Cakchiquel
MS   1970s   1979
140" x 42½"   (338cm x 108cm)
• *warp*: cotton, pair of singles; indigo; 45 epi (18 epc)
• *weft*: same as warp; indigo; 30 ppi (12 ppc)
Treadle-loomed; warp-predominant plain weave; 1 piece seamed together; *randa*; machine-sewn edges.

Randa typical of Xenacoj; series of half triangles; skirt wrapped around body so that the crossing of the *randas* is at the front center; provides a thick body protection; sturdy cloth used in many highland villages; indigo dyeing still practiced.

79–19
See **217, 220, 221**   Female Costume

huipil

Blouse

223

Sacatepéquez: Santa María de Jesús
Cakchiquel
MS   1970s   1979
25½" x 26½"   (65cm x 67cm)
• *warp*: cotton, 4 singles; indigo; 35 epi (14 epc)
• *weft*: same as warp; indigo; 25 ppi (10 ppc)
• *supplementary weft*: cotton, pearl cotton, silk; 7 singles and three 2-ply; red, green, and pink; over 2–10 warps
Backstrap-loomed, warp-predominant plain weave; two 4-selvedge pieces; two-faced supp. weft brocading; machine-stitched center and side seams; black velvet at cut-out head-hole and sleeves.

Iconography: lozenges.
　In the 1970s, **223** was the everyday style; a ceremonial style was still in use, and there was also a wedding *huipil* elaborately embroidered in silk by men. The silk used for supp. weft brocade in **223** represents an investment of $20, a major sum of money for a Mayan weaver. This style was worn in the 1930s (O'Neale 1945: frontispiece).

79–25
Anderson 1978:127–133
See **224, 225, 226**   Female Costume

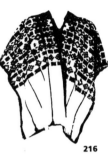

216

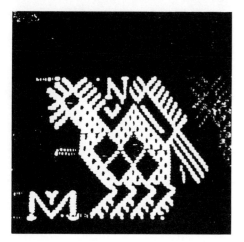

Detail 224

tzute

> ## Cloth, carrying

224

Sacatepéquez: Santa María de Jesús
Cakchiquel
MS 1970s 1979
43½" x 35½"   (111cm x 90cm)
- *warp*: cotton and pearl cotton, three 3-ply; red, blue, green, and multicolored; 45 epi (18 epc)
- *weft*: cotton and pearl cotton, 4 singles; red; 30 ppi (12 ppc)
- *supplementary weft*: cotton, silk, and synthetic, singles; multicolored; over 2–10 warps
Backstrap-loomed, warp-predominant plain weave; two 4-selvedge pieces; two-faced supp. weft brocading; warp and weft stripes; *randa*.

Iconography: three and four-legged animals, large and small stars; lozenges and stars create top and botton borders; an "M" in purple silk embroidered between two animals may be weaver's mark.
   A large, impressive cloth, highly valued by Santa María weavers; with a variety of colors and materials; there are several repaired areas in 224, lovingly executed with similar cloth from other *tzutes*; when asked about the use of synthetic yarn for supp. weft brocading, the weaver responded that it "covered well" and didn't lose color in washing. Synthetic yarn is generally available and cheap; brocading proceeds faster with these yarns, which tourists and entrepreneurs disdain.

79–26
Deuss 1981:45
See **223, 225, 226** Female Costume

faja

> ## Sash, female

225

Sacatepéquez: Santa María de Jesús
Cakchiquel
MS 1970s 1979
56" x 7"   (286cm x 17.5cm)
- *warp*: cotton, pair of singles; red, purple, green, and blue; 60 epi (24 epc)
- *weft*: same as warp; red; 25 ppi (10 ppc)
- *supplementary weft*: synthetic, silk, pearl cotton, and cotton, 2 and 3 singles and pair of 2-ply; multicolored and space-dyed; over 2–16 warps
Backstrap-loomed; warp-predominant plain weave; two-faced supp. weft brocading; warp stripes; cut warp ends worked into 32 braids.

Iconography: see 224; birds; different on each end of sash.
   Colors, materials, and iconography relate to 224. *Huipil* is tucked into wraparound skirt and held in place by sash; men still wear some costume elements in Santa María, such as a shirt which resembles make-up of 224 and 225, but a western-style suit jacket obscures this symbol of a traditional Mayan man.

79–27
See **223, 224, 226** Female Costume

corte or *morga*

> ## Skirt

226

Sacatepéquez: Santa María de Jesús
Cakchiquel
Museum Purchase 1980s 1983
94" x 45"   (236cm x 114cm)
- *warp*: cotton, pair of 2-ply; dark and light blue; 50 epi (29 epc)
- *weft*: same as warp; dark blue; 20 ppi (10 ppc)
Treadle-loomed, warp-predominant plain weave; warp stripes; *randas* join 2 widths and lengths to make a tube.

   Treadle-loomed cloth was being produced as a family operation in Santa María in 1978; women backstrap-wove while men wove on large treadle looms; cloth had been commissioned and upon completion was shipped directly to the United States; several different patterns are produced and worn in many highland villages including Santo Domingo Xenacoj, **222**, San Pedro Sacatepéquez, Guatemala, **239, 240**, Nahualá, **168**, and Chichicastenango, **132**, El Quiché. Western-style dresses and skirts are created out of this versatile cloth for sale to tourists, available in shops in the capitol.

83–21
See **223, 224, 225** Female Costume

huipil

> ## Blouse

227

Sacatepéquez: Sumpango
Cakchiquel
C&BS 1970s 1985
25" x 31"   (64cm x 80cm)
- *warp*: cotton, pair of 2-ply; red and multicolored; 45 epi (18 epc)
- *weft*: cotton, 8 singles; red; 20 ppi (8 ppc)
- *embroidery*: cotton and silk; four 2-ply; multicolored; over 2–52 warps
Backstrap-loomed, warp-predominant plain weave; two 4-selvedge pieces; warp stripes; *randa* at center and side seams; head-hole cut out.

Iconography: floral.
   Sumpango women embroider their *huipiles* with floral designs, separated by rows of chain stitch; *randas* joining the side and front seams and a satin-stitched front and neck opening combined with multicolored warp stripes gives an impression similar to the older style Patzún *huipil*, **193**. It is possible that the backstrap-loomed cloth comes from Xenacoj weavers.
   "They (Xenacoj) entirely supply the pueblo of Sumpango with clothes, as this last, though nearly equally ancient, was more a place of worship and the women never did any weaving" (Pettersen 1976:170). **227** was produced for sale.

85–166
Arriola Geng n.d.
See **228**

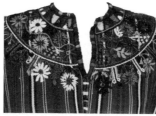

227

huipil

> ## Blouse

228

Sacatepéquez: Sumpango
Cakchiquel
C&BS 1970s 1985
22½" x 37"   (57cm x 94cm)
- *warp*: cotton, 2-ply; multicolored; 55 epi (22 epc)
- *weft*: cotton, 8 singles; red; 15 ppi (6 ppc)
- *supplementary weft*: cotton and pearl cotton, six 2-ply; multicolored; over 4–22 warps
- *embroidery*: pearl cotton
Backstrap-loomed, warp-predominant plain weave, two 4-selvedge pieces; two-faced supp. weft brocading; warp stripes; not joined at sides; *randa*; head-hole cut out.

Iconography: simple floral motifs.
   An unusual combination of two-faced supp. weft brocading combined with embroidery to create the traditional Sumpango *huipil* design; simple floral shapes are loom-produced, leaf and stem motifs embroidered. Another made-for-sale *huipil*. See **227** for comments.

85–167
See **227**

GUATEMALA

huipil

> ## Blouse

229

Guatemala: Chuarrancho
Cakchiquel
C&BS 1970s 1985
28" x 40"   (71cm x 101cm)
- *warp*: cotton, pair of singles; white and multicolored; 45 epi (18 epc)
- *weft*: same as warp; white; 30 ppi (12 ppc)
- *supplementary weft*: cotton, singles and 2-ply; purple and multicolored; over 3–4 warps
Backstrap-loomed, warp-predominant plain weave; two pieces, one a 4-selvedge piece, the other hand-sewn hems; two-faced supp. weft brocading; *randa*; head-hole cut out and folded under; held in place by whip stitch.

Iconography: a rich animal and geometric repertoire, shared by San Pedro Sacatepéquez, Guatemala, weavers, including double-headed eagles, little dogs, stars.
   229 is a ceremonial *huipil* worn outside the wraparound skirt, sometimes over an everyday *huipil*. Two-thirds of the garment is densely brocaded in predominantly purple, the ceremonial color. Motifs are divided by red bands and placed in mirror reflection over the central axis or center seam. Single geometric images appear on the lower third of the *huipil*; warp stripes at center seam add another dramatic design element. Made-for-sale.

85–165
Barrios 1983:41, 43, 59
See **230**

huipil

> ## Blouse

230

Guatemala: Chuarrancho
Cakchiquel
C&BS 1970s 1985
24" x 37"   (61cm x 94cm)
- *warp*: cotton, pair of singles; white; 40 epi (16 epc)
- *weft*: same as warp; white; 20 ppi (8 ppc)
- *supplementary weft*: cotton, singles and 2-ply; purple and multicolored
See **229** for fabrication and comments.

   Scale of animals larger than **229**, all two-legged; a single row of three-legged, animals with large tails are placed in mirror reflection on the lower third of the *huipil*; almost square head-hole. Made-for-sale.

85–164
See **229**

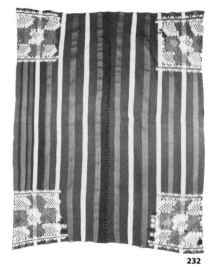

huipil
Blouse
231

Guatemala: San Juan Sacatepéquez
Cakchiquel
Museum Purchase 1970s 1980
23½" x 42"   (60cm x 106cm)
• *warp*: cotton, 2-ply; multicolored; 90 epi (36epc)
• *weft*: cotton, 6 singles; white; 10 ppi (4 ppc)
• *supplementary weft*: pearl cotton, four and six 2-ply; multicolored; over 8–36 warps
Backstrap-loomed, warp-predominant plain weave; two 4-selvedge pieces; two-faced supp. weft brocading; warp stripes; not joined at sides; *randa* at center, extended around head opening.

Iconography: large four-legged animals of mirror reflection in rows across the chest and shoulder areas.

Describing the San Juan Sacatepéquez *huipil* is complicated by the fact that several different types have been woven simultaneously; the everyday *huipiles* (**231**) have a basic format in common; they are composed of two pieces of fabric sewn together with a *randa*; sides are not sewn together but ends are tucked into the skirt and belt; sometimes a commercial blouse is worn underneath (Rowe 1981:50). The combination of red-yellow-mauve-brown stripes is typical of the 1960s and 1970s.

80–157
Pettersen 1976:167
See **232**   Female Costume

tzute
Cloth, carrying
232

Guatemala: San Juan Sacatepéquez
Cakchiquel
C&BS 1970s 1985
60" x 52"   (152cm x 132cm)
• *warp*: cotton, 3-ply; yellow, red, and lavender; 80 epi (32 epc)
• *weft*: cotton, 2-ply; red; 25 ppi (10 ppc)
• *supplementary weft*: cotton, three 3-ply; yellow, lavender, and green; over 4–8 warps
Backstrap-loomed, warp-predominant plain weave; two 4-selvedge pieces; two-faced supp. weft brocading; warp stripes; *randa*.

Iconography: four and two-legged animals, possibly birds and horses.

A large cloth sometimes called a *cargador*; supp. weft brocaded areas in four corners; images rendered upside-down on top so when folded can be seen right-side-up; lavender supp. weft band intersects top and bottom borders and contrasts with warp stripes. Woven-for-sale.

This kind (**232**) of *tzute* is generally used as a shawl, folded into a triangle, draped under the left arm and knotted on the right shoulder. Similarly slung it may be used to carry things or as a head cloth (Rowe 1981:54). Although only 12 kilometers from San Pedro Sacatepéquez, where weavers produce garments for other highland villages, San Juan women have maintained their own unique costume over time.

85–170
See **231**   Female Costume

232

huipil
Blouse
233

Guatemala: San Pedro Sacatepéquez
Cakchiquel
Museum Purchase 1970s 1983
22½" x 36"   (57cm x 92cm)
• *warp*: cotton, pair of singles; white, orange, purple, and green; 60 epi (24 epc)
• *weft*: same as warp; white, 25 ppi (10 ppc)
• *supplementary weft*: cotton, 6 singles; multicolored; over 4–6 warps
Backstrap-loomed, warp-predominant plain weave; two 4-selvedge pieces; single- and two-faced supp. weft brocading; warp stripes at edges; head-hole cut out; hand-sewn center seams; not joined at sides.

Iconography: zigzags, flowers, arches, stars, rectangles.

233 is an everyday *huipil*, woven-for-sale, a typical combination of single- and two-faced brocading; only a small part of the San Pedro weaver's iconographic repertoire is utilized; side seams are not joined so a commercial cloth blouse would be worn underneath; otherwise tucks are taken, side seams sewn, head hole cut out and bound with black velvet, as are the sleeves, for a form-fitting style, worn by young women (Barrios 1983:31). *Huipiles* are tucked into a wrap-around skirt and held in place by a belt; an apron completes the female costume.

83–73
Barrios 1983
See **234**

huipil
Blouse
234

Guatemala: San Pedro Sacatepéquez
Cakchiquel
Museum Purchase 1970s 1984
23½" x 38"   (60cm x 96cm)
See **233** for complete description.

Another woven-for-sale *huipil*; treatment of lower area differs from **233**; three rows of single-faced supp. weft geometric forms occupy one-half of the garment; there is a tie to close the head opening.

84–33
See **233**

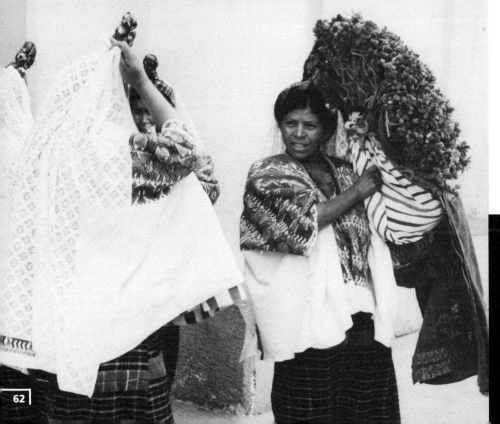

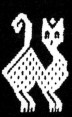

Cakchiquel women participating in *Cofradia* ceremonies. San Juan Sacatepéquez. 1976.
Photo by Clare Brett Smith. See **232**.

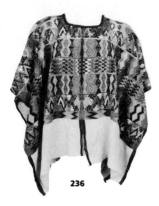

236

huipil

Blouse

235

Guatemala: San Pedro Sacatepéquez
Cakchiquel
Museum Purchase   1970s   1980
23" x 36"   (59cm x 92cm)
- *warp*: cotton, pair of singles; white; 60 epi (24 epc)
- *weft*: same as warp; white; 30 ppi (12 ppc)
- *supplementary weft*: cotton, 6 singles; multi-colored; over 4–6 warps
Backstrap-loomed, warp-predominant plain weave; two 4-selvedge pieces; single- and two-faced supp. weft brocading; warp stripes at edges; machine-stitched center seam; head-hole cut out; not joined at sides.

Iconography: geometric forms including six-sided or hexagonal blocks arranged in vertical rows.
Another version of the everyday *huipil*; see **233** for comments.

80–159
Barrios 1983:62
See **236**

huipil

Blouse

236

Guatemala: San Pedro Sacatepéquez
Cakchiquel
C&BS   1970s   1985
25½" x 36"   (64cm x 92cm)
- *warp*: cotton, pair of singles; white, green; 70 epi (26 epc)
- *weft*: same as warp; white; 25 ppi (10 ppc)
- *supplementary weft*: cotton, six 2-ply; multi-colored; over 4–12 warps
Backstrap-loomed; warp-predominant plain weave; two 4-selvedge pieces; single- and two-faced supp. weft brocading; warp wrapping; warp stripes; *randa*; head-hole cut out; side seams not joined.

Iconography: a variety of geometric forms including "water jars" (Morales Hidalgo 1982:21).
Warp wrapping at the end of each motif brings up a white warp that serves to outline the image; white background cloth serves as design element in some areas; **236** is a fiesta style, more elaborately brocaded than **233, 234, 235**; usually pearl cotton and fine embroidery yarn are used for this type of *huipil*; there are also special motifs (Barrios 1983:32).

85–156
Barrios 1983
See **235**

huipil

Blouse

237

Guatemala: San Pedro Sacatepéquez
Cakchiquel
C&BS   1970s   1985
24½" x 46"   (62cm x 116cm)
- *warp*: cotton, pair of singles; white and multi-colored; 45 epi (18 epc)
- *weft*: same as warp; white; 20 ppi (8 ppc)
- *supplementary weft*: cotton, 6 singles; purple and multicolored; over 4–6 warps
Backstrap-loomed, warp-predominant plain weave; two 4-selvedge pieces; two-faced supp. weft brocading; warp stripes; *randa*; head-hole cut out; not joined at sides.

Iconography: the tree-of-life motif dominates the chest area; animal and bird images including *chompipe muerto* (see **220**) and horses along with plant and flower motifs.
A ceremonial style, purple on white, with only two-faced brocading; colorful warp stripes at center seam, embroidered head opening, touches of color in supp. weft brocading contribute to a *huipil* of great visual interest. This style is always worn over an everyday *huipil*. An elaborate headdress completes the costume. *Chompipe muerto* or *de la fiesta* (of the fiesta) represents an offering made by the groom's parents to the bride's parents; the day of the wedding a bird is killed, stuffed, and adorned with flowers; it is placed in a basket with chocolate, liquor, and cigarettes, then carried to the bride's house and subsequently cooked and eaten with great care (Barrios 1983:67).

85–157
Barrios 1983
See **238**

huipil

Blouse

238

Guatemala: San Pedro Sacatepéquez
Cakchiquel
FS   1970s   1978
24½" x 41"   (62cm x 104cm)
- *warp*: cotton, 2-ply; white; 70 epi (24 epc)
- *weft*: cotton, 5 singles; white; 20 ppi (8 ppc)
- *supplementary weft*: cotton, five 2-ply; purple, light and dark green; over 2–8 warps
Backstrap-loomed, warp-predominant plain weave; three 4-selvedge pieces; two-faced supp. weft brocading; zigzag *randas*; head-hole cut out; side seams hand-sewn.

Iconography: double-headed eagle, tree-of-life, birds, three and four-legged animals.
A ceremonial *huipil* to be worn by those who serve the *cofradia* of the Virgin of the Rosary; **238** is modeled after the miniature *huipil* worn by the Virgin; the unusual feature is the construction; three instead of two 4-selvedge pieces are used; white background with clearly defined iconography in purple related to the diety; men participate in changing the clothes of the statue while women wash and prepare the clothes and accessories; this *cofradia* is the oldest documented one in San Pedro, over one hundred years in existence (Barrios 1983:54). The Virgin of the Rosary in the church has her own tunic from neck to foot woven in soft cotton by the virgins of the pueblo. Each will pay for the thread she uses and weave in her personal symbols, and work two to three hours daily (Pettersen 1976:164, 165).

78–262
See **237**

morga or *corte*

Skirt

239

Guatemala: San Pedro Sacatepéquez
Cakchiquel
Museum Purchase   1970s   1983
86" x 41"   (220cm x 105cm)
- *warp*: cotton, pair of singles; dark and light blues; 55 epi (22 epc)
- *weft*: same as warp; dark blue; 35 ppi (14 ppc)
Treadle-loomed; warp-predominant plain weave; 2 lengths joined by *randa* to make a tube.

This type of wraparound skirt is worn in many highland villages including San Juan Sacatepéquez, Santa María de Jesús, and Nahualá. One type of San Pedro *corte* or *morga* is woven in the municipality of El Tejar, Chimaltenango (Barrios 1983:43).

83–22
See **240**

morga or *corte*

Skirt

240

Guatemala: San Pedro Sacatepéquez
Cakchiquel
Museum Purchase   1970s   1983
88" x 46½"   (224cm x 118cm)
- *warp*: cotton, pair of singles; dark and light blues; 50 epi (20 epc)
- *weft*: same as warp; dark blue; 35 ppi (14 ppc)
See **239** for fabrication and comments.

83–23
See **239**

ESCUINTLA

tzute

Cloth, carrying

241

Escuintla: Palin
Pokomam
Museum Purchase   1970s   1985
14½" x 14½"   (37cm x 37cm)
- *warp*: cotton, 3-ply; white, red, and purple; 40 epi (16 epc)
- *weft*: cotton, pair of singles; white, red, and purple; 17 ppi (7 ppc)
- *supplementary weft*: cotton, eight 2-ply; red and purple; over 1–20 warps.
Backstrap-loomed, warp-predominant plain weave; one 4-selvedge piece; two-faced supp. weft brocading; machine-stitched selvedges.

Iconography: cats, dots, lozenge borders on four sides.
An especially small example, **241** may have been intended for ceremonial use or simply for sale.
The dots are characteristic of Palin weaving and are made by the supp. weft passing through an open plain-weave shed parallel to the ground weft; a little extra length of thread is allowed to stand out from the edge in a loop to heighten this effect; animal designs are woven on a closed shed; *tzutes* have white background and red borders on all four sides, an unusual arrangement in Guatemalan textiles. Because the weaving is warp-predominant the warpwise borders show more clearly than the weftwise ones (Rowe 1981:42,47). **241** has red and purple borders, both warp and weft, the favored colors characteristic of Palin textiles.

83–39
Rowe 1981:42–49

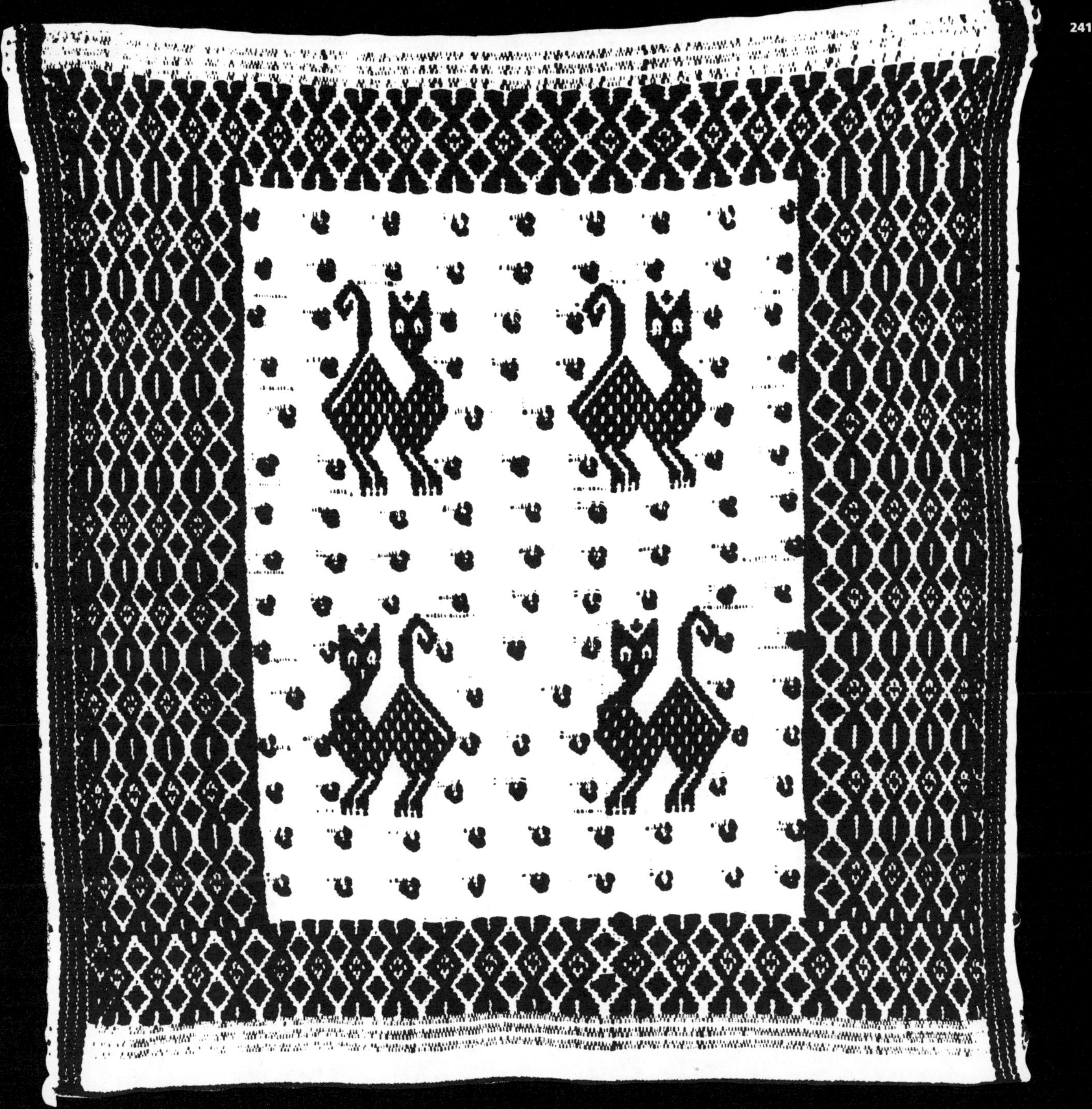

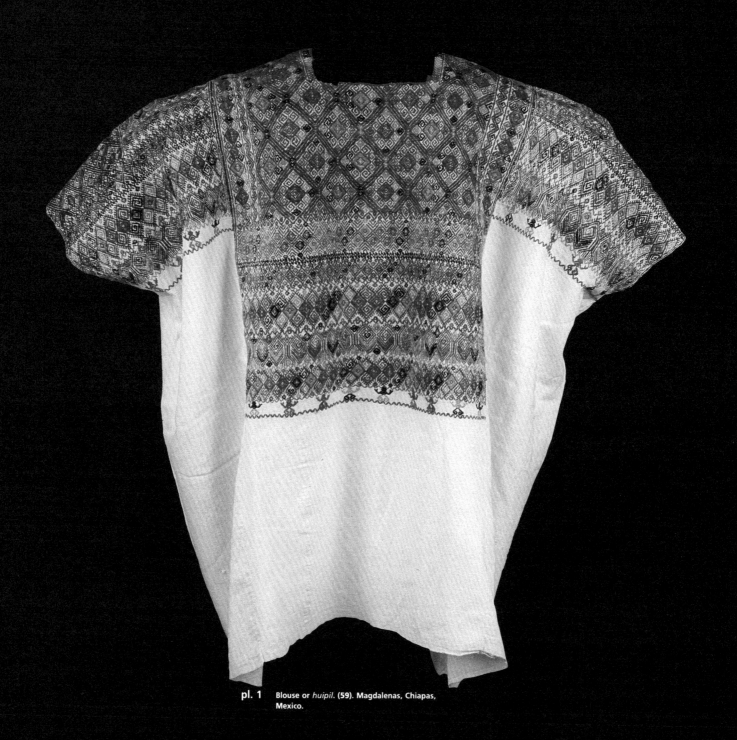

pl. 1   Blouse or *huipil*. (59). Magdalenas, Chiapas,
Mexico.

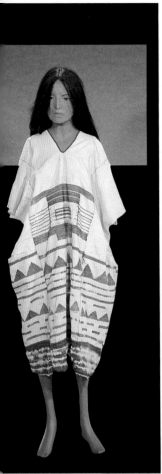

pl. 2
Wedding dress or *huipil*. **(83)**. Zinacantán, Chiapas, Mexico.

pl. 3
Pouch or *achuqalla* **(299)**. Lauramarka-Ocongate area, Cuzco, Peru.

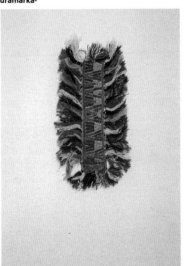

pl. 4
Male costume **(98, 99, 104–106)**. Todos Santos Cuchumatán, Huehuetenango, Guatemala.

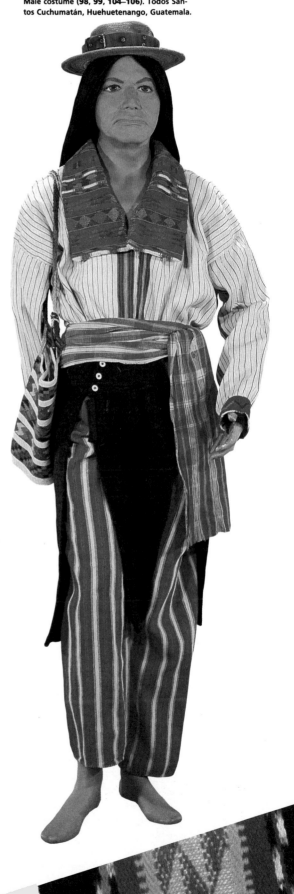

pl. 6

Female costume (246–248). Andahuaylas, Apurimac, Peru.

pl. 5

Uncut blouse or *huipil* (151). Quetzaltenango, Guatemala.

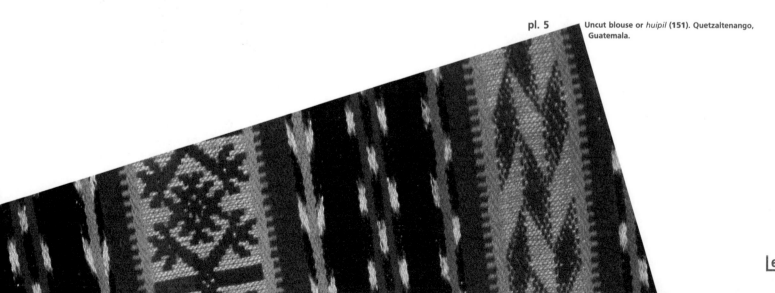

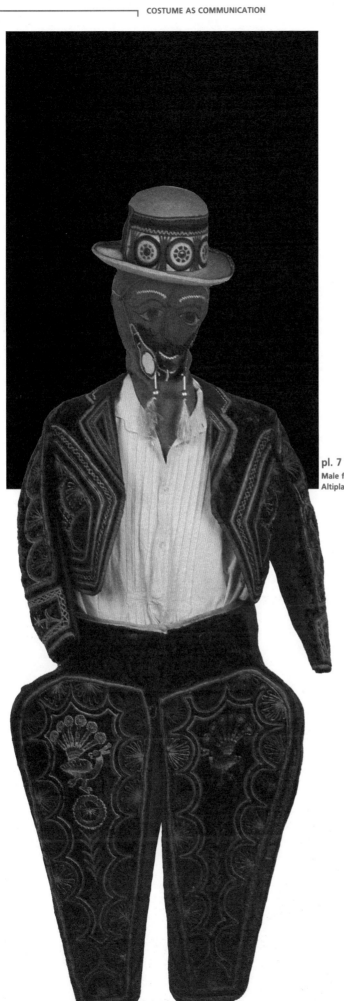

pl. 7
Male fiesta costume (273, 419, 422).
Altiplano, Peru and Bolivia.

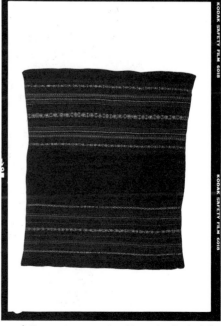

pl. 8   Overskirt or *aksu* (355). Challa region, Cocha-
              bamba, Bolivia.

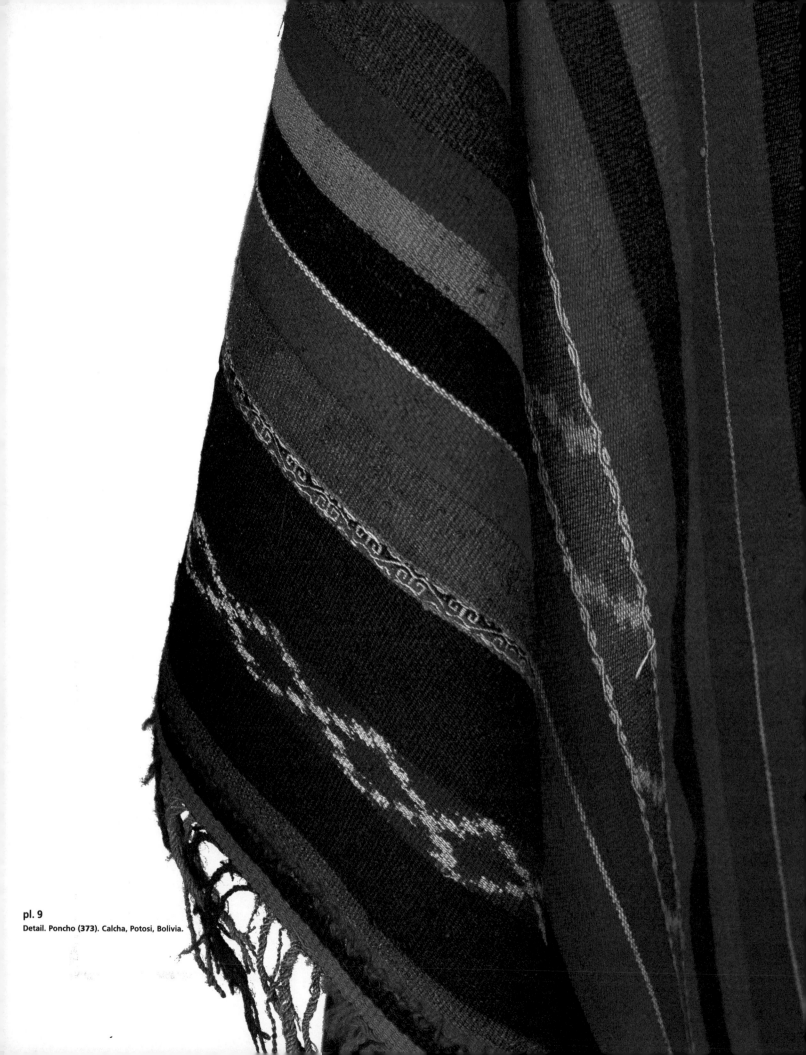

pl. 9
Detail. Poncho (373). Calcha, Potosi, Bolivia.

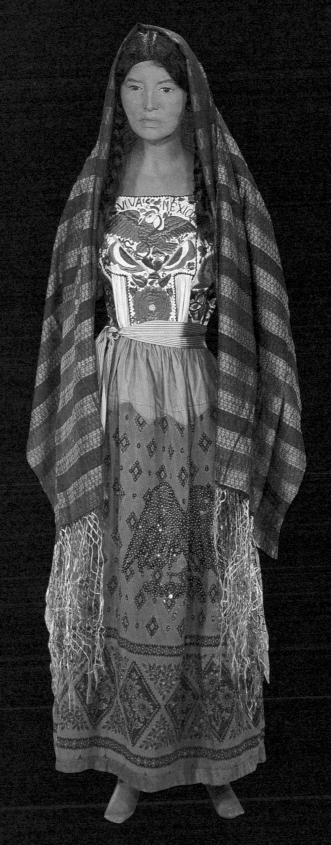

pl. 10
Female Costume, *China Poblana* (**21–24**). Mexico City, Mexico.

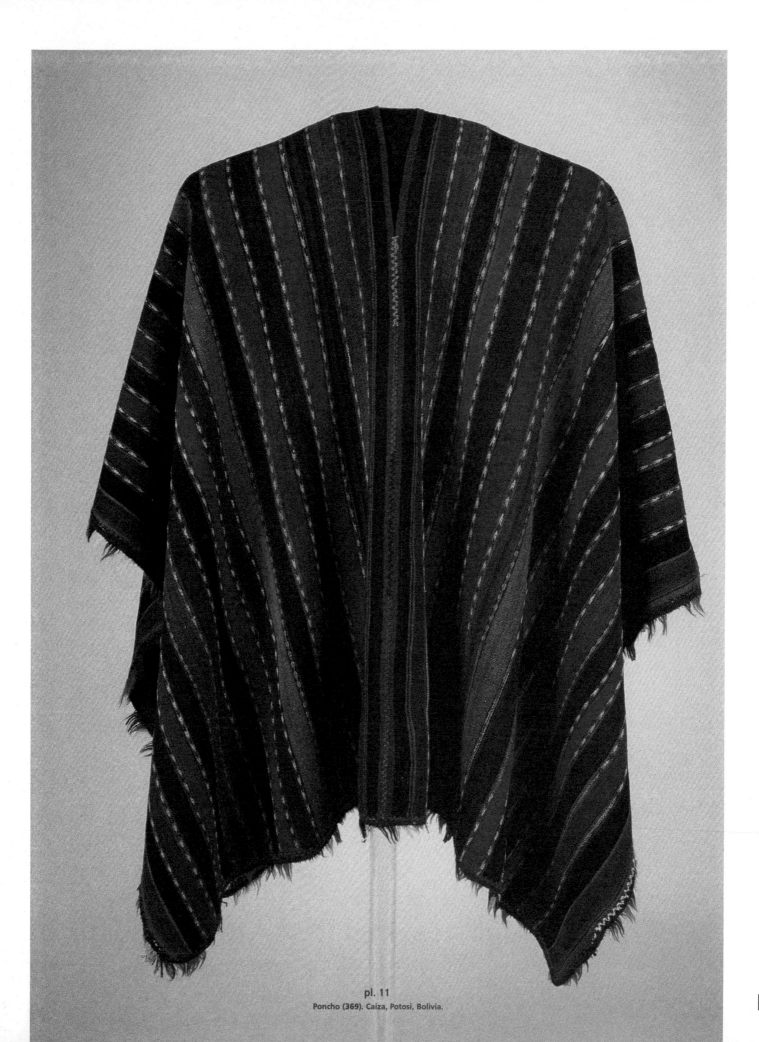

pl. 11
Poncho (369). Caiza, Potosi, Bolivia.

pl. 12   Female costume (177, 178, 184, 188). Male
costume (175, 179–182, 185, 187). Sololá, Sololá, Guatemala.

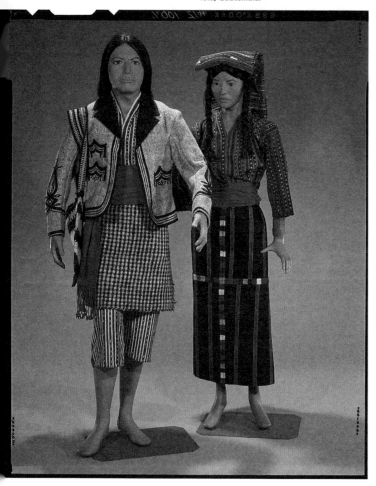

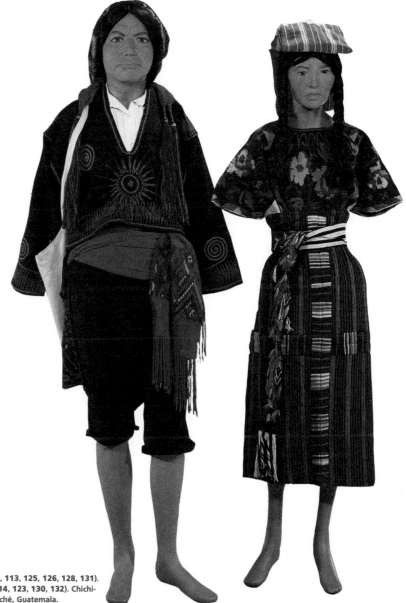

pl. 13
Male costume (112, 113, 125, 126, 128, 131).
Female costume (114, 123, 130, 132). Chichi-
castenango, El Quiché, Guatemala.

pl. 14   Details, Carrying cloths or *tzutes* (203, 204).
San Antonio Aguas Calientes, Sacatepéquez,
Guatemala.

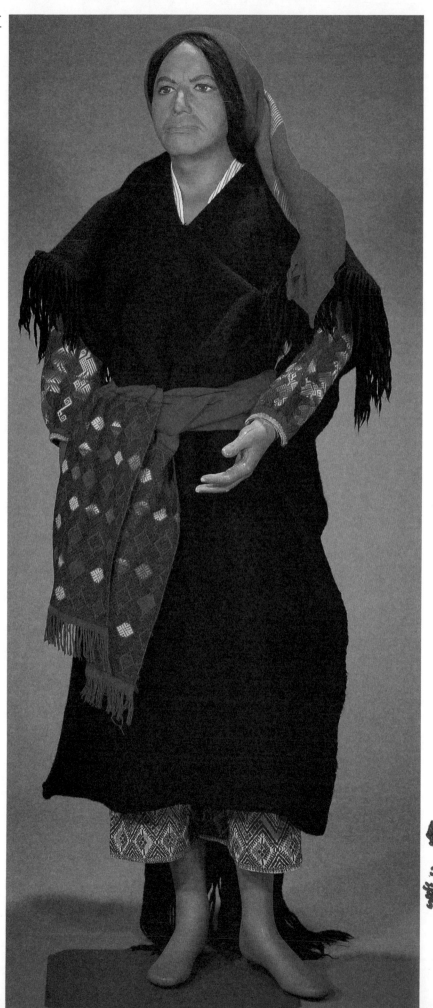

pl. 16   Male costume (159-163). San Martín Sacate-
          péquez (Chili Verde), Quezaltenango, Guate-
          mala.

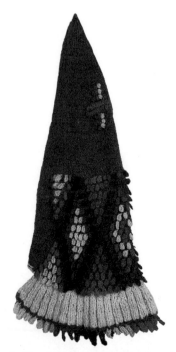

pl. 15   Cap or *chullo* (312). Acora, Puno, Peru.

pl. 17
Coca cloth or *unkhuña* (317). Ayaviri, Puno, Peru.

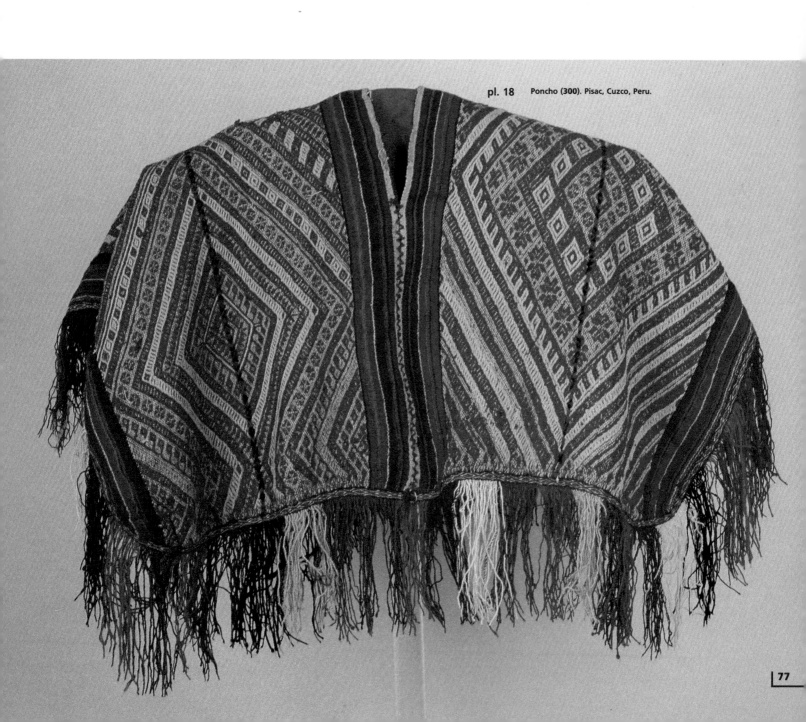

pl. 18   Poncho (300). Pisac, Cuzco, Peru.

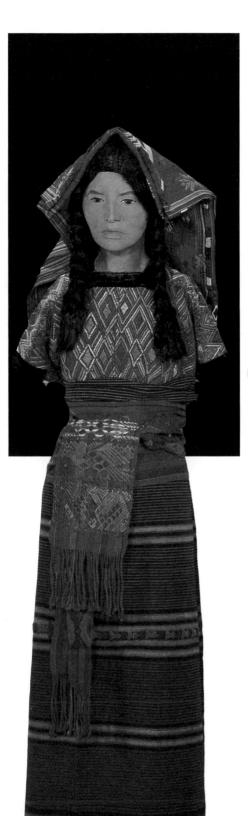

pl. 19   Female Costume (223–226). Santa María de
         Jesús, Sacatepéquez, Guatemala.

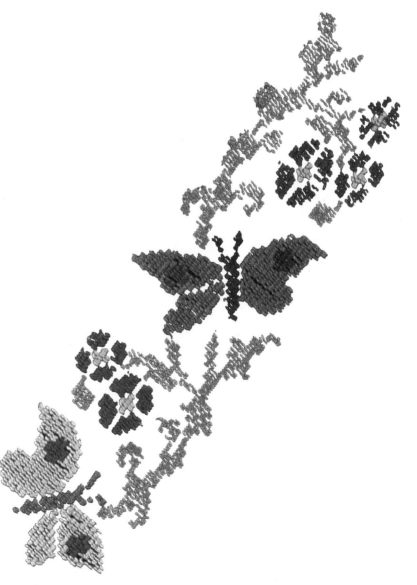

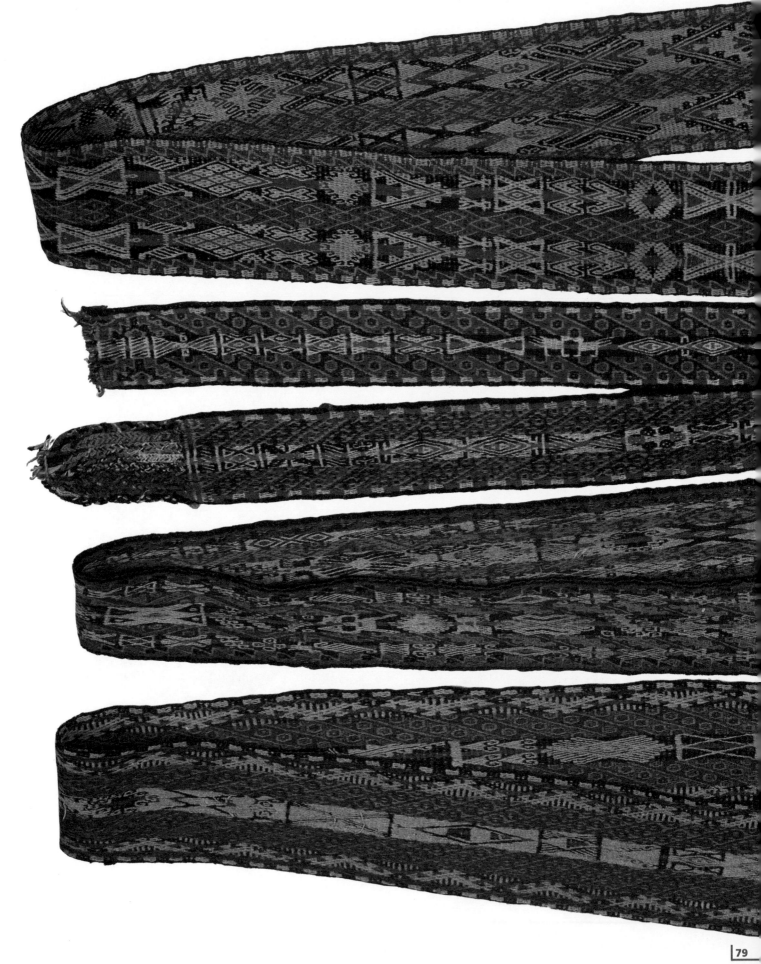

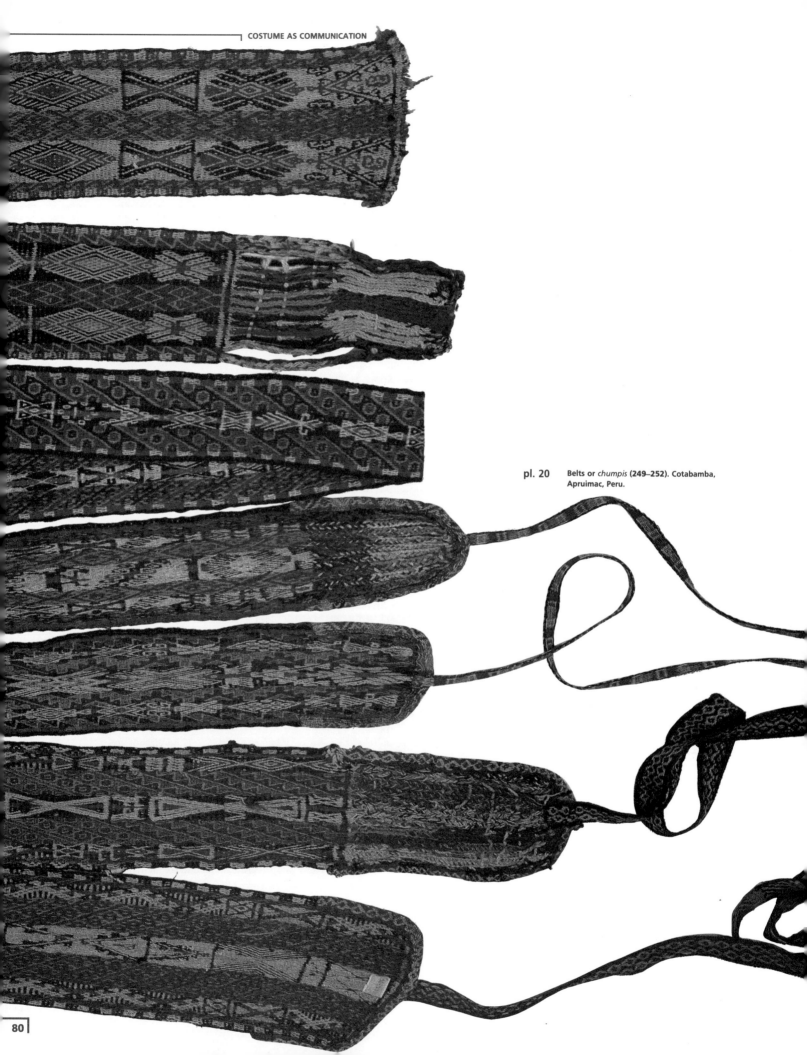

pl. 20   Belts or *chumpis* (249–252). Cotabamba,
Apruimac, Peru.

VI Threads of Time: Andean Cloth and Costume

by E.M. Franquemont

The Andean World

The Andes are perhaps the most unlikely home for one of the world's major civilizations. The area, totalling less than half the size of the United States, is built in longitudinal strips of extremes: a narrow coastal band of arid desert cut by short transverse river valleys, a central range of soaring alpine peaks and crashing valleys, and finally an expanse of dense Amazonian rain forest to the East. There is actually a fourth strip in the frigid Homboldt current that hugs the shoreline on its way north from the Antarctic, and it is this cold water that sets for the Andes extremes of climate that match the geography. Half of the year finds the coastal desert shrouded in dense fogs while the mountains are baked by strong sunshine; the other half of the year brings the desiccating sun to the coast and daily rains to the Sierra. While the challenges of this dramatic land have frustrated the efforts of modern state planners, pre-Columbian Andean people found a power here to fuel the development of sophisticated civilizations that followed strategies quite different from those of other parts of the world. Early in their history (ca. 3000 B.C.) coastal cultures drew upon abundant maritime resources and built huge adobe pyramids around dense urban populations without relying upon agricultural foodstuffs. Later Sierra-based societies such as those we know as Chavin (ca. 1000 B.C.), Huari, and Tiahuanaco (late first millenium A.D.) drew inspiration from jungle plants and animals for elaborate socioreligious movements that swept through both the mountains and the coastal regions to unify great masses of people. By the time of the European contact (A.D. 1532), Andean civilization had thoroughly set its distinctive character and was in its finest hour, the Inca Empire. At no time or place in the history of the preindustrial world had so many people been incorporated into a single political structure, and no nation had ever guaranteed the material needs of its population so effectively. The Inca command of engineering, mathematics, and human organization still reverberates to us through impressive monuments and institutions; and yet, the Inca accomplishment brings more questions and mysteries than answers and wisdoms. Andean culture reached its zenith without benefit of any of the foundations of western civilization, such as the arch, the wheel, written systems, or codified mathematics. The thrust of Andean knowledge and wisdom may have been lost forever in the turmoil of the Spanish conquest, but it has become increasingly clear that for those who would understand better this unique manifestation of human ingenuity, the answer lies with cloth.

The Ancient Andean World

The narrow strip of dry desert that is the coast of Peru is an archaeologists' paradise. The transverse river valleys and abundant maritime resources fostered cultural complexity, while the arid desert conditions assured that virtually everything left behind was preserved for inspection thousands of years later. Tombs yield naturally mummified bodies with deformed heads and tatooed skin, people whose life-styles and economics can be reconstructed from the fish bones, vegetable remains, textiles, and other wastes they discarded in the dry sterile sand around them. Yet, despite the unparalleled richness of the archaeological record on the Peruvian coast, the Andes have been slow to tell their story of human enterprise and cultural development. This history is obscure not because of lack of scholarship — since the end of the last century, talented researchers such as Max Uhle, Junius Bird, Julio C. Tello, and Alfred Kroeber invested great energy both in field studies and in constructing analytical frameworks. Nevertheless, the ancient Andean world was difficult to know because it fundamentally lacked history. Unlike other major preindustrial civilizations of China, the Near East, and Central America, there were no written systems on which to record the passage of time and historical events. Here there can be no Rosetta Stone or ingenious decipherment to unlock ancient records; rather we must deal with a cultural tradition based less on records and history than on abstract ideas.

Our understanding of the development of Andean culture came of age in the 1950s when John Rowe devised a method of reconstructing historical time through detailed analysis of the ceramic remains from Ica, a valley on the south coast of Peru. He was able to define a succession of time periods that allow the events of the ancient Andean world to be related to each other despite our general inability to tie them precisely to the absolute time frame of numbered years used to record western history. With this system it is possible to say that an event occurred during the Early Horizon and to know which events preceded, followed, or were contemporaneous with it, but in terms of absolute chronology, the best we can do is say that it most likely took place sometime in the seventh century B.C. Rowe's scheme is based on the recognition of three major pulsations of influences and energy that swept through the Andes, bringing a relatively large degree of cohesion and cultural uniformity. These were designated the Early, Middle, and Late Horizon; intervening time periods seemed to be characterized by greater regionalization and fragmentation.

Chronology for Ancient Peru (After Rowe)

Approximate Date	Period	Cultures	Events
1480–1532	Late Horizon	Inca	*Q'ompi* vs. *Awasqa*
			Cloth as State Commodity
900–1480	Late Intermediate	Chimu	Gauze Weaves
500–900	Middle Horizon	Huari	Fine Tapestry Shirts
		Tiahuanaco	
300 B.C.–500 A.D.	Early Intermediate	Nazca, Moche	Elaborate Plaiting
1400 B.C.–300 B.C.	Early Horizon	Chavin	Painted Cotton Fabrics
		Paracas	Introduction of Dyed Wool to Coast
			Embroidered Grave Cloths
2200 B.C.–1400 B.C.	Initial Period	Ancon	Invention of Heddle
3000 B.C.–2200 B.C.	Preceramic	Huaca Prieta	Twined Cotton Fabrics

Although Rowe's scheme has proven its utility for archaeologists and is the foundation for most subsequent research and analysis, it has some unsettling features. The most glaring is that each of the three major Horizons represent periods in which massive and unifying influences from the mountains held sway over the coastal people. During the Early Horizon, these influences came as a visionary religion and brought massive technological changes, such as the introduction of the heddle and true loom weaving. Middle Horizon societies, it can be argued, used this same religion to spread direct political and economic control. Finally, we know from historical sources that the Inca of the Late Horizon combined shrewd politics, intrigue, and an astounding productive capacity to dominate all of the Andes. Clearly the Sierra was the crucible for many of the most significant events in Andean prehistory, and yet we must model them based on their reflection in a small coastal valley. Is Andean history so trifurcate as events in Ica make it seem, or are the "intermediate" periods equally filled with major civilizations that for one reason or another failed to impact the south coast of Peru? The wealth of remains on the coast contrasted with scarcity of information from the wetter and more imposing Sierra leaves us little choice at present: we must base our interpretations mostly on events in an area that is probably marginal and subject to the forces that shaped the development of Andean culture.

The problems and pitfalls of this situation are nowhere more evident than they are in the study of the Andes' most important medium, cloth, whose history is almost entirely filled with the abundant and well-preserved fabrics from coastal contexts. Until the latter part of the Early Horizon (middle of the first millenium B.C.), these textiles are almost exclusively cotton and rely heavily upon structural decoration and painting rather than dyed colors. Twined fabrics dominate the Preceramic and Initial Periods, giving rise to the notion that common fish net manufacture may

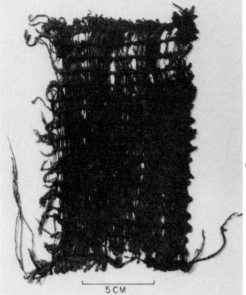

5 CM

have been the initial source of inspiration and expertise (Bird, Hyslop, and Skinner 1985; see fig. 22). Woolen yarns from alpacas and other camelids appear in quantity for the first time in graves of Paracas culture (late Early Horizon); these scarce and valued threads were used mostly for embroidery and almost certainly were traded to the coast from some as yet unidentified highland source. The spectacular bright colors of Paracas yarns offer the first hint of the existence of a highland tradition of woolen textiles, but the power of this shadowy technology is apparent in the single piece of early highland weaving extant, an elaborate shaped tapestry of Pucara culture at the beginning of the Early Intermediate Period (Conklin 1983). The fusion of highland and coastal traditions brought fiber arts to unparalleled heights of design and structural sophistication and defined the medium that has shaped the intellect and consciousness of Andean people into modern times.

Cloth in the Indigenous Andean World

For over 4000 years, the history of Andean civilization has been embedded in fiber; yet virtually all extant fabrics from the pre-Columbian Andes come from coastal contexts. The proliferation of plain cotton cloth in the archaeological sites of the dry coastal desert demonstrates an enormous productive capacity and shows that there was no difficulty supplying the needs of dense urban populations despite the extreme simplicity of the equipment used. But most remarkable is the fancy pattern cloth found in the tombs and the refuse of these ancient societies. Here are textiles executed with precision and skill in virtually every textile technique ever used anywhere on earth. Clearly, the ingenuity, creative drive, and sheer cultural energy invested by Andean peoples in cloth far exceeded any reasonable human impulse to simply elaborate and decorate the world. Convincing archaeological evidence argues that in the nonliterate cultures of the Andes cloth came to serve myriad functions, including roles as diverse as the embodiment of wealth, the vehicle of communication, and even the means of conceptualizing fundamental ideas.

Despite the work of Anna Gayton, Lila O'Neale, J.H. Rowe, John Murra, and others to point out the expanded role of textiles in Andean society, it has been difficult for contemporary western culture people to grasp how fiber could function as such a powerful and multifaceted receptacle of cultural meaning. This difficulty results in part from working with a literary model that expects the discrete visual designs of the cloth to represent words or verbal language in some way. In other words, we have been seeking to understand cloth as a kind of literature. While it may be true that Andean cloth functioned in this way in part, the painstakingly difficult or ingenious methods used by ancient weavers to accomplish things much more easily done in other ways argue that meaning is also conveyed by the structure of the cloth and the process of weaving itself (Conklin 1983). A checkerboard pattern like that shown in D'Harcourt, plate 2B (1962) could have been woven fairly easily with tapestry techniques, or with slightly more sophistication in doublecloth, both weaves at which Andean weavers excelled. Instead, the weaver used elaborate procedures with temporary cords called scaffolds to construct a checkerboard field in which each square is made of its own set of warps and wefts, and the continuity of fiber runs not in the direction of the warp or weft, but along the diagonal direction of the colors (ibid.: fig. 7). In this case, we might surmise that it was important that each square not only look different from its neighbors, but actually *be* different. Mary Frame (1986) argues that many of the abstract geometric designs of ancient fabrics are actually clever and faithful depictions of the way threads move to form the structure of fabrics, and that a system of codes and symbols was in use to allow the three-dimensional character of a weave to be rendered as a visual image on a flat surface of a fabric. Here not only the textile medium but actually the structure of the medium is in fact the message. Textile art of the ancient Andean people was not a representation of language and hence a poor cousin to writing, but rather the primary medium itself. The system of communication used not simply visual images but also structure, processes, tactile qualities, and fiber characteristics to encode meaning. Photographs and written descriptions of Andean cloth can present only the smallest facet of this rich system of communication. Few of us today have the technical expertise to understand and appreciate the scale of the Andean endeavor in cloth.

Most of the secrets of the ancient Andean textiles will never be unraveled for us – the system is too elaborate, the societies too distant, and the concerns of the people who made them too foreign to us. Nevertheless, the Spanish conquerors of the early sixteenth century have left at least a glimpse, however brief, at the workings of the Inca Empire and the kind of information that was important to Andean civilization. Many of these observations reflect their bias and interests as men and as conquerors, and they failed to understand much about social structure and in particular the role of women in the Andes. But the industrial revolution had not yet diluted their sense of cloth as treasure, and they left many observations about how the peoples of the Inca Empire used textiles. At the time of the Conquest, cloth was the most important material commodity of a society rich in gold, silver, and agricultural surplus (Murra 1962). The work of John Murra, J.H. Rowe, and others demonstrates that two distinct weaving traditions existed side by side in Inca times: Q'ompi, tradition of fine tapestry weaving probably produced by men who were full-time, state-supported specialists, and Awasqa, warp-faced and patterned cloth that was most likely produced in village contexts and served as an indicator of land-based social groups. Q'ompi cloth lingered briefly with the support of the Catholic church but basically disappeared with the destruction of the Inca state, while Awasqa has continued into the present. Rural Quechua- and Aymara-speaking weavers of the contemporary highland Andes are still at work in their distinctive local styles, maintaining and even innovating within modes of textile production that tie them to their pre-Columbian ancestors.

The Andes Today

The "Inca Nation," as J.H. Rowe (1946) aptly calls it, of these indigenous highland Andean people is today an integral but not integrated part of five different South American countries (Ecuador, Peru, Bolivia, and parts of Argentina and Chile). Quechua speakers by far dominate; only about two million Aymara-speaking people remain around Lake Titicaca. While Quechua language has been diffusing throughout the Andes since at least Inca times to engulf many smaller languages and some Aymara communities, it is easiest to refer to indigenous people by the language they speak since evidence connecting living societies with other languages and cultures is at best controversial at this point. Together, there are about 20 million indigenous highland people united by commonalities of economics, ecology, lifestyle, religion, world view, and language, yet they speak with no unified political voice. Their relationship with federal government varies from country to country, but improved transportation and the end of overtly exploitative Spanish colonial institutions in this century has brought almost all of these indigenous people into closer contact with western culture. As their awareness of these new contexts has grown, Quechuan and Aymara people are changing greatly as societies and as individuals. The most important of these changes sees people abandoning their ancient village identity in favor of greater participation in the money economy and life in cities and towns; this has spawned a kind of pan-Andean class consciousness with its own distinctive culture. In response to the dynamics of these changes, sociologists have devised many different ways of referring to the contemporary

Andean person, including such words as *Mestizo* (a person of mixed Spanish and Indian blood), and *Cholo* (an Indian attempting to use *Mestizo* culture). All require value judgments and assumptions by the classifier. The situation is further complicated by folks who dress and behave as indigenous village people most of the time but assume *Cholo* or *Mestizo* posture upon entering a city. Here, however, we are fortunate, since the major defining quality of identity is still clothes; we can sidestep the complexities of ethnicity in the contemporary Andes by considering textiles themselves to designate village Quechuan or Aymara people depending upon language of the users and makers, or as characterizing urban Andean culture. This simple but wholly adequate set of classifiers, of course, obscures a great deal of fuzzy areas between the categories, but reflects the emerging Andean reality and the shift from village identity to a growing involvement with larger political and economic structures.

In the past two decades, a major arm of fieldwork has come to focus at last on the Andean weavers themselves, their ways of work, and the functions of their remarkable products in contemporary Andean life. Many recent researchers (e.g. Meisch, Zorn, and the Franquemonts) have recognized that this is an essentially experiential domain and have emphasized learning through fingers by developing competency with the Andean textile process. More than an anthropological entree, this has allowed them to meet the Andean mind at work in this complex nonverbal medium. The growing body of ethnographic information suggests that the contemporary Andean world is itself an elaborate fabric constructed on many distinctly different and separate parts with varying skills, techniques, styles, and local culture. At one level, cloth serves as part of an "ethnic code" (C. Franquemont 1986) that communicates local village identity and participates in local ritual use. Most of these local costumes were heavily influenced by the Europeans during the eighteenth century, but the system still functions to define local land-based social groups that are certainly indigenous in origin. Dress strengthens in-group solidarity and sets clear contrasts with others; some evidence suggests, that even within each group, nuances of costume characterize small land-defined subgroups. These local styles and traditions function in a complex manner for new techniques, patterns, and materials diffuse quite easily throughout the area but do not affect the underlying style definitions (E.M. Franquemont 1984). What these essential components of local costume and style are has not yet been addressed by systematic research. These area-defined local styles are the individual warps of the fabric and are held together by strong threads of economics, religion, language, and history. The correspondingly important roles played by cloth at this level were probably occupied in pre-Columbian times by the now extinct *Q'ompi* tapestries. Cloth is used all over the Andes to indicate ritual; the simple act of laying a piece of fabric on the ground transforms common earth into a ritual *mesa* (table) for curing, divination, or celebration. Pan-Andean pilgrimages such as *Qollur Rit'i* represent another unifying vector of Andean life. Hundreds of thousands of indigenous people converge annually upon a mountain peak south of Cuzco in a massive adoration of glacial snow and its symbolic extensions. Most devotees wear their village costumes but make special fabrics for use in ritual games. Some of these fabrics are made of magical left-spun yarns or are miniature versions of garments in daily use. Other participants at *Qollur Rit'i* shed their normal personalities and assume ritual roles by wearing a standard set of costumes that are understood throughout the Peruvian Andes.[5] Common economic concerns and conditions also unite Andean people and are reflected in the cloth they use. While rural people hold to traditions of costume that emphasize their village identity, urbanized Quechua and Aymara dress to indicate their socioeconomic class and their reliance upon the money economy. Their

5 Dwight Heath's notes accompanying this collection indicate that the Bolivian fiesta of Alasitas (Jan. 24) is similar in character.

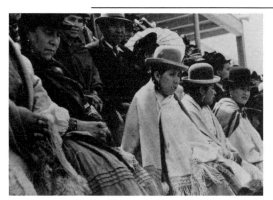

Fig. 23
Urban Andean women. 1920–1930. Herbert J. Spinden Photo Archives, Haffenreffer Museum of Anthropology.

6 The male weaver from Anta pictured in A.P. Rowe 1975 is weaving in the style of Cuzco's San Jeronimo prison.

clothes are manufactured in small shops from machine-made fabrics which are sold in the major urban markets. As a result, urban Andeans dress in similar ways throughout Peru and Bolivia. The women, who are the backbone of the urban Andean society, are especially distinctive in a costume that includes a starched white straw hat, layers of skirts and aprons, a blouse with appliqué lace, flesh tone hose, shoes, and a machine-made shawl of some kind (see fig. 23; 243, 244, 245). Industrial products like these, designed and manufactured expressly for the indigenous consumer, are often overlooked because they do not fit our notions of art. Yet these are a major and perhaps growing part of the contemporary Andean textile traditions. In a similar way, rural men seem to be shedding their village identity in favor of an emerging class consciousness that is pan-Andean. This change is reflected in their adoption of a plain coffee-colored poncho that is not specific to any local area (E.M. Franquemont 1984). Thoroughly urbanized Andean men shift to denims and windbreakers and completely eschew the felt hat that is ubiquitous to rural settings. Should they wear a poncho, it is handwoven of brightly colored synthetic yarns.

"Macro" styles in Andean dress unite people from many local culture areas into a coherent class identity. They are probably recent phenomena, due in part to the growth of transportation, media, western economic systems. Macro trends ripple through the Andes in mysterious ways, but certainly one pressure toward homogenization of the Andean textile tradition along class lines is exerted by the local jails. Incarcerated men earn a living by contract weaving in a generalized style that fills the textile needs of urban and upwardly mobile rural Andeans who no longer weave and are separating themselves from their communities in favor of greater participation in the money economy. Such work is done on a contract basis: the customer brings the yarns or the prepared warp to be woven by the prisoner in the style which he knows. Since few men have textile skills when they enter jail, they are taught to weave by their fellow prisoners in this generalized style (272). Not only are textiles in the prison-style common in almost all communities of the Cuzco region, but many men continue to practice these new skills and aesthetics when they return to their communities.[6]

The material functions of cloth as indicator of identity, class, or economic status are only one layer of meaning, and perhaps the most superficial. In a much more profound sense, the fiber arts still form an experience base that is fundamental and universal to the Andean reality, even for those who are outside the productive process. All people, even men, understand cloth and how it is made. In some way, the mechanics of fiber and its potential for structure, design, and color constitute a metaphor, a model so powerful that it can communicate more than art and aesthetics, more than village identity and economic status but also ideas that can be used to understand much of human experience. The basic ideas of Andean spinning and weaving are also used to conceptualize the natural world, agricultural processes, social relations, house-building techniques, and even soccer strategy. It would be wrong to say that Andean weaving is a symbol of these other domains; rather it is a tangible expression of many of the fundamental concepts of Andean life, and the vehicle through which these concepts are learned. The fiber art of the Andes continues to represent a philosophy built of visual and tactile ideas rather than verbal ones, a philosophy that finds no parallel in contemporary western society but powers the engine of Andean creativity.

Technology

The traditional Andean weaver today works with the simplest of equipment, a labor-intensive process, and materials that are for the most part

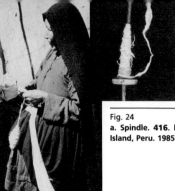

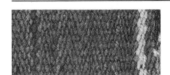

Fig. 24
a. Spindle. 416. b. Woman spinning, Taquile Island, Peru. 1985. Photo by Margot Schevill.

Fig. 25
Herringbone effect created by alternating Z and S-plied yarns.

7 The collector of this piece, Gale Hoskins, reports that this is a fabric for mourning and that both the amount of counterspinning and the presence of pink weft yarn indicate magical status.

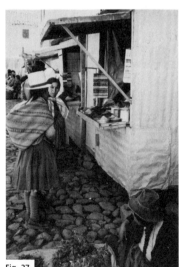

Fig. 27
Dye trader. Cuzco, Peru. 1986. Photo by E.M. Franquemont.

readily at hand. Drop spindles, really nothing more than shaped and weighted sticks (see fig. 24), spin sheep and camelid fibers into three sizes: *nanu* (fine, about 3500 yards/pound singles), *regular* (about 1600 yards/pound singles), and *raku* (600 yards/pound singles). Each of these sizes is customarily made into a Z-spun, S-two-ply yarn for weaving, although the *regular* size is often used in *bayeta* (balanced plain weave) and *jerga* (balanced twill) floor loom yardage as a single strand (E.M. Franquemont 1983). Yarn is occasionally spun in the opposite direction. This S-spun, Z-plied yarn, called by Quechuan people *lloq'e*, or left-handed, has attracted attention of many researchers because of its use in ritual and magical life (Goodell 1969; see fig. 25). This association is undeniably important, but *lloq'e* yarns are also used in other ways. The weavers of certain styles like to place stripes of counterspun yarns near the side selvedges of the cloth to help keep the corners from curling. Weavers from Q'ero, near Paucartambo, Peru, use counterspun stripes to create a kinetic quality in a plain-woven field that is difficult to achieve through color striping alone (**303**). One remarkable example of Andean counterspinning is a *phullu* (woman's wrap) from Juli, Puno, Peru (**323**). The threads in each lease alternate spin direction throughout the plain-weave Pampa section (see fig. 26 for the warp plan). The counterspun yarns lying next to each other wedge together into V-form pairs that have a remarkable resemblance to knitted stitches.[7] Chinchero weavers favor *lloq'e* yarns as the weft for belts because they believe they are stronger, and in at least one Andean community (Patacancha, Distrito de Ollantaytambo, Cuzco, Peru), almost all fabrics are routinely made of *lloq'e* yarns. These uses of *lloq'e* yarns show practical and aesthetic considerations, but it may well be that these are ultimately still based upon the magical properties attributed to backwards-spun yarn.

Dyed colors have always played a vital role in the elaboration of most Andean handwoven textiles, and the dye industry so well developed early in Andean prehistory persisted until recent times. Ancient dyers used madder, cochineal, and a form of indigo as well as many other plant substances, but the methods by which they worked are unknown. This indigenous dye technology was threatened and mostly lost with the advent of the cheap chemical dyes beginning in the second half of the nineteenth century. Today it is difficult to find people who control any aspect of it. Some contemporary dyers in the Andes are now working with European vegetable dye technology that has been introduced in the past few decades, but the soft and muted tones they produce were probably never part of the Andean palette. As in the rest of the world, the use of indigo to make a variety of blue shades persisted longest because an effective substitute was not developed until the 1930s. Cochineal as a versatile red dye is still in use in parts of the Andes, but there is no comprehensive study to date of indigenous Andean production and dyeing methods. The Andean textile tradition was particularly vulnerable to new synthetic dyestuffs because the vegetable dyes had been traded throughout the Andes in prepared, easy-to-use form for centuries. Those who produced and processed the dyestuff were not necessarily those who actually used them on fiber. The dye trader is still a well-recognized part of the Andean textile landscape today (see fig. 27). While for the most part his wares are now chemically based, this role probably has ancient roots in a large scale Andean trade network. Although the vegetable dye industry appears to have disappeared in this century, traces still remain but have not yet been studied in any detail. Despite their dependence upon cheap synthetic dyes this network now brings them, Andean people have not lost their respect for natural dyes and may still hoard *umas* ("heads") of powdered indigo that have been stored for more than thirty years awaiting an appropriate occasion.

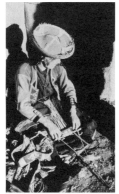

Fig. 28
Backstrap weaver. Chincheros, Cuzco, Peru. 1986. Photo by Margot Schevill.

Z = S-spun, Z two ply yarns
S = Z-spun, S two ply yarns

.... **Z S Z S Z S Z S** .... shed roll
.... **Z S Z S Z S Z S** .... heddle

Fig. 26
Warp plan for a *phullu* from Juli, Puno (323) showing distribution of left- and right-spun yarns in two leases. Drawing by E.M. Franquemont.

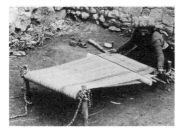

Fig. 29
Staked loom weaver. Songo, Cuzco, Peru. 1975. Photo by Catherine J. Allen.

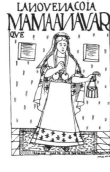

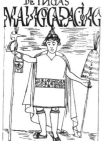

Fig. 30
Male and female Incan costume. Drawings by Guaman Poma de Ayala.

In most of the Andes, the technology of weaving is extremely simple. The loom itself is nothing more than a series of shaped sticks and small ties that use a continuous warp and applied heddle to produce four-selvedge cloth. A simple, narrow, *hakima* strip loom is used by little girls to learn the principles of their craft. A multiloop heddle is applied to one side of the cross and a shed loop holds the other. By manipulating these shedding devices alternately, the weaver produces a basic warp-faced plain weave. For design bands such as that shown in the figure, she considers this plain weave as a raw product from which complex patterns can be picked up by hand. Larger looms follow the same principles (**359**), although to accomodate scale some different equipment is necessary, such as a bone pick (*ruk'i* or *wich'una*) and a shed roll in place of the shed loop (see fig. **28**). This basic equipment is widespread throughout the contemporary Andes, but strangely, there seem to be at least two completely different ways of operating it to produce similar cloth. Many weavers from Cuzco south into Bolivia stretch their loom out between four stakes and work with fixed tension on the web, while others use body tension systems that allow them to change tension to facilitate different parts of the process (A.P. Rowe 1975; see fig. **29**). These differences seem to represent broad geographical and cultural divisions in the textile traditions that are still very poorly studied and understood. The true equipment for working either system, however, is not the loom but rather the mental agility of the weavers who find in the simple looms no mechanical limits to their creative vision and traditional skills. Either way of weaving can be used to produce very elaborate patterning in warp-faced cloth through adroit and surprisingly fast manual manipulation. The range of techniques employed by ancient and contemporary Andean weavers is truly astounding and has been thoroughly surveyed by Ann Pollard Rowe in her book *Warp Patterned Weaves of the Andes*.

There are two major types of warp patterned cloth made in the Bolivian and Peruvian Andes today. The loom in figure 28 shows rudimentary complementary warp patterning in which all the threads that form the pattern also form the structure of the cloth (A.P. Rowe 1977a:53–80). This type of patterning was in wide use in pre-Columbian times and can be quite extensive and complex (**318**). In more recent times, elaborate supplementary warp patterning has come into vogue in much of the area. This is simpler to understand and faster to accomplish, for the yarns of the design are not part of the structure of the fabric itself (**297**; A.P. Rowe 1977a:ch. 7). While local village styles may call for one or the other of these types of patterning, both are common throughout the area, from Cuzco south. Bolivian weavers also use multiharness arrangements to produce double cloth (**382**; Cahlander 1985:pl. 7), and other more bizarre, complex loom technologies have been reported from the contemporary Andes (E.M. Franquemont 1983; Cahlander, Franquemont, and Bergman 1981). Despite Rowe's survey of the textiles themselves, much work still remains to be done to elucidate the methods actually used by Andean weavers to create these fabrics.

Fabrics and Garments of the Contemporary Andes

The 4-selvedge cloth produced by Andean weavers has always been used uncut, with no tailoring beyond seaming panels together. In Inca times, most men wore only a knee-length shirt called an *unkhu* that may have been held with a belt; the *poncho* so characteristic of today's Andes is actually a colonial period import. Women wore a skirt or dress with a belt, and a *lliklla* wrapped about the shoulders and pinned with an ornamental *tupu* or a needle (see fig. 30). Most Andean people, however, came under repressive dress codes during the eighteenth century, which forever altered cloth-

8 These words are of Spanish origin but have come to be a part of everyday Quechuan language.

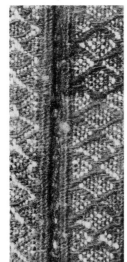

Fig. 31
Golón made in Chincheros, Cuzco, Peru. Photo by E.M. Franquemont.

Fig. 32
The heddle plan for fig. 31. Drawing by E.M. Franquemont.

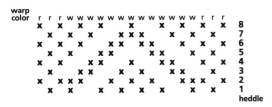

```
warp
color  r  r  r  w  w  w  w  w  w  w  w  w  w  w  w  w  r  r  r
       x  x  x  x     x        x  x  x  x  8
          x  x  x     x  x  x     x  x  x  7
       x  x  x     x  x     x  x     x  x  x  6
          x  x     x  x        x  x     x  x  5
       x  x     x  x        x  x     x  x  4
          x  x  x     x     x     x  x  3
       x  x  x  x     x     x     x  x  x  x  2
          x  x     x     x  x     x  x  1
                                         heddle
```

The weft is red with *kantunga* blocks of green 2 cm. wide about 28 cm. apart

ing styles through the introduction of such garments for women as the *pollera*[8] (pleated full skirt), the *jabon* (waist-length jacket), the *montera* (saucer-shaped hat with a basketry frame), and for men, trousers and the *tablera* (coat with tails). Even in the most remote parts of the Andes, contemporary costume represents the fusion of indigenous traditions of uncut decorated cloth with Spanish tailored garments, providing a visual gestalt of the history of the area.

Andean traditional dress styles are surprisingly varied, but there is a shared basic inventory of textile categories. The smallest woven fabrics are *hakimas* (straps) and *watanas* (a thing for tying; **421**), strips of patterned cloth made mostly by little girls and used for many purposes. Slightly larger bands are *chumpis* (belts) used by both men and women as belts (see **249**, and pl. 20) or as straps for swaddling babies (**407**). *Unkhuña* (small cloth; see **317** and pl. 17) is a small square or rectangular cloth made of a single warp that is used to carry coins, coca leaves, or lunch and as a surface for coca divination. For warmth, men wear a *poncho* (see **300** and pl. 18) that they also use as a general purpose cloth. It is usually made of two identical 4-selvedge panels. The corresponding women's garment is the *llijlla* (wrap) (**297**). It is also made of two identical 4-selvedge panels that are seamed together and usually represents the pinnacle of the weaver's skills in any style. Men and women both carry packs made of a *k'eparina* (a thing for carrying; **272**) which may be a special cloth or simply an older *llijlla*. Pants and a shirt complete the men's costume, while women wear a variety of skirts, underskirts, vests, jackets, and blouses (see **390–396**, a complete woman's costume from Tarabuco, Bolivia). A number of other fabrics are also important to Andean life, including *sogas* (braided llama ropes), *warakas* (slings; **361**), *chuspas* (coca bags; **265**), and *costales* (produce sacks; **307**). There is no really complete inventory of the complex of cloth in use in an Andean Sierra village available, but Adelson and Takami's catalogue, *Weaving Traditions of Highland Bolivia* (**1978**), beautifully represents the range of local costumes of traditional Bolivia.

Among the fabrics that are still poorly reported are the complex hair ties (**294, 295**), cloth edgings, or *golones* (skirt borders). These small and easily overlooked fabrics are often quite ingenious in design and technology, employing discontinuous wefts, intersecting warps, and complex multiheddle loom procedures. *Golones* of various kinds are present in many of the textiles in the Haffenreffer Museum collections. These strips of complex balanced weave probably began in imitation of some Iberian fabric and are commonly used in the Cuzco area as skirt borders (**287**) or as bag straps (A.P. Rowe 1977a: fig. 14). Depending on local style, the *golon* varies in width from under three centimeters to over ten centimeters and ranges in technique from 2/2 straight or bird's-eye twill to a thirteen-harness compound weave. The *golon* made in Chincheros uses eight heddles with a complex arrangement (see figs. 31 and 32), and is the only multiheddle fabric produced in the town. The warp is wound as a simple figure-eight pattern that the weaver reorganizes into eight leases and installs heddles so that she can weave the pattern with no further pick up. The weave itself combines twill lines with plain weave blocks but is usually dominated by the color patterning in the weft. In Chincheros this patterning is organized into registered color zones in a system called *kantunga*; in other areas the colors are more ambitiously arranged to form diamonds, zigzags, or other designs that require discontinuous wefts. Rowe (1977a: fig. 14) reports examples in which *kantunga* color shifts are accomplished through ikat of a single continuous weft thread. In recent years, the *golon* has come to be a piece of handwoven trim that can be applied to almost any machine-made fabric to give it an "Andean" look for sale to tourists (**278–280**).

Urban indigenous people acquire their garments through purchase, trade, or by contracting with a specialist for their manufacture. In most cases, their clothes are made in small shop situations by other indigenous people from purchased yardage and then sold in market stalls; often the vendor is also the producer. Some shops specialize in producing fancy fiesta clothes of velvet with sequins, mirrors, embroidery, or other embellishments (see pl. 7). Many rural towns also manage to support a specialist male weaver who makes *bayeta* and *jerga* yardage on a European treadle loom. These specialists are usually the poorest members of a community and do part-time work at their looms on a contract basis in order to supplement the meager output of their agricultural enterprise.

The Collection

The Andean textiles presented here from the Haffenreffer Museum of Anthropology reflect the ethnographic emphasis of the Museum and its major collectors. Among the real strengths of the collection are the exhaustive and provocative field notes made by Dwight Heath of Brown University, who acquired one of the first major components in mid-1960s.[9] These notes provide not only details of the object and the circumstances of its acquisition, but also interesting asides, such as:

[349] Woman's blouse. Sp.: Blusa. This distinctive style is made and worn by Negro women in the Yungas region. Although cut and manner of weaving are similar to Aymara blouses [400, 401], stylized floral embroidery is distinctive of Negroes who occupy a few small endogamous enclaves in predominantly Aymara area. (Poor grade everyday blouses of Aymaras are also muslin, but with simpler ornamentation like [354].) The rest of Negro dress is almost identical with that of Aymaras.

The result is that the cloth speaks to us of Bolivian society in a way that technical analysis of the object alone could never hope to achieve. Here we learn of a population of black people who speak a highland Indian language in the Bolivian lowlands! Heath concentrated upon acquiring for the museum examples of the everyday cloth he saw in the markets and in use around him, as well as examples of fabrics and garments he knew to be representative of specific economic function, social conditions, or historical moment. There are, to be sure, excellent examples of traditional *awasqa* cloth expressing village identity, such as several fine pieces from the Charazani area (334). But equally compelling are such strange fabrics as a quilted handwoven mule pad and strap (339) and an enormous coca harvest bag (351) that have functions in a radically different context. Another major component of the Haffenreffer collection comes from the work of former Museum director Jane Dwyer and her husband Edward Dwyer of Rhode Island School of Design. As archaeologists their attention was focused on style and technology. They worked mostly by commissioning Quechuan friends to find or produce items of interest. A number of other collectors have also collaborated in a smaller way, but their work has been confined to the major textile trading centers of Cuzco, Juliaca, Puno, and La Paz where the textiles are far removed from their original context and intent, and must stand essentially alone. In recent years the Museum has acquired through purchase from dealers a number of excellent examples of cloth from just over the horizon of contemporary times; such fabrics have been termed "Aymara Weavings" (Adelson and Tracht 1983), although equating textile styles with linguistic groups is risky business in the Andes. These outstanding pieces of art (e.g. 314, 315) are notable not so much for the weaving, which tends to be fairly simple and sparse, but more for the remarkable spinning, vegetable dyeing, and all over design sense. It is, to be sure, a delight to come across such lovely objects in the collection but in another way it is also somewhat disturbing that they are merely objects. The collectors' notes do at times relay some

9 About one quarter of Heath's collection consists of textiles and related objects. Comparably perceptive observations cover other artifacts made of ceramic, wood, leather, vegetable, and other materials.

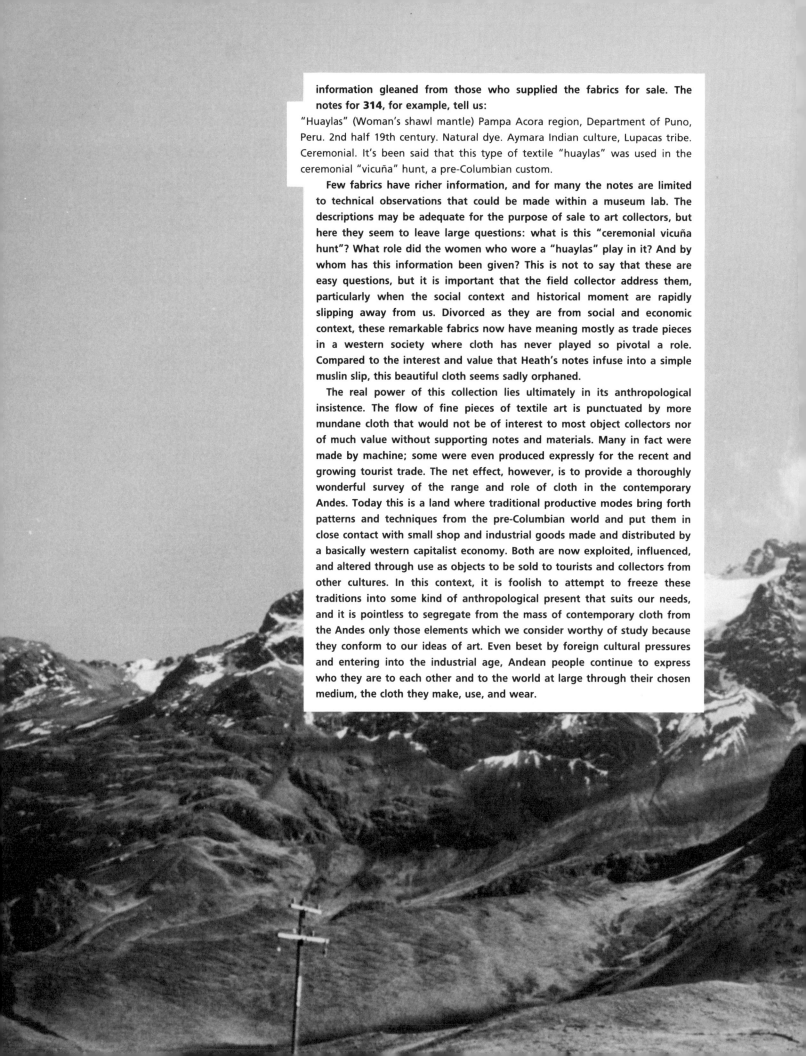

information gleaned from those who supplied the fabrics for sale. The notes for **314**, for example, tell us:

"Huaylas" (Woman's shawl mantle) Pampa Acora region, Department of Puno, Peru. 2nd half 19th century. Natural dye. Aymara Indian culture, Lupacas tribe. Ceremonial. It's been said that this type of textile "huaylas" was used in the ceremonial "vicuña" hunt, a pre-Columbian custom.

Few fabrics have richer information, and for many the notes are limited to technical observations that could be made within a museum lab. The descriptions may be adequate for the purpose of sale to art collectors, but here they seem to leave large questions: what is this "ceremonial vicuña hunt"? What role did the women who wore a "huaylas" play in it? And by whom has this information been given? This is not to say that these are easy questions, but it is important that the field collector address them, particularly when the social context and historical moment are rapidly slipping away from us. Divorced as they are from social and economic context, these remarkable fabrics now have meaning mostly as trade pieces in a western society where cloth has never played so pivotal a role. Compared to the interest and value that Heath's notes infuse into a simple muslin slip, this beautiful cloth seems sadly orphaned.

The real power of this collection lies ultimately in its anthropological insistence. The flow of fine pieces of textile art is punctuated by more mundane cloth that would not be of interest to most object collectors nor of much value without supporting notes and materials. Many in fact were made by machine; some were even produced expressly for the recent and growing tourist trade. The net effect, however, is to provide a thoroughly wonderful survey of the range and role of cloth in the contemporary Andes. Today this is a land where traditional productive modes bring forth patterns and techniques from the pre-Columbian world and put them in close contact with small shop and industrial goods made and distributed by a basically western capitalist economy. Both are now exploited, influenced, and altered through use as objects to be sold to tourists and collectors from other cultures. In this context, it is foolish to attempt to freeze these traditions into some kind of anthropological present that suits our needs, and it is pointless to segregate from the mass of contemporary cloth from the Andes only those elements which we consider worthy of study because they conform to our ideas of art. Even beset by foreign cultural pressures and entering into the industrial age, Andean people continue to express who they are to each other and to the world at large through their chosen medium, the cloth they make, use, and wear.

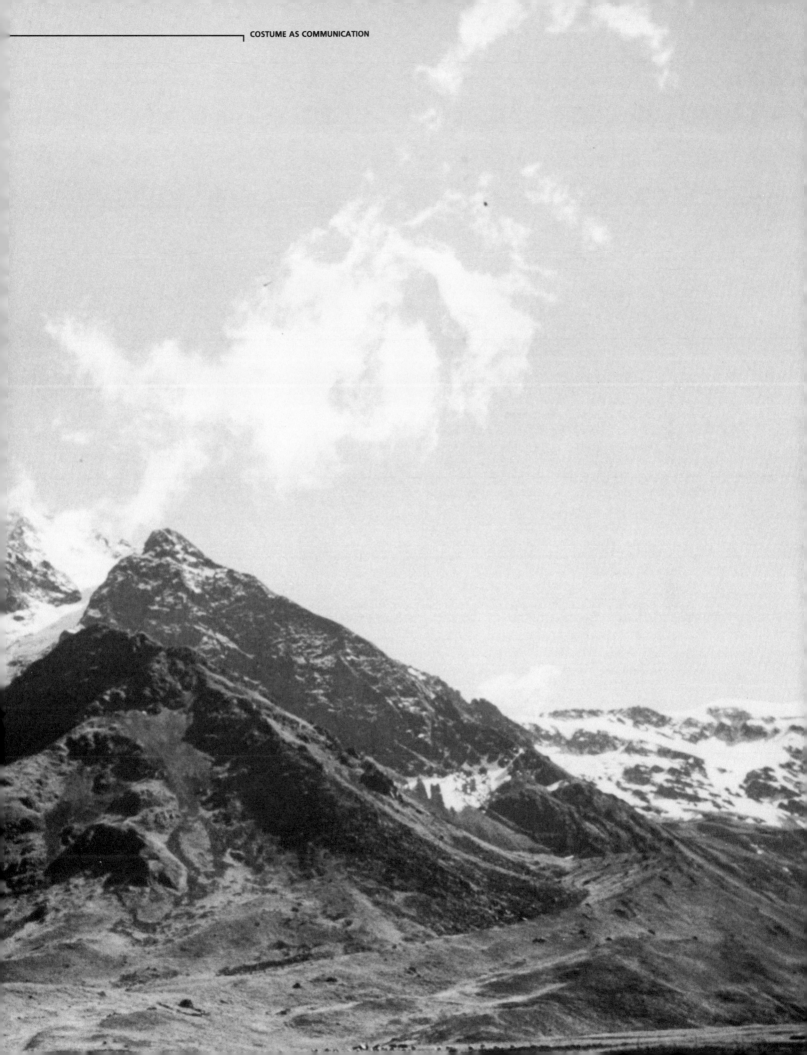

Catalogue data will follow this format:

Native name
> **Object**
> _____

Entry number
> Department: Region, town, or village
> Linguistic affiliation
> Source
Dimensions: inches and centimeters
• Yarn make-up
Fabrication
> **Iconography**
> **Comments**

Haffenreffer Museum number
References cited
See **Internal References** to textiles in the collection

Entry Number is the catalogue number and the textile is referred to by this number within the text.

The object is identified in English and then in the *native language*. In the Andes textiles are often known in three languages: Spanish, Quechua, and Aymara. Unless otherwise indicated with a (Q.) or (A.) the language used is Spanish.

Department refers to the state of origin.

Region, town, or village is where the textile was purchased or manufactured, if known. Exact identification is often difficult in the Andes so in some citations more than one is offered. Initials follow indicating the source for the identification.

Source indicates the name or the initials of the donor, the collection date if known, and the museum accession date, which often postdates the acquisition.

Dimensions are presented with the length first, then the width. Sleeve measurements are not included. For *hats*, the depth of the crown indicates the length, the diameter of the brim is the width. For *skirts*, width relates to the approximate waist measurement, although many skirts do not have waistbands. For *ponchos*, or *ponchitos*, the length is from shoulder to hem, one-half of the actual length, since this textile is always seen on the body.

Yarn make-up includes several indices: the type of yarn, ply, spin, color, and warp and weft count or sett. Camelid and sheepswool are the most common fibers in use, but in recent time *dralon*, a synthetic fiber, has become popular for weavings among urban Andeans. Ply and spin are indicated. Synthetic dyed yarn is most common and not indicated while natural dyed yarn is indicated. Camelid and sheepswool are generally used in natural colors unless otherwise indicated.

The warp and weft count or sett is given in inches and centimeters: epi and epc mean ends (warps) per inch and centimeter; ppi and ppc mean picks (wefts) per inch and centimeter; gauge for knitted textiles is spi and spc, which mean stitches per inch and centimeter.

Fabrication describes the weaving process and putting-together of the textile including cut-and-sew tailoring if present.

Iconography is included when appropriate.

Comments derive from field notes, personal communication, textile analysts, consultants, primary and secondary sources, and the initials of the contributor are placed within parentheses after the statement. E.M. Franquemont analyzed each Andean textile and provided comments. Annie Fisher is responsible for the first draft of the format and contributed to the comments as well. Otherwise the voice is the author's.

The flow of the catalogue section follows textile provenience from the northwestern state of the Central Andes of Peru to the southern states of Andean Bolivia (see map).

Initials indicate the following.

JA	Jeff Appleby	S&BG	Sidney and Barbara Greenwald	GH	Gale Hoskins
BB	Barry Bainton	B&EH	Barbara and Edward Hail	CL	Cynthia LeCount
E&JD	Edward and Jane Dwyer	DH	Dwight Heath	JP	Jone Pasha
AF	Annie Fisher			IS	Irene Saletan
EF	Edward M. Franquemont			MS	Margot Schevill

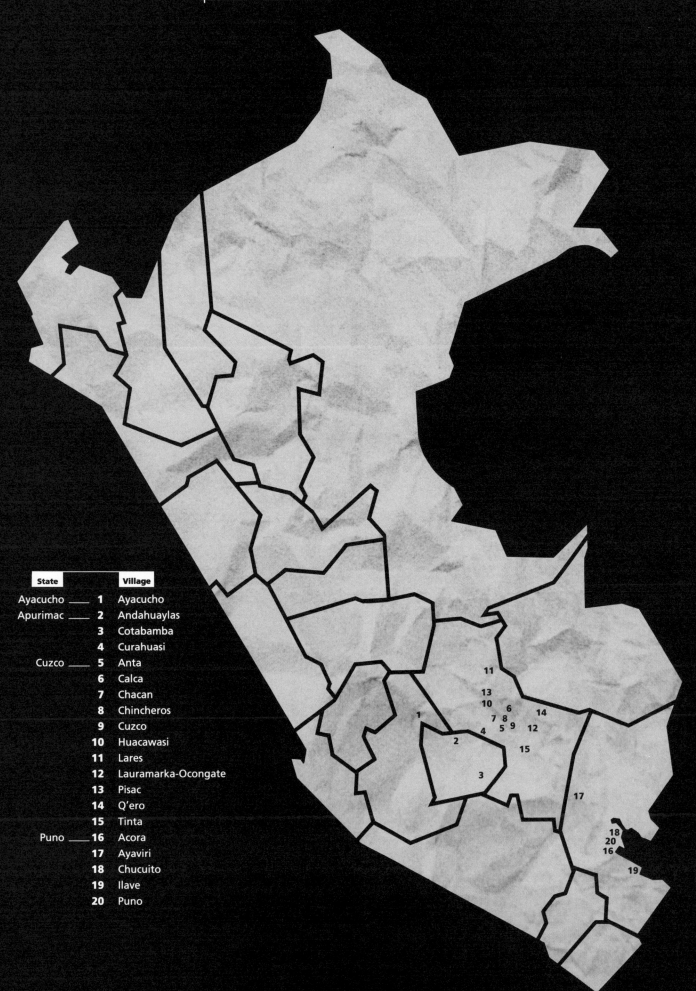

State		Village
Ayacucho ——	**1**	Ayacucho
Apurimac ——	**2**	Andahuaylas
	3	Cotabamba
	4	Curahuasi
Cuzco ——	**5**	Anta
	6	Calca
	7	Chacan
	8	Chincheros
	9	Cuzco
	10	Huacawasi
	11	Lares
	12	Lauramarka-Ocongate
	13	Pisac
	14	Q'ero
	15	Tinta
Puno ——	**16**	Acora
	17	Ayaviri
	18	Chucuito
	19	Ilave
	20	Puno

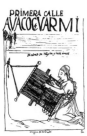

Quechuan backstrap weaver. Drawing by Guaman Poma de Ayala.

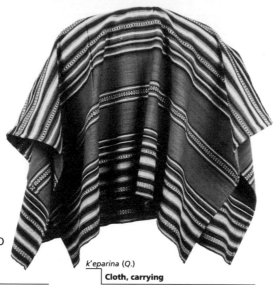

243

AYACUCHO

frazada

Blanket, or wall hanging

242

Ayacucho: Ayacucho
Quechua
S&BG 1970s 1973
66" x 57"   (167cm x 134cm)
• *warp*: sheepswool, 2-ply handspun; white; 8 epi (3 epc)
• *weft*: sheepswool, single handspun; purple, orange, and yellow; 6 ppi (2.5 ppc)
Warp-faced plain weave and interlocking tapestry woven on a floor loom. Edges finished by sewing 2 warps together.

Iconography: sun image.
A Peace Corps–inspired project for sale to tourists; by the mid-1970s natural dyes and pre-Columbian designs were being utilized by Ayacucho weavers to make rugs of all sizes; a thriving folk art industry (Plunkett, pers. com. 1986).

73–19

k'eparina (Q.)

Cloth, carrying

243

Ayacucho
Quechua/Spanish
BB 1960s 1967
39" x 43"   (98cm x 107cm)
• *warp*: cotton, acrylic; 2-ply machine-spun; multicolored, primarily pinks and reds; 34 epi (13.5 epc)
• *weft*: cotton, 2-ply machine-spun; red; 22 ppi (9 ppc)
Warp-faced plain weave, 2-color complementary warp weave. Woven as one piece on a four-harness treadle loom, cut in half and sewn together by hand. Warp stripes.

Common to urban Andean women. Woven in a shop situation by a professional weaver (EF). Carrying cloths are woven in San Pedro de Cajas, Junin, on treadle looms and sold all over Peru. In the 1980s dralon has replaced cotton (Plunkett, pers. com. 1986).

67–6570
See **244, 245, 272, 420**

k'eparina (Q.)

Cloth, carrying

244

Ayacucho
Quechua/Spanish
BB 1960s 1967
43" x 23"   (108cm x 58.5cm)
• *warp*: cotton, 2-ply machine-spun; multicolored, primarily deep red; 36 epi (14.5 epc)
• *weft*: cotton, 2-ply machine-spun; red; 22 ppi (8.8 ppc)
See **243** for fabrication and comments.

Probably just half of a finished carrying cloth (EF).

67–6574
See **243, 245, 272, 420**

k'eparina (Q.)

Cloth, carrying

245

Ayacucho
Quechua
BB 1960s 1967
43½" x 22½"   (110cm x 57cm)
• *warp*: cotton, acrylic; 2-ply machine-spun; multicolored, primarily deep red; 20 epi (8 epc)
• *weft*: cotton, acrylic; 2-ply machine-spun; red; 20 ppi (8 ppc)
See **243** for fabrication.

One section of a carrying cloth. A good example of Andean symmetry. The sides are balanced around a central axis, but each half is not a perfect mirror reproduction of the other. Each half contains several internal axes of symmetry (AF, EF).

67–6575
See **243, 244, 272, 420**

APURIMAC

blusa

Blouse

246

Apurimac: Andahuaylas
Quechua/Spanish
BB 1960s 1967
19½" x 17"   (49cm x 43cm)
Commercial rayon satin, machine-sewn into tailored blouse, reinforced with commercial cotton muslin. Hand-smocked, embroidered and decorated with sequins, ribbon, buttons and machine-made lace.

Worn typically by urban Andean women for special occasions. Made by professional seamstresses and for sale in market (EF).

67–6586
See **247, 248** Female Costume and **400**

montera

Hat

247

Apurimac: Andahuylas
Quechua
BB 1960s 1967
4" x 14"   (10cm x 36cm)
Blue wool felt hat, decorated with a scalloped edge and a green ribbon.

Felt comes from Arequipa (EF).

67–6585
See **246, 248** Female Costume

pollera

Skirt

248

Apurimac: Andahuaylas
Quechua/Spanish
BB 1960s 1967
30" x 33"   (76cm x 84cm)
Machine-woven yellow wool cloth, heavily brushed and felted; white cotton commercial cloth, sewn into gathered skirt. Decorated with 2 horizontal tucks, and elaborate floral embroidery done with multicolored cotton floss.

Probably worn by urban Andean women for special occasions (EF).

67–6587
See **246, 247** Female Costume and **414, 415**

chumpi (Q.)

Belt

249

Apurimac: Cotabamba
Quechua
E&JD 1970s 1978
62" x 2½"   (153cm x 6.5cm)
• *warp*: alpaca, sheepswool; 2-ply handspun; white and multicolored; 30 epc (12 epc)
• *weft*: alpaca, 2-ply handspun; white and multicolored; 10 ppi (4 ppi)
Warp-faced plain weave, warp stripes, 3-color complementary warp weave. One 4-selvedge cloth, finished one end with heading cord, the other with eight 5-loop braids. Bound with rolled warp-faced plain weave edging, possibly woven on a treadle loom.

Iconography: geometric forms.
Very similar to belts woven in Challwahuacho; this piece may in fact be from that town. Uses repeating motives (EF).

78–6 A
Rowe 1977a:83
Cason and Cahlander 1976:143–144
See **250, 251, 252**

chumpi (Q.)

Belt

250

Apurimac: Cotabamba
Quechua
E&JD 1970s 1978
71" x 5"   (178cm x 12cm)
• *warp*: alpaca, sheepswool; 2-ply handspun; white and multicolored; 50 epi (20 epc)
• *weft*: camelid, 2-ply handspun; tan; 15 ppi (6 ppc)
Warp-faced plain weave, warp stripes, 2- and 3-color complementary warp weave. One 4-selvedge cloth, finished one end with heading cord, the other with 15 braids, stitched together. The whole thing bound with treadle-woven *golon* strip, and strips added to each end as a tie.

See 249 for iconography and comments.

78–7
Rowe 1977a:24,83
Cason and Cahlander 1976:143–144
See **249, 251, 252**

chumpi (Q.)

| Belt |

251

Apurimac: Cotabamba
Quechua
E&JD   1970s   1978
63" x 6"   (158cm x 10cm)
• *warp*: sheepswool, 2-ply handspun; multicolored; 75 epi (30 epc)
• *weft*: camelid, 2-ply handspun; tan; 11 ppi (6 ppc)
Warp-faced plain weave, warp stripes and 2- and 3-color complementary warp weave. Finished one end with heading cord, other end with fifteen 5-loop braids.

   The 3-color complementary warp weave used in this belt produces a two-sided piece. There is no right or wrong side, but both sides show a design. There is some repetition of geometric design motifs (EF).

78–18
See **249** for references.
See **249, 250, 252**

chumpi (Q.)

| Belt |

252

Apurimac: Cotabamba
Quechua
E&JD   1970s   1978
64" x 3"   (162cm x 7.5cm)
• *warp*: alpaca, 2-ply handspun; white, multicolored; 100 epi (40 epc)
• *weft*: alpaca, 2-ply handspun; tan; 18 ppi (8 ppc)
Warp-faced plain weave, warp stripes and 2- and 3-color complementary warp weave. Edge rolled over on itself. Ends finished with eleven 5-loop braids, sewn together and applied *hakima* (Q.) ties.

   See 249 for iconography and comments.

78–306
Rowe 1977a:83
Cason and Cahlander 1976:104–105
See **249, 250, 251**

honda, waraka (Q.)

| Sling |

253

Apurimac: Curahuasi
Quechua
BB   1960s   1967
64" x 2" (at cradle) x ½" (cord).   (160cm x 5cm at cradle, 1cm at cord).
Camelid, 2-ply handspun; white and brown.

   Cradle: slit tapestry woven. Cord: 24 strand round braid with diamond or *ñawi* pattern. Wrapped and embroidered with white llama wool at one end with finger loop. Applied tassel at other end (EF).

67–6588
Cahlendar 1980:21, 32, 55, 45
See **344, 361**

llijlla (Q.)

| Shawl |

254

Cuzco: Anta
Quechua
E&JD   early 20th cent.   1978
34" x 37"   (85cm x 93cm)
• *warp*: alpaca, 2-ply handspun; natural dyed multicolored and black; 70 epi (28 epc)
• *weft*: alpaca, 2-ply handspun; black; 21 ppi (8.5 ppc)
Warp-faced plain weave, warp stripes, 2-color complementary warp weave and 2-color supplementary warp weave. Woven as two 4-selvedge panels and seamed down center by hand. Needle holes indicate that it was originally edged with a *ribete*, now lost.

   Iconography: geometric forms.
   The two panels are identical except for one pattern which switches position. This shawl shows wear from having been folded for a long period, perhaps in someone's hope chest (EF).

78–28
See **255**

llijlla (Q.)

| Shawl |

255

Cuzco: Anta
Quechua
E&JD   early 20th cent.   1978
33" x 34"   (83cm x 86cm)
• *warp*: alpaca, 2-ply handspun; black and natural dyed multicolored; 54 epi (21.5 epc)
• *weft*: alpaca, 2-ply handspun; brown; 18 ppi (7 ppc)
Warp-faced plain weave, warp stripes, 2-color supplementary warp weave and 3-color complementary warp weave. Woven as two identical 4-selvedge cloths, seamed together by hand with zigzag stitch in center. Applied complementary warp-woven *ribete*.

   Iconography: geometric forms.
   This piece has been darned several times, using synthetic yarn (EF).

78–16
See **254**

chuspa (Q.)

| Bag |

256

Cuzco: Calca (JA) or Lares (EF)
Quechua
JP   1970s   1974
5" x 3"   (12cm x 8cm)
sheepswool, alpaca, 2-ply handspun; green, red, black, white; 13 spi (5 spc)
Knit: stockinette stitch, *pica-pica* scalloped edge, color patterning. Applied fringes and braided cord. Knit from top to bottom.

   Odd shape. Used to carry small items such as coins (EF).

74–164
See **299, 327, 410**

biyetta

| Cloths, embroidered |

257

Cuzco: Chacan
Quechua
BB   1960s   1967
12½" x 19"   (32cm x 48.5cm)
• *warp*: sheepswool, single handspun; purple; 18 epi (7.2 epc)
• *weft*: sheepswool, single handspun; purple; 16 ppi (6.5 ppc)
Balanced warp-faced plain weave. Handwoven bayeta on a treadle loom, cut edges. Embroidered with brightly colored wool yarn.

   Iconography: human, animal, plant forms, rural scenes.
   Peace Corps project (BB).

67–6559
See **258–262**

biyetta

| Cloths, embroidered |

258–262

Cuzco: Chacan
Quechua
BB   1960s   1967
Same information as **257**.

   Color of the bayeta changes, often natural, sometimes dyed one color. Names of the artists are frequently embroidered onto the piece (AF). These cloths are being produced in Chijnaya, Puno; a folk art industry that has evolved employing most residents, who moved from Taraco on the shores of Lake Titicaca in 1967 when water level got dangerously high; now being embroidered with natural colored yarns (Plunkett, pers. com. 1986).

67–6560–6564

llijlla (Q.)

| Cloth, shoulder |

263

Cuzco: Chincheros
Quechua
JP   1970s   1986
36½" x 40½"   (91cm x 101cm)
• *warp*: sheepswool, 2-ply handspun; brown and multicolored, primarily red; 26 epi (11 epc)
• *weft*: alpaca, 2-ply handspun; brown; 10 ppi (4 ppc)
Warp-faced plain weave, warp stripes, and 2- and 3-color complementary warp weaves. Woven as two 4-selvedge pieces and seamed by hand. Crossed-warp *ribete* woven onto edge.

   Iconography: geometric forms.
   Edge is badly frayed.

85–793
Franquemont and Franquemont n.d.

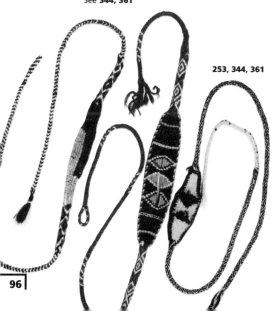

253, 344, 361

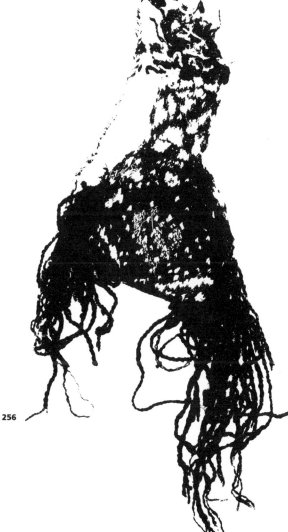

256

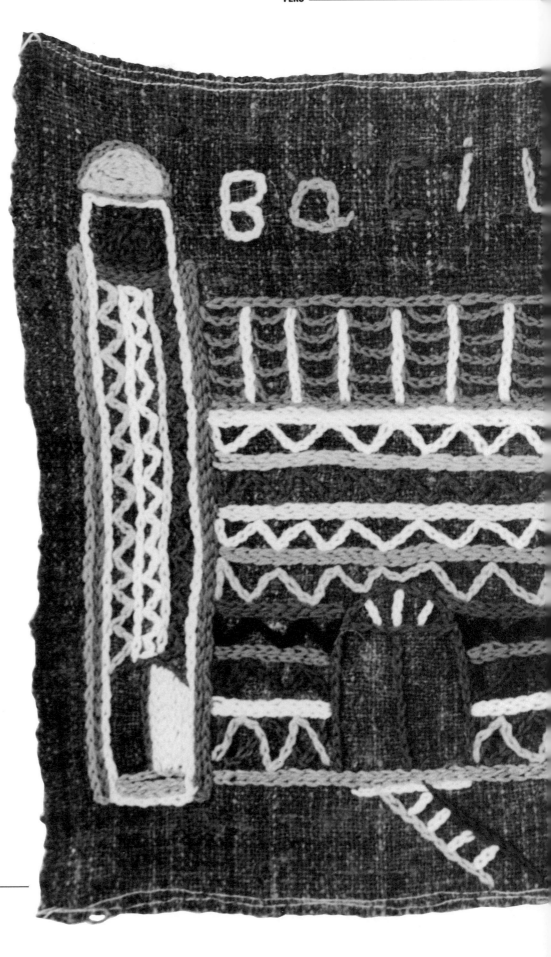

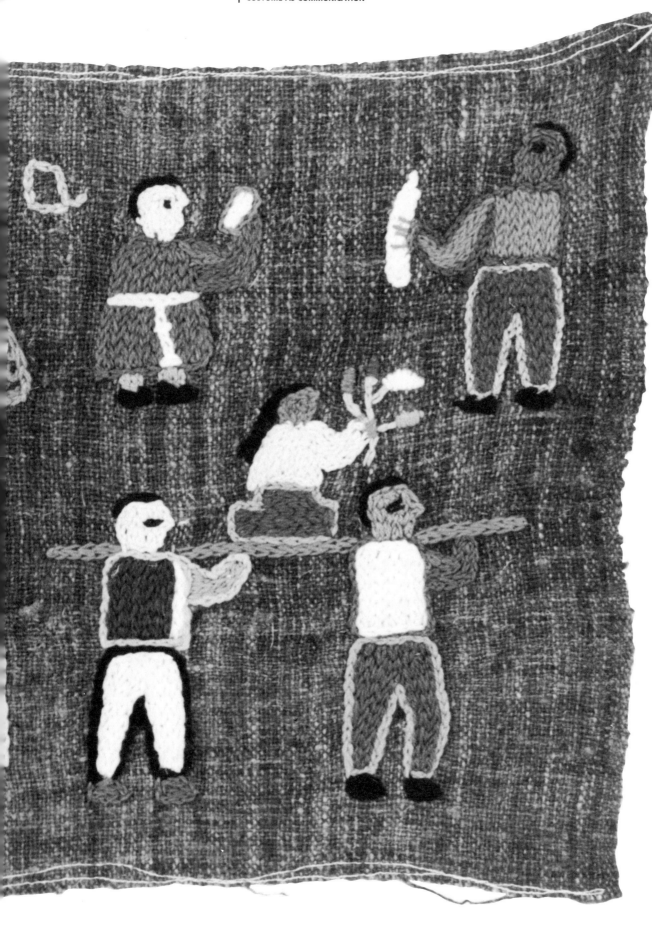

chumpi awana (Q.)
| Loom, belt

264
Cuzco: Chincheros
Quechua
E&JD 1970s 1978
39" x 2"   (98cm x 5cm)
• **warp**: sheepswool, 2-ply; dralon; machine-spun and overspun by hand; multicolored; 60 epi (32 epc)
• **weft**: sheepswool, 2-ply; dralon; machine-spun and overspun by hand; white; 11 ppi (7ppc)
Loom made of wooden lease and heddle sticks, string heddle loops and string heading cords rather than loom bars. Half-finished belt is warp-faced plain-woven with warp stripes and 2-color complementary warp weave.

> **Iconography:** lozenges and x's.
> A belt loom of this sort is usually used by teenage girls in Chincheros (EF).

78–1
Rowe 1977a:75
Franquemont and Franquemont n.d.

chuspa (Q.)
| Bag, coca

265
Cuzco: Cuzco
Quechua
JP 1970s 1974
8" x 8.8"   (20cm x 22cm)
• **warp**: alpaca, sheepswool, 2-ply handspun; brown, white, red, and blue; 52 epi (20.8 epc)
• **weft**: alpaca, 2-ply handspun; tan; 14 ppi (5.6 ppi)
Warp-faced plain weave, 3-color complementary warp weave. Woven as one 4-selvedge cloth, folded and hand-sewn into small bag. Applied wool complementary warp weave strap, and tubular crossed-warp weave edge binding; applied tufts of fringe.

> **Iconography:** round forms divided into six sections.
> Complementary warp bands are rather loose and sloppy, possibly made with sale to tourists in mind (EF).

74–166
Rowe 1977a:43

Quechuan woman and child. Chincheros, Cuzco, Peru, 1920–1930. Herbert J. Spinden Photo Archives, Haffenreffer Museum of Anthropology.

chullo (Q.)
| Cap

266
Cuzco: Cuzco
Quechua/Spanish
E&BH 1970s 1979
7" x 10"   (14.5cm x 22.5cm)
alpaca, 2-ply handspun; brown and white; 4 spi (1.5 spc)
Knit: stockinette and garter stitches, color patterning. Knit on straight needles in the round. Finished with crochet edge and tassel.

> **Iconography:** animal and half-triangular forms.
> Both the soft spun alpaca and the llama patterns indicate that this cap was probably knit for sale to tourists (AF).

79–47

chullo (Q.)
| Cap

267
Cuzco: Cuzco
Quechua/Spanish
E&BH 1970s 1979
9½" x 7½"   (23cm x 20cm)
sheepswool, 2-ply handspun; multicolored; 6 spi (2.5 spc)
Knit: stockinette stitch, color striping and patterning. Finished with a crochet edge and tassel.

> **Iconography:** letters and diamond shapes.
> The inscription "Cuzco" on the side of the hat shows that it was probably made for sale to tourists as a souvenir (AF).

79–48
See **268, 269**

chullo (Q.)
| Cap

268
Cuzco: Cuzco
Quechua/Spanish
E&JD 1970s 1981
9" x 6"   (23cm x 15cm)
sheepswool, 2-ply handspun; multicolored; 7 spi (3 spc)
See **267** for fabrication and comments.

> **Iconography:** *1975* knitted into cap flaps.

81–83
See **267, 269**

chullo (Q.)
| Cap

269
Cuzco: Cuzco
Quechua/Spanish
E&JD 1970s 1981
13" x 7½"   (33cm x 19cm)
sheepswool, 2-ply handspun; multicolored; 7 spi (3 spc)
See **267** for fabrication and comments.

> **Iconography:** *Cuzco* knitted into cap flaps.

81–84
See **267, 268**

chullo (Q.)
| Cap

270
Cuzco: Cuzco
Quechua
Museum Purchase 1970s 1981
15" x 10"   (39cm x 28cm)
alpaca, sheepswool; 2-ply handspun; brown, multicolored; 8 spi (3 spc)
Knit: stockinette and garter stitches, color stripes and patterning. Started at bottom with zigzag *pica-pica* edge. Finished with knit tassel. Knit on straight needles in the round.

> **Iconography:** human and geometric figures.
> A very nice example of Andean knitting combining brightly colored wool and natural alpaca (AF).

81–87
See **271**

chullo (Q.)
| Cap

271
Cuzco: Cuzco
Quechua
Museum Purchase 1970s 1981
15" x 10"   (39cm x 28cm)
sheepswool, 2-ply handspun; multicolored and white; 7.5 spi (3 spc)
For fabrication see **270**, probably made by same knitter (IS).

81–88
See **270**

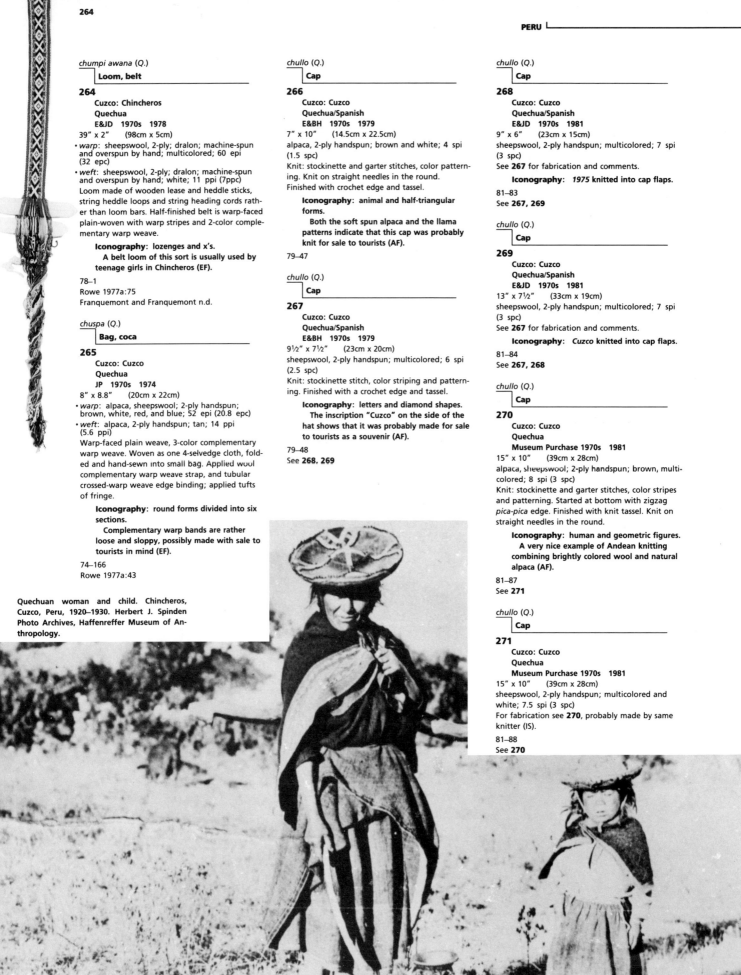

k'eparina (Q.)
| Cloth, carrying

272
Cuzco: Cuzco
Quechua
E&JD 1970s 1979
41½" x 43½"   (105cm x 110cm)

• *warp*: sheepswool and alpaca; 2-ply handspun; multicolored and tan; 24 epi (9.5 epc)
• *weft*: llama, 2-ply handspun; tan; 7 ppi (3 ppc)
Warp-faced plain weave, warp stripes and 2-color complementary warp weave. Woven as a single 4-selvedge panel, cut in half and seamed together by machine widthwise.

Iconography: *mayo k'enko* (Q.) or meandering river pattern.

The visibly knotted warp threads in this piece indicate that it was not woven by a master weaver. The color patterning of many multicolored warp stripes separated by very narrow white stripes is typical of the textiles woven by men in San Jeronimo prison in Cuzco. This "prison style" is becoming more and more common in the Cuzco area as prisoners learn to weave from each other in order to pay for their food, which is not provided by the prison (EF). Indigenous female weavers also provide prison weavers with prepared warps and pay them to execute the weaving (Callañaupa, pers. com. 1985).

79–196

montera
| Hat

273
Cuzco: Cuzco
Quechua
S&BG 1970s 1973
5" x 12"   (13cm x 30.5cm)
White felt with a wide cloth band, decorated with couched multicolored synthetic yarn. Brim bound with commercial cotton cloth, also decorated with synthetic yarn.

Worn by women for special occasions (EF). Hats are produced by specialists, usually a family operation; felt purchased, forms made, decoration added; women wholesale hats in Puno market (Plunkett, pers. com. 1986).

73–12

273

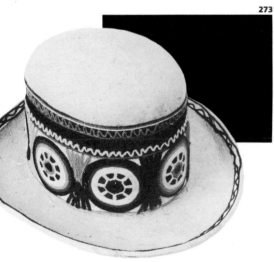

montera
| Hat

274
Cuzco: Cuzco
Quechua/Spanish
S&BG 1970s 1973
3½" x 11½"   (8cm x 29cm)
Red and black bayeta over a straw form. Decorated with multicolored *golon* strips and straps.

Worn by traditional Quechuan and urban Andean women. Acts as a symbol of ethnicity for those who are no longer living completely within their traditional societies. Frequently the women who sell goods to tourists in Cuzco wear hats of this sort, partially as advertising. Hats like 274, 275, 276, 277 are made by a man and his family in Chincheros (EF).

73–15
See **278, 288**   Female Costume

montera
| Hat

275
Cuzco: Cuzco
Quechua/Spanish
S&BG 1970s 1973
3" x 13"   (8cm x 34cm)
See **274**; variation in color of bayeta utilized.

73–16

montera
| Hat

276
Cuzco: Cuzco
Quechua/Spanish
E&BH 1960s 1969
3" x 13½"   (7.5cm x 34cm)
See **274**.

69–10585
See **279, 285, 289**   Female Costume

montera
| Hat

277
Cuzco: Cuzco
Quechua
E&JD 1960s–1970s 1972
3½" x 11"   (9cm x 28cm)
See **274**.

Part of a costume for a 10-year-old girl. Made by seamstresses, probably for sale to tourists (EF). Complete costume worn for *fiestas* (Plunkett, pers. com. 1986).

72–2367 A
See **280, 286, 287**   Girl's Costume

saco
| Jacket

278
Cuzco: Cuzco
Quechua/Spanish
S&BG 1970s 1973
17" x 14"   (43cm x 35cm)
Treadle-woven yellow bayeta machine-sewn into short jacket. Trimmed with rickrack and *golon* strips.

73–17
See **274, 288**   Female Costume

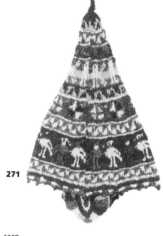

271

saco
| Jacket

279
Cuzco: Cuzco
Quechua/Spanish
E&BH 1960s 1969
17" x 17"   (43cm x 43cm)
See **278**

This costume was made by specialists in a shop situation either for use by urban Andean women in the Cuzco area or for sale to tourists. Reflects a Peruvian national image of what Quechuan people are, more than their own sense of ethnicity (EF).

69–10581
See **276, 285, 289**   Female Costume

saco
| Jacket

280
Cuzco: Cuzco
Quechua/Spanish
E&JD 1960s 1972
12" x 12"   (31cm x 31cm)
See **278**.

72–2367 C
See **277, 286, 287**   Girl's Costume

awana (Q.)
| Loom

281
Cuzco: Cuzco
Quechua
BB 1960s 1967
35½" x 21"   (90cm x 53cm)

• *warp*: sheepswool, alpaca; 2-ply handspun; multicolored; 32–52 epi (13–21 epc)
• *weft*: sheepswool, llama; 2-ply handspun; dark and bright red; 14 ppi (6 ppc)
• *loom*: wood sticks, respun commercial cotton thread heddles, braided llama tie straps.
Warp-faced plain weave, warp stripes, and 3-color complementary warp weave.

The textile on this loom is a partially woven *llijlla* (Q.) half. The loom is a horizontal loom and is set up by driving four pegs into the ground and stretching the loom between them. The shed rod is missing (EF). Bought from weaver on the road to the Inca Baths outside of Cuzco (Bainton, pers. com. 1986).

67–6593
Adelson and Tracht 1983:40

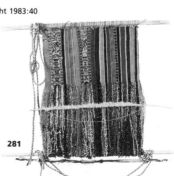

Quechuan women at Sacsahuaman, Cuzco, Peru. 1920–1930. Herbert J. Spinden Photo Archives, Haffenreffer Museum of Anthropology.

Detail 272

281

Poncho

282

Cuzco: Cuzco
Quechua
BB purchase   1960s   1967
26½" x 57"   (67cm x 145cm)
• *warp*: sheepswool, 2-ply handspun; black, pinks, and purples; 38 epi (15 epc)
• *weft*: sheepswool, 2-ply handspun; black; 9 ppi (3.5 ppc)
Warp-faced plain weave, warp stripes. Woven as 2 identical 4-selvedge pieces. Seamed together by hand. Bound with plain-woven red and white band with multicolored weft fringe.

> The collector of this piece reported this as a "dress" poncho from outside the city of Cuzco (BB), however E.M. Franquemont thinks this was woven for sale to tourists.

67–6583
See **342**

Poncho

283

Cuzco: Cuzco
Quechua
BB   mid 20th cent.   1967
32¼" x 56"   (82cm x 142cm)
• *warp*: sheepswool, 2-ply handspun; white, black, and multicolored; 26 epi (10.5 epc)
• *weft*: sheepswool, 2-ply handspun; white, black; 13 ppi (5 ppc)
Warp-faced plain weave, warp stripes, two 4-selvedge pieces hand-seamed and bound with plain-woven tubular strip around edges and at neck.

> Poncho used for everyday and work by Andean men (BB).

67–6592

---

k'eparina (Q.)
Shawl

284

Cuzco: Cuzco
Quechua/Spanish
S&BG   1970s   1973
45½" x 43"   (115 x 109cm)
• *warp*: acrylic, 2-ply machine-spun; white; 23 epi (9 epc)
• *weft*: acrylic, 2-ply machine-spun; multicolored primarily bright pink; 50 ppi (20 ppc)
Weft-faced plain weave, weft stripes and complementary weft weave. Woven on a treadle loom. Hemmed by machine.

> This piece, a treadle-loomed version of a traditional *llijlla* (Q.) is unusual in that it is weft-rather than warp-faced. Made for use by urban Andeans or for sale to tourists, probably in a shop situation (EF, AF).

73–11
See **243, 244, 245**

llijlla (Q.)
Shawl

285

Cuzco: Cuzco
Quechua/Spanish
E&BH   1960s   1969
30½" x 16½"   (77cm x 42cm)
Red bayeta, machine hemmed and trimmed with *golon* strips.

69–10583
See **279, 276, 289**   Female Costume

llijlla (Q.)
Shawl

286

Cuzco: Cuzco
Quechua/Spanish
E&JD   1960s–70s
25" x 11"   (63cm x 27cm)
See **285**. Yellow bayeta.

72–2367 D
See **277, 280, 287**   Girl's Costume

---

pollera
Skirt

287

Cuzco: Cuzco
Quechua/Spanish
E&JD   1960s   1972
15" x 17"   (38cm x 43cm)
Black wool bayeta, machine-sewn into gathered skirt. Waistband plaid, treadle-woven cloth. Decorated with rickrack, ribbon, and *golon* strips.

72–2367 B
See **277, 280, 286**   Girl's Costume

pollera
Skirt

288

Cuzco: Cuzco
Quechua
S&BG   1970s   1973
21" x 72"   (53cm x 184cm)
Black bayeta sewn into a full skirt. Trimmed with *golon* strips.

73–18
See **274, 278**   Female Costume

pollera
Skirt

289

Cuzco: Cuzco
Quechua/Spanish
E&BH   1960s   1969
21½" x 73"   (54cm x 182cm)
See **288**. Yellow bayeta.

69–10584
See **276, 279, 285**   Female Costume

chaleco
Vest

290

Cuzco: Cuzco
Quechua/Spanish
S&BG
18" x 18"   (46cm x 46cm)
Dark blue bayeta, red collar, trimmed with *golons*, rickrack, tailored, machine-stitched.

> Made for sale to tourists; also worn by Quechuan men in some communities for fiestas.

73–9

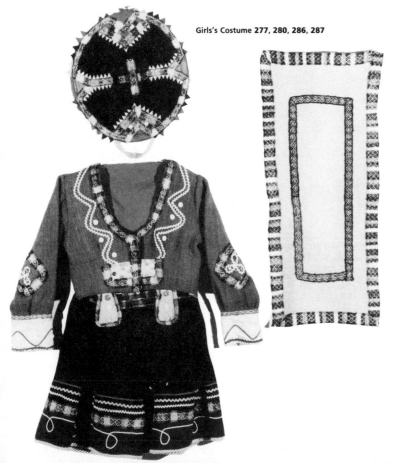

Girls's Costume 277, 280, 286, 287

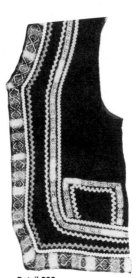

Detail 290

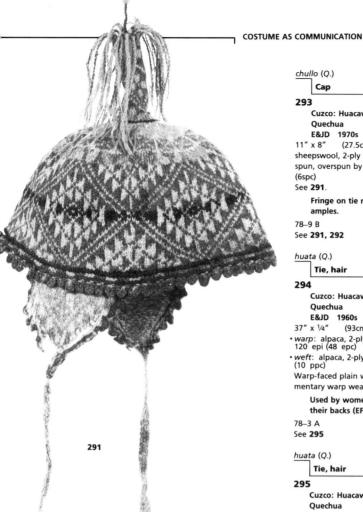

291

chullo (Q.)

> **Cap**

291

    Cuzco: Huacawasi
    Quechua
    JP 1960s 1974
6" x 9"   (15cm x 23cm)
sheepswool and alpaca; 2-ply handspun; red and black; 12 spi (5 spc)
Knit: stockinette stitch, color patterning, knit on double-pointed straight needles from bottom up, starting with scalloped *pica-pica* edge. Ear flaps knit separately and applied to finished cap. Applied tassels and braided ties (IS). The design on the main section is very similiar to the designs on *llijllas* (Q.) from Huacawasi (EF). Andean knitting is invariably done with 5 double-pointed needles, generally by men in Bolivia, women in Peru (CL).

74–163
Rowe 1977a:41
See **292, 293**

chullo (Q.)

> **Cap**

292

    Cuzco: Huacawasi
    Quechua
    E&JD 1970s 1978
10½" x 8"   (26.5cm x 22cm)
sheepswool, alpaca; 2-ply handspun; primarily red; 10 spi (4spc)
See **291**.

    Applied tassel and complementary warp-woven *hakima* (Q.) ties.

78–9 A
See **291, 293**

chullo (Q.)

> **Cap**

293

    Cuzco: Huacawasi
    Quechua
    E&JD 1970s 1978
11" x 8"   (27.5cm x 20.5cm)
sheepswool, 2-ply handspun; dralon, machine-spun, overspun by hand; primarily red; 15 spi (6spc)
See **291**

    Fringe on tie more elaborate than other examples.

78–9 B
See **291, 292**

huata (Q.)

> **Tie, hair**

294

    Cuzco: Huacawasi
    Quechua
    E&JD 1960s 1978
37" x ¼"   (93cm x .5cm)
• *warp*: alpaca, 2-ply handspun; reds and white; 120 epi (48 epc)
• *weft*: alpaca, 2-ply handspun; white; 25 ppi (10 ppc)
Warp-faced plain weave, warp stripes and complementary warp weave. Applied twisted fringe.

    Used by women to tie their braids behind their backs (EF).

78–3 A
See **295**

huata (Q.)

> **Tie, hair**

295

    Cuzco: Huacawasi
    Quechua
    E&JD 1970s 1978
51" x ¼"   (132cm x .5cm)
• *warp*: alpaca, 2-ply handspun; multicolored; 120 epi (48 epc)
• *weft*: alpaca, 2-ply handspun; white; 25 ppi (10 ppc)
Warp-faced plain weave, warp stripes and 2-color complementary warp weave. Intersecting warps at each end, also woven in 2-color complementary warp weave.

    A beautifully woven *huata* (Q.), with transverse warps (EF).

78–4
See **294**

llijlla (Q.)

> **Shawl**

296

    Cuzco: Lares
    Quechua
    E&JD 1960s 1978
39½" x 45½"   (99cm x 114cm)
• *warp*: sheepswool, 2-ply handspun; multicolored; 34 epi (13.5 epc)
• *weft*: alpaca, single handspun; brown; 13 ppi (5 ppc)
Warp-faced plain weave, warp stripes, 2-color supplementary warp weave. Woven as two identical 4-selvedge pieces, seamed together by hand.

    Iconography: large diamond patterns.
    Extremely good terminal finish; working stripes in middle of each pattern section; the two halves are slightly different sizes; the patterns on each half are slightly offset because of this (EF).

78–14
See **297**

llijlla (Q.)

> **Shawl**

297

    Cuzco: Lares
    Quechua
    E&JD 1960s 1978
34½" x 44"   (86cm x 110cm)
• *warp*: sheepswool, 2-ply handspun; multicolored, primarily reds; 32 epi (13 epc)
• *weft*: camelid, 2-ply handspun; dark brown; 15 ppi (6 ppc)
Warp-faced plain weave, warp stripes, and supplementary warp weave. Woven as two identical 4-selvedge panels and seamed with decorative zig-zag stitch. Uses counter-spun yarns in the plain woven sections.

    Iconography: large diamond patterns.
    The pattern sections are divided by plain woven stripes and contrasting color stripes within the supplementary woven areas. Creates the effect of a series of pattern stripes rather than a large overall pattern as in other Cuzco pieces. Very good technical control, although the *llijlla* (Q.) has been repaired several times (EF).

78–12
See **296**

chuspa (Q.)

> **Bag, coca**

298

    Cuzco: Lauramarka (JA)
    Quechua
    JP 1970s 1974
7" x 5½"   (18cm x 14cm)
• *warp*: sheepswool, 2-ply handspun; multicolored; 32 epi (13 epc)
• *weft*: llama, 2-ply handspun; brown; (11 ppi, 4.5 ppc)
Warp-faced plain weave, warp stripes, 2-color complementary warp weave, applied strap, also 2-color complementary warp weave, and tubular edge binding. Applied fringe.

    Iconography: geometric forms.
    Design is woven in registered blocks (EF).

74–165

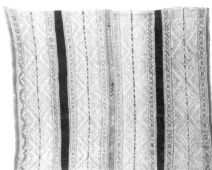

297

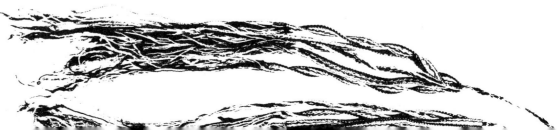

295

achuqalla (Q.)

Pouch

299

Cuzco: Lauramarka - Ocongate area
Quechua
JP 1970s 1974
11" x 2½"   (27.5cm x 6.5cm)
• *warp*: alpaca, single handspun; multicolored and white; 112 epi (44.8 epc)
• *weft*: alpaca, single handspun; white; 28 ppi (11.2 ppc)
Warp-faced plain weave, and 2-color complementary warp weave. Applied fringe. Woven as one 4-selvedge cloth and seamed at sides. Embroidered at random places with red wool, possibly to cover mistakes in the pick-up pattern.

Iconography: zigzag forms.
Pouches of this shape, although often referred to as flute pouches, are used to carry any small objects such as coins. The item is put in the bottom, and the top of the bag rolled over several times and tied with a cord (Rowe, pers. com. 1985). The name "achuqalla" is also used for a ferret that lives in the walls and roofs of houses throughout the Cuzco area. It probably refers to the long thin shape, but the fuzzy edges are also reminiscent of the animal. The animal is associated with luck (both good and bad) and there is a belief that money will multiply within the bag. It is not a costume piece. A visual onomatopoeia (EF).

74–167
See **256, 327, 410**

Poncho

300

Cuzco: Pisac
Quechua
E&JD 1960s 1978
18" x 35"   (46cm x 87cm)
• *warp*: sheepswool, 2-ply handspun; primarily red and white; 50 epi (20 epc)
• *weft*: alpaca, single handspun; dark brown; 12½ ppi (5 ppc)
Warp-faced plain weave, warp stripes and 2-color supplementary warp weave. Woven as two 4-selvedge panels and hand-seamed with zigzag stitch. Bound with applied complementary warp weave *ribete*, with secondary weft fringe. Corners turned under.

Iconography: large overall diamond patterns.
Designs are typical of the Department of Cuzco. One narrow color stripe goes down the center of the pattern area. Geometric motifs on fringe band called *loraypo* (Q.). This poncho is generally extremely well woven, especially in the terminal zone (EF).

78–230
Rowe 1977a:40–42
See **301, 302**

Poncho

301

Cuzco: Pisac
Quechua
E&JD 1960s 1978
14½" x 36½"   (37cm x 91cm)
• *warp*: sheepswool, 2-ply handspun; multicolored, primarily red and white; 70 epi (28 epc)
• *weft*: alpaca, single handspun; brown; 19 ppi (7.5 ppc)
See **300**. Working stripes in center of diamond patterns.

78–13
See **300, 302**

Poncho

302

Cuzco: Pisac
Quechua
E&JD 1960s 1978
15" x 37½"   (38cm x 93cm)
• *warp*: sheepswool, 2-ply handspun; multicolored, primarily reds and white; 66 epi (26.5 epc)
• *weft*: alpaca, single handspun; sheepswool, 2-ply handspun; brown and white; 17 ppi (7 ppc)
See **300**. Complementary warp-woven *ribete* with supplementary weft fringe applied to edge. The edge is applied in such a way to make the corners slightly rounded without turning under the fabric edge (EF).

78–11
See **300, 301**

llijlla (Q.)

Shawl

303

Cuzco: Q'ero
Quechua
E&JD 1960s 1978
30" x 24½"   (76cm x 62cm)
• *warp*: sheepswool, alpaca; 2-ply handspun; multicolored, primarily red and overdyed black; 60 epi (24 epc)
• *weft*: camelid, 2-ply handspun; dark brown; 20 ppi (8 ppc)
Warp-faced plain weave, warp stripes, 3-color complementary warp weave. Uses counter-spinning in plain woven sections. Woven as two identical 4-selvedge panels and seamed with decorative zigzag embroidery.

Iconography: diamonds and lozenges.

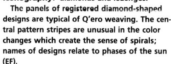

The panels of registered diamond-shaped designs are typical of Q'ero weaving. The central pattern stripes are unusual in the color changes which create the sense of spirals; names of designs relate to phases of the sun (EF).

78–8
Rowe 1977a:86, pl. VI
Cohen 1957
Silverman-Proust 1986

chuspa (Q.)

Bag, coca

304

Cuzco: Tinta
Quechua
BB 1960s 1967
10½" x 5½"   (26cm x 14cm)
• *warp*: sheepswool, 2-ply handspun; multicolored, primarily red and black; 45 epi (18 epc)
• *weft*: camelid, 2-ply handspun; tan; 13 ppi (5 ppc)
Warp-faced plain weave, warp stripes and 3-color complementary warp weave. Woven as one 4-selvedge piece, folded and hand-seamed to make a bag. Complementary warp weave *hakima* (Q.) strap added to finished bag.

Iconography: geometric forms in blocks.
This bag shows another kind of pattern symmetry. There are two patterns used, *ch'-aska* (Q.), star and *chhili* (Q.), scalloped effect in center. On the reverse side of the bag, the patterns switch position so that the central design on this side becomes the border pattern on the other and vice-versa; a "Yin-Yang" cloth representing the dual universe in balance (EF).

67–6589
E.M. Franquemont 1986

chuspa (Q.)

Bag, coca

305

Cuzco: Exact location unknown
Quechua
BB 1960s 1967
5" x 4"   (12cm x 9cm)
• *warp*: sheepswool, single handspun; multicolored; cotton, multiple machine-spun; white; 12–22 epi (5–9 epc)
• *weft*: sheepswool, 2-ply handspun; white; 16 ppi (6.5 ppc)
Two warp-faced strips joined to 2 balanced weave strips; warp-faced bands of supplementary warp weave. The warp-faced plain weave sections have warp and weft stripes creating a plaid. Stitched closed at bottom loosely. Applied fringe and *golon* strip. Strap is a 3-strand braid.

This bag is an interesting collage of fabrics. It was probably assembled in Cuzco by an urban Andean from bits of old garments for sale to tourists (EF). One fragment is in the style of Tinta ponchos (JA). Plaid, treadle-woven cloth utilized in ponchos made for export in 1970s.

67–6590

frazada

Blanket

306

Cuzco: Exact location unknown
Quechua
BB 1960s 1967
56" x 31"   (142cm x 131cm)
• *warp*: alpaca, sheepswool, 2-ply handspun; black, white, pinks, and reds; 28 epi (11 epc)
• *weft*: alpaca, 2-ply handspun; grey and white plied together; 7 ppi (3 ppc)
Warp-faced plain weave, warp stripes, two 4-selvedge panels, hand-seamed together.

Used for household use all across the Andes. Quechuan name for yarn plied of two different colored threads: *muro q'aytu* (EF). The collector reported that this piece is an unfinished bag (Bainton, pers. com. 1986).

67–6581

costal

Sack, grain or potato

307

Cuzco: Exact location unknown
Quechua
BB mid 20th cent. 1967
59" x 21"   (147cm x 54cm)
• *warp*: llama, 2-ply handspun; brown and black; 14 epi (6 epc)
• *weft*: llama, 2-ply handspun; brown; 10 ppi (4 ppc)
Warp-faced plain weave, warp stripes, two 4-selvedge cloths, sewn together at the center, and then along side selvedges to make a sack.

This home produced sack is unusually long and narrow; probably meant to be carried by llamas (EF).

67–6584
Cason and Cahlander 1976:20
See **308, 352, 398, 399**

costal

Sack, grain

308

Cuzco: Exact location unknown
Quechua
BB 1960s 1967
37" x 20"   (93cm x 50cm)
• *warp*: llama, sheepswool, 2-ply handspun; black, brown, white; 26 epi (10.5 epc)
• *weft*: llama, 2-ply handspun; tan and white; 11 ppi (4.5 ppc)
Warp-faced plain weave, warp stripes; one 4-selvedge piece folded and hand-seamed to make sack.

Bag used to carry grain or potatoes (EF).

67–6591
Cason and Cahlander 1976:20
See **307, 352, 398, 399**

LIMA

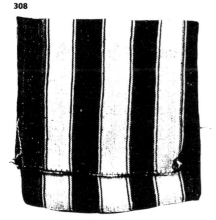

309

muñecas

| Dolls

309–310

Lima: Lima, place of purchase
Spanish
S&BG   1970s   1973
10" x 4"   (25cm x 10cm)
Carved and painted wooden dolls: male and female. The female has a baby doll on her back. Costumes made of scraps of bayeta, wool yarn, and
golon strips.

> Clothing is in romantized Quechuan style
> from Cuzco (EF). Most dolls made in Cuzco
> (Plunkett, pers. com. 1986). Male doll holding
> a *varna*, the mayor's silver-headed staff.

73–3 and 4
See **311**

muñecas

| Dolls

311

Lima
Spanish
E&JD   1970s   1980
A: 9½" x 3"   (24cm x 8cm)
B: 9" x 3"   (23cm x 8cm)

> Tourist dolls, which show a national image of
> Quechuan people rather than their own eth-
> nicity (AF). Female dolls are spinning.

80–103 A and B
See **309–310**

PUNO

chullo (Q.)

| Cap

312

Puno: Acora
Quechua
Museum Purchase   1970s   1981
21" x 8 ¼"   (53cm x 21cm)
alpaca, sheepswool; 2-ply handspun; white and
multicolored; 4 spi (1.5 spc)
Knit: stockinette and rib stitches, crochet or hand-
knot loops, stitched or knitted onto cap: color sequence creates triangular shapes, cross on upper
half (IS).

> Known as a "virgin cap"; worn until marriage
> when bowler derby replaces it (Plunkett,
> pers. com. 1986).

81–89
See **313**

chullo (Q.)

| Cap

313

Puno: Acora
Quechua
Museum Purchase   1970s   1981
19" x 8"   (49cm x 20.5cm)
sheepswool, alpaca; 2-ply handspun; brown,
white, and black; 6 spi (2.5 spc)

85–40
See **312**

308

---

unkhuña (Q.)

| Cloth, coca

314

Puno: Acora
Aymara
GH   late 19th cent.   1985
31" x 32½"   (79cm x 82cm)
• *warp*: alpaca, 2-ply handspun; natural dyed multicolored; 64 epi (25.5 epc)
• *weft*: alpaca, 2-ply handspun; brown; 17 ppi
(7 ppc)
Warp-faced plain weave, warp stripes and 2-color
complementary warp bands. Woven as one
4-selvedge cloth and bound with tubular crossed-
warp band.

> This type of *unkhuña* (Q.) is called a "toj'jo
> ccuto." This name refers to the chain stitch
> striping, made with warp stripe effects, and
> means pattern that returns on itself. Inside
> patterns mostly *mayo k'enko* (Q.),
> meandering river. The tubular binding is not
> complete but is finished in a braid (EF). The
> Aymara shamans, *Yatiris*, place offerings of
> food, coca leaves, cups of alcohol on *incuñas*
> to *pachamama*, Earth Mother (GH).

85–9
Adelson and Tracht 1983:116–123, fig. 44
See **317, 328, 341**

---

huallas (A.)

| Shawl

315

Puno: Acora
Aymara
GH   2nd half 19th cent.   1985
41½" x 41½"   (105cm x 105cm)
• *warp*: alpaca, 2-ply handspun; brown and natural
dyed blue and pink; 36 epi (14.5 epc)
• *weft*: alpaca, 2-ply handspun; brown; 17 ppi
(7 ppc)
Warp-faced plain weave, warp stripes. Woven as
two identical 4-selvedge panels and seamed together at center. Bound with applied crossed-
warp tubular band.

> All natural dyes. It has been said that this
> type of textile was used in the ceremonial
> "vlcuña hunt," a pre-Columbian tradition.
> Worn by women in the Lupacas tribe of Ay-
> mara speakers (GH).

85–8
Adelson and Tracht 1983:82

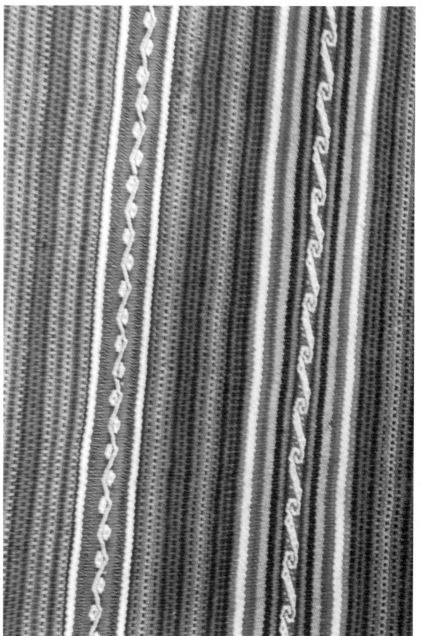

Detail 314

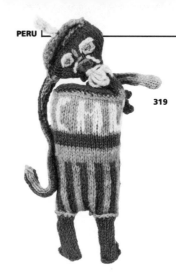

319

chumpi (Q.)

| **Belt**

316

Puno: Ayata (JA), purchased at Ilave market (BB)
Aymara
BB 1960s 1967
48" x 4"   (119cm x 9cm)
• *warp*: sheepswool, 2-ply handspun; multicolored; 46 epi (18.5 epc)
• *weft*: llama, 2-ply handspun; brown; 7 ppi (3 ppc)
Warp-faced plain weave 2-color complementary warp weave, twill effect with double weft in places. Finished one end with heading cord, the other with eight 3-strand braids.

Woven woolen belts used by men and women (BB).

67–6573
See **329**

unkhuña (Q.)

| **Cloth, coca**

317

Puno: Ayaviri (JA)
Quechua
Malagua early 20th cent. 1977
14½" x 16½"   (36.5cm x 42cm)
• *warp*: alpaca, 2-ply handspun; synthetic, multi-ply machine-spun; tans and pink, blue, green; 58 epi (23 epc)
• *weft*: alpaca, 2-ply handspun; tan; 18 ppi (7 ppc)
One 4-selvedge cloth. Warp-faced plain weave with supplementary warp weave strips. Decorated with applied machine-braided tassels and wrapped cords. Edges finished with pink and red embroidery.

This piece is unusual in its combination of finely woven handspun alpaca and machine made elements (AF).

77–23
Adelson and Tracht 1983:116–123
See **314, 328, 341**

chumpi (Q.)

| **Belt**

318

Puno: Ayaviri (JA)
Quechua
E&JD 1970s 1978
59" x 5"   (147cm x 12cm)
• *warp*: sheepswool, 2-ply handspun; white and multicolored, primarily red; 28 epi (12 epc)
• *weft*: camelid, 2-ply handspun; white; 11 ppi (5 ppc)
Warp-faced plain weave, warp stripes and 2-color complementary warp weave. Finished one end with warp loops, the other with fourteen 3-strand braids.

Iconography: horses and large diamond shapes.

78–10

muñeca

| **Doll**

319

Puno: Chucuito
Quechua/Aymara
BB 1960s 1967
8" x 3"   (20cm x 7cm)
sheepswool, 2-ply handspun; multicolored; 8 spi (3 spc)
Knit: stockinette stitch, color patterning, pieces knit separately and joined with crochet stitch. Face details crochet stitched. Built over wire form and stuffed.

Made as a Peace Corps crafts project (BB). Knitted images have become a folk art industry for export. (Plunkett, pers. com. 1986).

67–6513
See **320, 321**

burro

| **Toy, burro**

320

Puno: Chucuito
Quechua/Aymara
BB 1960s 1967
3" x 5"   (7cm x 11.5cm)
alpaca, 2-ply handspun; brown and tan; 5 spi (2 spc)
Knit: stockinette stitch. Body is one piece with legs and ears knit separately and added on. Eyes and nose embroidered with colored wool yarn. Tail braided.

67–6515
See **319, 321**

| **Toy, fish**

321

Puno: Chucuito
Quechua/Aymara
BB 1960s 1967
7" x 2"   (17cm x 6cm)
sheepswool, 2-ply handspun; multicolored; 7 spi (2.5 spc)
Knit: stockinette and garter stitch, color patterning, body knitted on straight needles in the round, fins knitted onto body. Stuffed with soft filling. Braided strap.

67–6518
See **319, 320**

frazada

| **Blanket**

322

Puno: bought at Ilave market
Aymara
BB 1960s 1967
69" x 57"   (172cm x 142cm)
• *warp*: sheepswool, 2-ply handspun; multicolored, primarily pink; 20 epi (8 epc)
• *weft*: sheepswool, 2-ply handspun; tans and browns, 7.5 ppi (3 ppc)
Warp-faced plain weave, warp stripes, two 4-selvedge pieces, hand-seamed together.

Used for everyday, blankets like this are found in any Quechuan or Aymara house. But the formal organization is the same as that of fancier cloth with both an overall axis of symmetry along the center seam and several internal axes in each half (EF).

67–6594

phullu (A.)

| **Cloth, shoulder, ceremonial**

323

Puno: Ilave (JA)
Aymara
GH 1900s 1985
39" x 29"   (102cm x 75cm)
• *warp*: alpaca, 2-ply handspun; black, over-dyed black, purple, and multicolored; 76 epi (32 epc)
• *weft*: alpaca, 2-ply handspun; red; 21 ppi (10 ppc)
Warp-faced plain weave, warp stripes and 2-color complementary warp weave. Counter-spun yarn utilized in black warp-faced plain weave sections, in stripes of one thread each.

**Iconography: double-headed eagle, a European-influenced design, appears in warp pattern sections along with geometric forms.
Worn on head or over shoulder by women during periods of mourning; pink-colored wefts have special significance (GH).**

85–6
Adelson and Tracht 1983:91
Yorke 1980:13

318

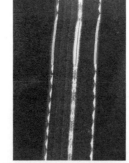

Detail 323

saco

Jacket

324

Puno: bought at Ilave market
Quechua/Aymara
BB 1960s 1967
15" x 15"   (37.5cm x 37.5cm)
• *warp*: sheepswool, single handspun; white;
22 epi (9 epc)
• *weft*: sheepswool, single handspun; black; 22 ppi
(9 ppc)
Broken twill weave, woven on a four-harness treadle loom, cut, tailored, and machine-sewn into a
short jacket. Hemmed with muslin, and commercial tape, embroidered with black handspun wool.

Hispanic-style short jackets of this sort are
worn frequently by women in the central
Andes. This piece, made very carefully, was
probably the work of a specialist (AF).

67–6566

pollera

Skirt

325

Puno: bought at Ilave market
Quechua/Aymara
BB 1960s 1967
20" x 160"   (50cm x 400cm)
Machine-woven deep red wool cloth, machine-
stitched into full gathered skirt. Waistband
smocked and bound with commercial tape. Lined
with blue muslin. Decorated with 3 rows of tucks.

67–6571
See **412, 413**

camisa

Undergarment

326

Puno: bought at Ilave market
Quechua/Aymara
BB 1960s 1966
39" x 13"   (130cm x 44cm)
Commercial muslin sewn into long-sleeved slip.
Embroidered around neck with colored wool, sim-
ple patterns.

See 354.

67–6568
See **354**

chuspa (Q.)

Bag ∗

327

Puno: Puno (MS)
Quechua
Musuem purchase 1980s 1985
6" x 4"   (15cm x 11cm)
sheepswool and alpaca; 2-ply handspun; brown
and tan; 12 spi (5 spc)
Knit: garter and stockinette stitches, color patterning, knit on straight needles in the round.
Trimmed with crochet edging.

Iconography: bull and geometric motifs.

85–10
See **256, 299, 410**

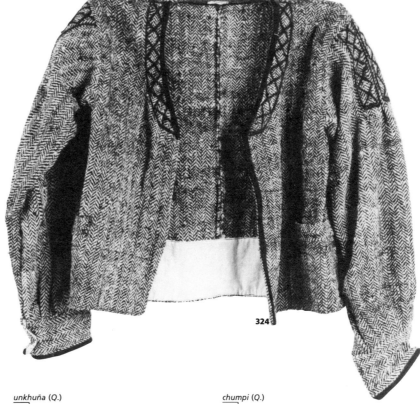

324

unkhuña (Q.)

Cloth, ceremonial

328

Puno: Puno
Quechua/Aymara
BB 1960s 1967
19" x 19"   (51cm x 51cm)
• *warp*: alpaca, sheepswool; 2-ply handspun;
brown, tan, red, and blue; 38 epi (15 epc)
• *weft*: camelid, 2-ply handspun; tan; 14 ppi
(5.5 ppc)
Warp-faced plain weave, warp stripes and 2-color
complementary warp weave. Woven as one
4-selvedge piece, bound with applied
crossed-warp band.

Iconography: *tanka ch'oro* (Q.) or forked diagonal.
BB reports this piece as an *unkhuña* (Q.),
used to carry coca leaves, food, or to place ritual objects on during ceremonies (BB). But
from its size and weight, E. M. Franquemont
thought this to be a pad for a pack mule. The
stripes are irregular, probably because of
warps breaking (EF).

67–6558
Zorn 1986
Rowe 1977a:102
Adelson and Tracht 1983:116–123
See **314, 317, 341**

chumpi (Q.)

Belt

329

Puno:
Quechua/Aymara
BB 1960s 1967
53" x 3½"   (133cm x 3.5cm)
• *warp*: sheepswool, 2-ply handspun; multicolored;
50 epi (20 epc)
• *weft*: llama, 2-ply handspun; brown; 7.5 ppi
(3 ppc)
Warp-faced plain weave, 2-color complementary
warp weave, twill effect with double weft in
places. Finished one end with heading cord, other
end with thirteen 3-strand braids.

Fairly heavy weight belt, worn by both sexes.
Color gradations work to create an overall ef-
fect typical of Aymaras near Lake Titicaca
(EF). Used like rope or strap to bundle up
wood for carrying (Bainton, pers. com. 1986).

63–6572
See **316**

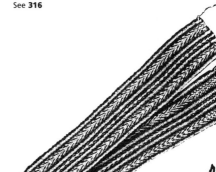

329

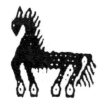

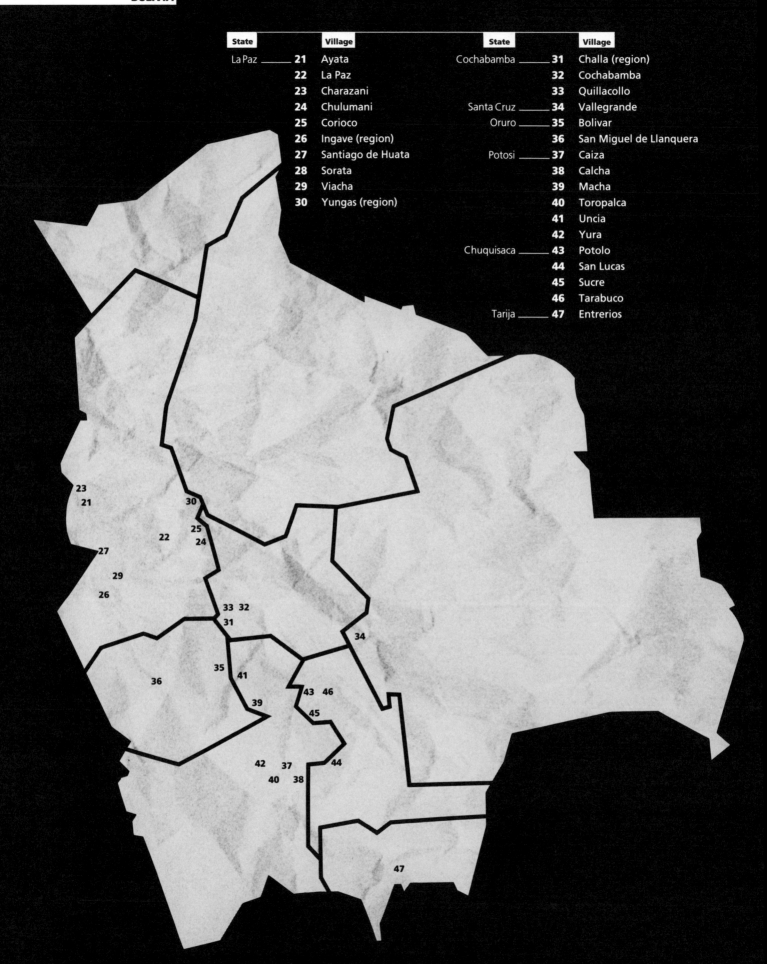

State		Village		State		Village
La Paz	21	Ayata		Cochabamba	31	Challa (region)
	22	La Paz			32	Cochabamba
	23	Charazani			33	Quillacollo
	24	Chulumani		Santa Cruz	34	Vallegrande
	25	Corioco		Oruro	35	Bolivar
	26	Ingave (region)			36	San Miguel de Llanquera
	27	Santiago de Huata		Potosi	37	Caiza
	28	Sorata			38	Calcha
	29	Viacha			39	Macha
	30	Yungas (region)			40	Toropalca
					41	Uncia
					42	Yura
				Chuquisaca	43	Potolo
					44	San Lucas
					45	Sucre
					46	Tarabuco
				Tarija	47	Entrerios

LA PAZ

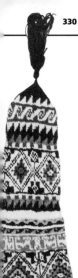

llucho (A.)

Cap

330

> **La Paz: Ayata**
> **Aymara**
> **DH 1960s 1966**
> 29" x 9"   (74cm x 9cm)
> sheepswool, 2-ply; multicolored and white;
> 5.5 spi (2 spc)
> Knit: stockinette and garter stitches, *pica-pica*
> edge, color patterning, and tassel at peak.

> **The colors, specific designs and the unusually long shape of this cap are all distinctive of the community of Ayata. (DH).***

66–4199

Poncho

331

> **La Paz: Ayata**
> **Aymara**
> **DH 1950s 1966**
> 29½" x 54"   (75cm x 134cm)
> • *warp*: sheepswool, 2-ply handspun; multicolored, (primarily red); 60 epi (24 epc)
> • *weft*: sheepswool, 2-ply handspun; white; 12 ppi (5 ppc)
> Warp-faced plain weave and 3-color supplementary warp weave. Woven as two 4-selvedge panels, seamed together by hand. Fringed complementary warp weave band applied to edge. Corners turned under.

> **Iconography: blocks and geometric forms.**
> The small geometric design bands and the fringed edge are distinctive of Ayata. An exceptionally well-woven poncho. Ponchos are gradually being replaced by overcoats (DH).

66–4186
Rowe 1977a:43
Adelson and Takami 1978:12

bolsa de lana

Bag *

332

> **La Paz: Charazani**
> **Quechua/Aymara**
> **DH 1960s 1966**
> 11½" x 14½"   (28.5cm x 36cm)
> • *warp*: alpaca, 2-ply handspun; natural multicolored; 40 epi (16 epc)
> • *weft*: alpaca, 2-ply handspun; brown; 15 ppi (6 ppc)
> Warp-faced plain weave with 2-color complementary warp weave; tubular edge; 5 pom-poms added; strap belt-loomed.

> **The collector of this bag said it is very similar to the shoulder bags carried by the Callawayas, itinerant medicine men, to carry herbs, amulets, and other paraphernalia (DH). But, because the yarn used is not tightly overspun, but instead is soft, and not very durable, this bag may have been woven for sale to tourists (EF).**

66–4168
Bastien 1978
Girault 1969

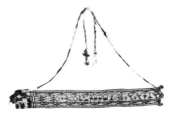

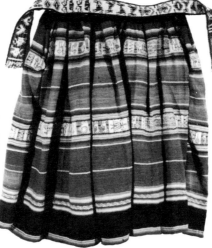

333–335

chumpi (Q.)

Belt

333

> **La Paz: Charazani**
> **Quechua/Aymara**
> **DH 1960s 1966**
> 54" x 2½"   (137cm x 6.5cm)
> • *warp*: sheepswool, camelid; 2-ply handspun; multicolored; 92 epi (36 epc)
> • *weft*: alpaca, 2-ply handspun; dark brown; 13 ppi (5 ppc)
> Warp-faced plain weave double cloth, finished with multi-loop braids on one end.

> **Iconography: human, animal, and geometric forms.**
> This sash was woven to be worn wrapped around the waist of Aymara women. The figurative designs are a regional characteristic of Charazani, as is the fine weaving. Charazani women are said to be among the best weavers in Bolivia because their husbands, the itinerant Callawayas, are absent for long periods of time leaving them with more responsibilities, but fewer children (DH).

66–4169
Cahlander 1985:pl. 7
Girault 1969

wincha (Q.) *llautu* (Q.)

Headband

334

> **La Paz: Charazani**
> **Quechua/Aymara**
> **DH 1910s 1966**
> 15" x 2"   (37cm x 5cm)
> • *warp*: alpaca 2-ply handspun; red and white; 152 epi (61 epc)
> • *weft*: alpaca, 2-ply handspun; white; 25 ppi (10 ppc)
> Warp-faced plain weave single weft double cloth with the warp ends wrapped. Trimmed with tassels and glass beads.

> **Iconography: human, animal, and geometric forms.**
> This finely woven headband, made in the early 20th century, was worn traditionally by Callaway medicine men during specific rites (DH). However Charazani women also traditionally wore such headbands.

66–4258
Wasserman and Hill 1981:pl. 3
Cason and Cahlander 1976:31
Girault 1969
Adelson and Takami 1978:31

pollera

Skirt *

335

> **La Paz: Charazani**
> **Quechua/Aymara**
> **DH 1960s 1966**
> 25" x 105½"   (62cm x 264cm)
> • *warp*: sheepswool, 2-ply handspun; multicolored, primarily red; cotton, multi-ply machine-spun; white; 30–88 epi (12–35 epc)
> • *weft*: alpaca, 2-ply handspun; light brown; 17 ppi (7 ppc)
> Warp-faced plain weave, 2-color complementary warp weave and double cloth. Woven in one 4-selvedge panel, gathered into a full skirt with the warp horizontal; hand-stitched seams.

> **Iconography: human, animal, and geometric forms.**
> This is an exceptional example of a dress skirt, worn only on special occasions by women in Charazani. Everyday skirts are less full and do not have pattern bands and stripes (DH).

66–4185
Adelson and Tracht 1983:112,113

chumpi (Q.)

Belt

336

> **La Paz: Charazani (JA)**
> **Quechua/Aymara**
> **DH 1960s 1966**
> 36" x 2"   (90cm x 4.5cm)
> • *warp*: sheepswool, 2-ply handspun; primarily red, blue, and white; 44 epi (17.5 epc)
> • *weft*: camelid, 2-ply handspun; brown; 19 ppi (7 ppc)
> Warp-faced plain weave, double cloth. Finished one end with heading cord, the other end with warp loops.

> **Iconography: animal and geometric forms.**
> Woven and worn by women to support skirts (DH).

66–4268
Wasserman and Hill 1981:pl. 4
Cason and Cahlander 1976:77–81

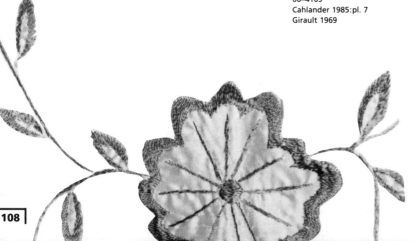

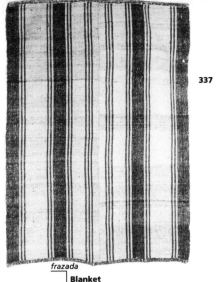

337

frazada

| **Blanket**

337

    La Paz: Chulumani
    Quecha/Aymara
    DH   1960s   1966
71" x 52"   (180cm x 132cm)
• *warp*: sheepswool, 2-ply handspun; white and black; 7 epi (3 epc)
• *weft*: sheepswool, 2-ply handspun; white and grey; 9 ppi (3.5 ppc)
Warp-faced plain weave; color stripes; single warp cut in half and hand-seamed.

    This fairly coarse textile was woven for utilitarian purposes. It is quite similar to the *costales* or bags used to carry potatoes (EF).

66–4036
See **345**

llajqa (A.)

| **Blanket, baby**

338

    La Paz: Coroico
    Aymara
    DH   1960s   1966
30½" x 28½"   (76cm x 71cm)
Commercial peach rayon cloth, hand embroidered with dark orange thread; lined with muslin.

    This elaborate cloth would have been used to wrap a baby on festive occasions. Cloths such as these are made by specialists (DH). Because the pattern is slightly asymmetrical, it was probably not drawn out before the actual embroidery was done (EF).

66–4180

estera y radera

| **Pad and crupper**

339

    La Paz: Coroico
    Aymara
    DH   1960s   1966
47½" x 20"   (121cm x 51cm) crupper 7½" wide (19cm)
• *warp*: Crupper: llama, 2-ply handspun; natural multi-colors; 28 epi (14 epc); cotton, single handspun; white; 46 epi (18 epc). Pad: vegetal fiber, single machine-spun; 26 epi (14 epc)
• *weft*: Crupper: llama, 2-ply handspun; tan; 8 ppi (5 ppc); cotton, single handspun; white; 46 ppi (18 ppc). Pad: vegetal fiber, single machine-spun; 9 ppi (5 ppc)
Crupper: three layers of cloth quilted together by hand with handspun llama wool. Top layer is llama, plain woven with warp stripes creating horizontal and vertical stripes. Middle layer, probably plain woven vegetal fiber, added for strength and thickness. Bottom layer, treadle-woven white cotton bayeta. The quilting causes the upper llama layer to pucker. Pad: constructed out of commercial sack: twill-woven, with threads in pairs. Badly soiled and printed with "CMB La Paz, ST" (AF).

    This pad would have been used over another pad and held in place with the help of the crupper which passes under the animal's tail. Mules are still the primary means of transport for Aymaras in the mountainous jungles of the Yungas region (DH).

66–4216

awayo (Q.)

| **Shawl**

340

    La Paz: Ingave region (JA)
    Quechua
    GH   early 20th cent.   1980
40½" x 33"   (102cm x 82cm)
• *warp*: alpaca, 2-ply handspun; natural multi-colored dyes, primarily pink and blue; 58 epi (26 epc)
• *weft*: alpaca, 2-ply handspun; tan; 19 ppi (7 ppc)
Warp-faced plain weave, warp stripes and 2-color complementary warp weave. Woven as two identical 4-selvedge pieces, seamed together by hand. Bound with applied plain woven tubular edging.

    Iconography: small geometric forms.

80–87
Wasserman and Hill 1981:pl. 7
Adelson and Tracht 1983:94
Cason and Cahlander 1976:126
See **366**

339

unkhuña (Q.)

| **Cloth, ceremonial**

341

    La Paz: Lake Titicaca region
    Aymara
    RISD Transfer: Lisle Estate   1960s   1985
18" x 17"   (46cm x 43cm)
• *warp*: alpaca, sheepswool, 2-ply handspun; multi-colored and white; 46 epi (18.5 epc)
• *weft*: alpaca, sheepswool, 2-ply handspun; tan; 19 ppi (7.5 ppc)
Warp-faced plain weave, warp stripes and 2-color complementary warp weave. Woven as one 4-selvedge cloth, bound with tubular edging and applied tassels at corners.

    Iconography: animal and geometric motifs.
    The terminal zones are especially long, taking up almost one-third of this piece; soiled with wax deposits. Used for ritual purposes (EF).

85–482
Adelson and Tracht 1983:116–123
See **314, 317, 328**

| **Poncho**

342

    La Paz: Lake Titicaca region
    Aymara
    DH   1960s   1966
26" x 58½"   (66cm x 148cm)
• *warp*: sheepswool, 2-ply handspun; black, reds, and pinks; 28 epi (11 epc)
• *weft*: sheepswool, 2-ply handspun; black; 13 ppi (5 ppc)
Warp-faced plain weave, narrow warp stripes. Woven as two identical 4-selvedge panels, seamed together by hand and the corners turned under. Reinforced around the edges with black wool yarn.

    The predominately dark color is typical of Aymaras on the east coast of Lake Titicaca. The narrow color bands identify the wearer as a former *jilicata* (A.) or headman. Badly worn, but carefully darned (DH).

66–4269
See **282**

ponchito

| **Poncho, miniature**

343

    La Paz: Santiago de Huata
    Aymara
    DH   early 20th cent.   1966
16" x 22"   (41cm x 55cm)
• *warp*: alpaca, 2-ply handspun; black, white, and red; 80 epi (32 epc)
• *weft*: alpaca, 2-ply handspun; black; 19 ppi (7.5 ppc)
Warp-faced plain weave, warp stripes, woven in one 4-selvedge piece, with a hole cut for the neck. Bound with a plain woven tubular *ribete*, weft threads pulled out to make a sparse fringe.

    Worn by Aymara headmen; other symbols of office are distinctive whip and sash (DH).

66–4284
Adelson and Tracht 1983:68–69; 61
See **367**

343

Detail 340

honda, waraka (Q.)

Sling

344

La Paz: Santiago de Huata
Aymara
DH   1960s   1966
59" x 1½" (at cradle) x 2½" (at narrowest braid)
147cm x 4cm (at cradle) x 6cm (at narrowest braid)
camelid, 2-ply handspun; brown, black, white.
Cradle: slit tapestry weave. Wide braid: 24-strand
round braid, in diamond pattern. Narrow braid:
8-strand square braid in herringbone pattern. Finished one end in a loop, the other end in a tassel.

**Used with stones for herding sheep, hunting
small game, or occasionally as offensive
weapon. A pre-Columbian survival used by
both sexes, all ages, among most Andean Indians (DH).**

66–4264
Cahlander 1980:35, 64
See **253, 361**

frazada

Blanket *

345

La Paz: Sorata
Aymara
DH   1960s   1966
7' x 4'   (214cm x 130cm)
• *warp*: sheepswool, 2-ply handspun; grey; 14 epi
(5.5 epc)
• *weft*: sheepswool, 2-ply handspun; grey; 8 ppi
(3 ppc)
Warp-faced plain weave; woven as one 4-selvedge
piece then cut in half and sewn together widthwise; random color mixing.

A typical Aymara blanket (DH).

66–4035
See **337**

awayo (Q.)

Mantle

346

La Paz: Sorata
Quechua
DH   1960s   1966
30½" x 33"   (76.5cm x 83cm)
• *warp*: sheepswool, alpaca, 2-ply handspun;
brown, orange, and red; 50 epc (20 epc)
• *weft*: alpaca, 2-ply handspun; brown; 15 ppi
(6 ppc)
Warp-faced plain weave, warp stripes and complementary warp weave. Woven as two identical
4-selvedge cloths. Sewn together by hand.

**This piece is unusual in its combination of col-
or and motif. It was probably made by a woman from Charazani (utilizing typical method
and motifs) but living near Sorata (of which
the colors and overall proportions are typical)
(DH). Or possibly from Calamarka (JA).**

66–4270

montera

Hat

347

La Paz: Viacha
Aymara/Spanish
DH   1960s   1966
4½" x 12"   (11.5cm x 30.5cm)
Felt, painted yellow, trimmed with commercial rib-
bon and cord.

**This style of derby hat is typical of urban An-
dean women in Bolivia. The origin of this
style is unclear; although it appears in illustrations from as early as 1850. One story has
it derived from riding habit of English rail-
road and embassy staff in late 19th century,
another suggests introduction by an anony-
mous "Yankee Trader" (DH). In the early part
of this century hats of this sort were imported from England, now they are made within
the country; worn only by women (JA).**

66–4067
See **273** for comments.

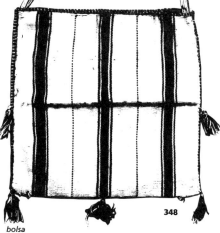

bolsa

Bag

348

La Paz: Yungas region
Aymara
DH   1960s   1966
13½" x 14"   (35cm x 36cm)
• *warp*: cotton, 2-ply handspun; white; wool, 2-ply
handspun; green; 45 epi (18 epc)
• *weft*: cotton, 2-ply handspun; white; 15 ppi
(6 ppc)
Warp-faced plain weave, warp stripes, woven as
one 4-selvedge cloth, folded and trimmed with *ribete* and 5 green-and-white tassels. Applied strap
woven out of commercially spun white, pink, yellow, and blue cotton.

**This tightly woven bag was woven by
women for use by men in the few small endogamous Black enclaves that are scattered
throughout the predominantly Aymara Yungas region. The use of locally grown cotton
and simple color decoration is distinctive of
this work (DH).**

66–4202

blusa

Blouse

349

La Paz: Yungas region
Aymara
DH   1960s   1966
22½" x 17½"   (56cm x44cm)
Commercial cotton muslin, machine-stitched into
long-sleeved blouse and hand embroidered with
multicolored rayon thread.

**This blouse, embroidered with stylized
flowers is typical of the Black women who
live in a few small endogamous enclaves in
the predominately Aymara Yungas region.
The rest of the typical Black dress is very similar to that of Aymara women (DH).**

66–4182

cinchon

Girth for pack mule

350

La Paz: Yungas Region
Aymara
DH   1960s   1966
• *warp*: llama, 2-ply handspun; natural
multi-colors; 26 epi (14 epc); cotton, single handspun; white; 30 epi (16 epc)
• *weft*: llama, 2-ply handspun; tan; 8 ppi (5 ppc);
cotton, single handspun; white; 30 ppi (16 ppc)
Three layers of cloth quilted together by hand
with heavy 2-ply cotton. Top layer is llama, plain
woven with weft-faced stripes. Middle layer, probably plain woven vegetal fiber, added for strength
and thickness. Bottom layer, treadle-woven white
cotton *bayeta*. The quilting causes the upper
llama layer to pucker. One end lashed with vegetable fiber cords to a wooden buckle.

**Used together with a pad and crupper (339)
by Aymaras in the Yungas region for transportation (DH).**

66–4291

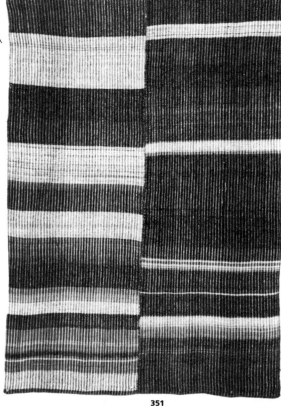

351

saca para manejar coca

Sack, coca

351

La Paz: Yungas region
Aymara
DH   1960s   1966
77½" x 56"   (194cm x 140cm)
• *warp*: llama, single handspun; various natural colors; 23 epi (9epc)
• *weft*: llama, single handspun; various natural colors; 19 ppi (7.5 ppc)
Balanced 2/2 twill, warp and weft stripes, woven
on a treadle loom, cut and sewn vertically to create a very large bag.

**This extremely large bag was made to carry
coca leaves (the "green gold" of the Yungas
region) in bulk. The leaves must be collected,
spread to dry before being pressed into
bales. This tough, large bag allows relatively
easy handling of the crop (DH).**

66–4219

alforja

Bag, saddle

352

La Paz: Yungas region
Aymara
DH   1960s   1966
48½" x 24"   (123cm x 61cm)
• *warp*: llama, 2-ply handspun; various natural colors; 26 epi (10 epc)
• *weft*: llama, 2-ply handspun; various natural colors; 12 ppi (5 ppc)
Warp-faced plain weave, warp stripes. Woven as
one 4-selvedge piece, folded to make 2 large
pockets. Edged with a 10-strand braid.

**This saddle bag would have been draped
over pads on pack mules by Aymaras. Such
bags are usually used for masses of small
items (e.g. coca leaves, oranges, tangerines,
etc.). The fabric is very similar to that used
for potato sacks (DH).**

66–4218
See **307, 308**

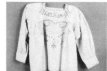

349

354

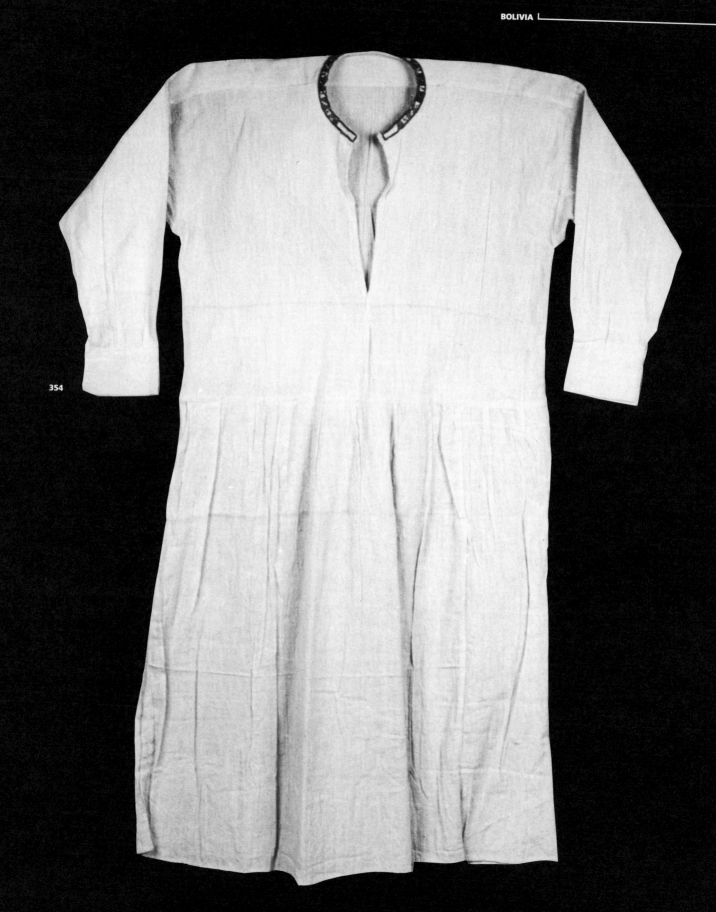

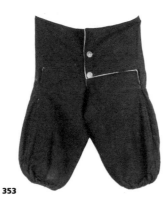

353

pantalón

| Trousers |

353

La Paz: Yungas region
Aymara
DH 1960s 1966
20½" x 14"   (52cm x 32cm)
Black wool factory-made "drill" cloth, lined with
homespun warp-faced plain weave tan *bayeta*
cloth, cut and sewn into trousers.

> This distinctive knicker style of trousers with
> false pockets and buttoned fly was once
> worn by male Aymaras in the Yungas region,
> but since the beginning of the century,
> factory-made clothing has replaced this style
> completely. Impossible to find small-crowned,
> broad-brimmed Panama hat that "went with"
> such trousers (DH).

66–4221
Collier, de Rick, and Berger 1981:fig. 14

camisa

| Undergarment |

354

La Paz: Yungas region
Aymara
DH 1960s 1966
40" x 23"   (102cm x 58.5cm)
• *warp*: cotton, single handspun; white; 50 epi
(20 epc)
• *weft*: cotton, single handspun; white; 40 ppi
(16 ppc)
Plain woven muslin, machine stitched into simple
long-sleeved slip. Embroidered around neck with
brightly colored wool.

> This type of coarse slip is the only kind of un-
> dergarment worn by women in highland Bo-
> livia and is only found in the Yungas region.
> Even this simple garment is ornamented with
> embroidery (DH).

66–4181
See **326**

COCHABAMBA

aksu (Q.)

| Overskirt |

355

Cochabamba: Challa region
Quechua/Aymara
GH 1900s 1985
41½" x 48½"   (105cm x 123cm)
• *warp*: alpaca, 2-ply handspun; dark brown, reds,
and purples; 56 epi (22.5 epc)
• *weft*: alpaca, 2-ply handspun; tan; 18 ppi (7 ppc)
Warp-faced plain weave, warp stripes, and 2-color
complementary warp weave. Woven as two
4-selvedge pieces, balanced, though not perfectly
symmetrical. Sewn together by hand and bound
with crossed-warp tubular edging.

> **Iconography: bird, floral, and geometric
> forms.**
>   All natural dyes except for one orange. This
> ceremonial textile was woven by Aymaras
> who now speak Quechua in a bilingual fringe
> area (GH).

85–7
Adelson and Tracht 1983:102–109, fig. 40

chumpi (Q.)

| Belt |

356

Cochabamba: Cochabamba
Quechua
DH 1960s 1966
52" x 2½"   (130cm x 6.5cm)
• *warp*: sheepswool, 2-ply handspun; multicolored,
primarily lime green, pinks, and white; 30 epi
(12 epc)
• *weft*: sheepswool, 2-ply handspun; lime green;
15 ppi (6 ppc)
Warp-faced plain weave and double cloth.

> **Iconography: female figures holding hoops,
> four rounded forms joined by diagonals.**
>   This style is typical of the city of Cochabam-
> ba (DH).

66–4267

frazada

| Blanket * |

357

Cochabamba: Cochabamba region
Quechua
DH 1960s 1966
77" x 58"   (193cm x 145cm)
• *warp*: sheepswool, 2-ply handspun; multicolored;
16 epi (6.5 epc)
• *weft*: sheepswool, 2-ply handspun; dyed red;
12 ppi (5 ppc)
Warp-faced plain weave, warp stripes; two
4-selvedge pieces hand-seamed.

> This household blanket was probably woven
> by a professional weaver on a floor loom
> (EF). Its bright colors are typical of the Que-
> chuas who live south of Cochabamba (DH).

66–4204

montera

| Hat |

358

Cochabamba: Cochabamba region
Quechua
DH 1960s 1966
6" x 15"   (15cm x 39cm)
Tan felt with a black fabric band

> This style of hat is worn by both sexes.
> People are sheepherders and subsistence
> farmers living in isolated homesteads.
> Women wear it with the brim turned up (as
> in this example), men with the brim turned
> down (DH).

66–4050
Adelson and Takami 1978:12

awana (Q.)

| Loom |

359

Cochabamba: Cochabamba region
Quechua
DH 1960s 1966
42" x 30½"   (109cm x 75cm)
• *warp*: sheepswool, 2-ply handspun; multicolored;
48 epi (19 epc)
• *weft*: sheepswool, 2-ply handspun; pink, red, and
white; 10 ppi (4 ppc)
Wood loom bars, metal heddle rod with wool heddle string. Heading cords are lashed to each loom
bar. Cloth is warp-faced plain weave, warp stripes
and 2-color complementary warp weave.*

> This loom which holds an almost completed
> *llijlla* (Q.) half, is used upright. Weaving is
> done by women, when they are not helping
> in fields or herding sheep (DH).

66–4053
Adelson and Tracht 1983:40

Poncho

| Poncho |

360

Cochabamba: Cochabamba region
Quechua
DH 1960s 1966
38½" x 53"   (98cm x 133cm)
• *warp*: llama, 2-ply handspun; brown; 20 epi
(8 epc)
• *weft*: llama, 2-ply handspun; brown; 11 ppi
(4.5 ppc)
Warp-faced plain weave. Woven as 2 pieces on a
treadle loom, cut on 3 sides, hemmed with handwoven tape and sewn together by hand. Folded
collar was woven separately and applied.

> This heavy poncho, worn only by men and
> during daylight hours only by *jilicatas* (A.)
> (headmen), is unusual for a Bolivian poncho
> because it has a collar (DH). Collared ponchos
> are found in Ecuador (EF). Brushed with cock-
> lebur to create deep nap.

66–4061

honda, *waraka* (Q.)

| Sling |

361

Cochabamba: Cochabamba region
Quechua
DH 1960s 1966
58" x 2½" (at cradle)½" (at narrow
braid).   (145cm x 6cm [at cradle] .9cm [at
narrow braid].)
Camelid, 2-ply handspun; primarily orange, and
blue
Cradle: slit tapestry. Wide braid: 32-strand, 3-color
in diamond pattern. Narrow braid: 6-strand,
3-color, uses 4 extra strands, which float in the
middle of the braid for bulk, and switch with the
braided strands for color variation.

> **Bright colors typical of Cochabamba Valley
> (DH).**

66–4274
Cahlander 1980:21,31,73
See **253, 344**

pantalón de bayeta

| Trousers, wool |

362

Cochabamba: Cochabamba region
Quechua
DH 1960s 1966
40½" x 13"   (101cm x 33cm)
• *warp*: sheepswool, single handspun; black;
24 epi (9.5 epc)
• *weft*: sheepswool, single handspun; black; 18 ppi
(7 ppc)
Warp-faced plain weave woven on a treadle loom,
cut and sewn into trousers, lined with muslin;
pockets.

> Worn by men throughout the Andes, but
> dark colors are prefered in Cochabamba (DH).

66–4271

Detail 356

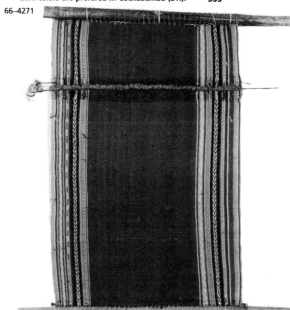

359

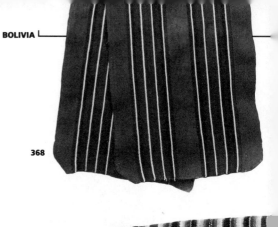

368

chumpi (Q.)

Belt

363

Cochabamba: Quillacollo
Quechua
DH 1960s 1966
75½" x 2"   (189cm x 4.5cm)
• *warp*: sheepswool, 2-ply handspun; multicolored,
primarily red; 40 epi (16 epc)
• *weft*: sheepswool, 2-ply handspun; red; 13 ppi
(5.2 ppc)
Warp-faced plain weave, warp color patterning to
create horizontal and vertical stripes. One end
finished with heading cord, the other with two
3-strand braids.

66–4259

SANTA CRUZ

cobija caballar

Blanket, saddle

364

Santa Cruz: Vallegrande
Spanish
DH 1960s 1966
26½" x 23"   (63cm x 58.5cm)
• *warp*: sheepswool, 2-ply handspun; orange, yellow, white, and brown; 23 epi (9 epc)
• *weft*: sheepswool, 2-ply handspun; white; 7 ppi
(3 ppc)
Warp-faced plain weave, warp stripes, one
4-selvedge cloth, heavily felted from use.

**Used by cowboys in the eastern lowlands
(DH).**

66–4263

Poncho

365

Santa Cruz: Vallegrande
Spanish
DH 1960 1966
33" x 49"   (84cm x 124cm)
• *warp*: cotton, 2-ply machine-spun; natural or natural dyed browns; 56 epi (22.5 epc)
• *weft*: cotton, 2-ply machine-spun; brown; 18 ppi
(7 ppc)
Warp-faced plain weave with subtle warp stripes
woven on a treadle loom, cut and sewn into a
poncho. Edges bound with plain woven, warp-
faced strip.

**The Spanish-speaking communities in the re-
gion of Vallegrande are marginal to both the
Quechuan/Aymara highlands and the Camba
tropical plains. This garment shows the distinctive combination of a highland garment
(poncho) with a more lowland plant (cotton).
Perhaps the only Andean region where the
poncho is made of cotton. Worn by cowboys
over western dress (DH).**

66–4261

ORURO

awayo (Q.)

Shawl

366

Oruro: Bolivar (JA)
Aymara/Quechua
GH late 19th cent. 1980
31½" x 39"   (79cm x 97cm)
• *warp*: alpaca, 2-ply handspun; natural dyed multicolored, primarily pink and blue; 76 epi (30 epc)
• *weft*: alpaca, 2-ply handspun; natural dark
brown; 20 ppi (8 ppc)
Warp-faced plain weave, warp stripes, 3-color
complementary warp weave. Woven as 2 identical
panels, sewn together by hand. Bound with
crossed-warp tubular strip.

Iconography: geometric forms.

80–89
See **340**

Detail 366

---

ponchito

Poncho, miniature ∗

367

Chuquisaca: Tarabuco (JA)
Quechua
DH 1960s 1966
16" x 17½"   (41cm x 45cm)
• *warp*: sheepswool, 2-ply handspun; multicolored
primarily reds; 42 epi (21 epc)
• *weft*: sheepswool, 2-ply handspun; 18 ppi
(7.2 ppc)
Warp-faced plain weave, warp stripes and color
patterning. Woven in two 4-selvedge panels,
seamed together with zigzag embroidery. Woven
fringed band applied to edge.

66–4179
See **343**

chalina de jilicata (A.)

Scarf

368

Oruro: San Miguel de Llanquera
Aymara
DH early 20th cent. 1966
63" x 14"   (161cm x 35cm)
• *warp*: alpaca, 2-ply handspun; natural browns
and natural dyed red, green, blue, yellow; 64 epi
(25 epc)
• *weft*: alpaca, 2-ply handspun; browns; 15 ppi
(6 ppc)
Warp-faced plain weave, warp stripes to create
vertical stripes, one 4-selvedge piece.

**The collector of this piece reported that this
is an extremely wide sash, worn only by jilica-
tas (A.) (DH). Another collector, J. Appleby,
thought that it was a chalina or scarf.∗**

66–4178
Adelson and Tracht 1983:111

POTOSI

Poncho, man's ceremonial

369

Potosi: Caiza
Quechua
GH 1940s 1985
35½" x 55½"   (90cm x 141cm)
• *warp*: alpaca, 2-ply handspun; multicolored;
54 epi (28 epc)
• *weft*: alpaca, 2-ply handspun; brown; 14 ppi
(6 ppc)
Warp-faced plain weave, warp stripes and 3-color
complementary warp weave. Woven in two
4-selvedge strips, and sewn together with zigzag
embroidery. Edges are bound with a plain woven
binding with weft fringes, also attatched with zigzag embroidery.

Iconography: small geometric motifs.
   **This poncho was worn by a local leader as
a symbol of office (GH). Its beauty comes
from the juxtaposition of many plain-woven
stripes with narrow pattern bands. The terminal zones, which are balanced diagonally
across the back and front of the garment, are
very long, probably as much for visual appeal
as for ease in weaving (AF).**

85–4
Adelson and Tracht 1983:pl. 14

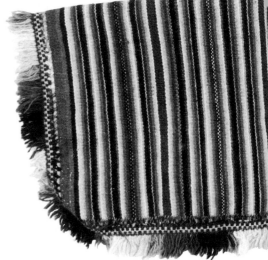

367

chumpi (Q.)

Belt

370

Potosi: Calcha
Quechua
GH 1970s 1984
186" x 1½"   (465cm x 3.5cm)
• *warp*: alpaca, 2-ply handspun; multicolored;
65 epi (26 epc)
• *weft*: alpaca, 2-ply handspun; tan; 25 ppi
(10 ppc)
Warp-faced plain weave and 2-color complementary warp weave. One end finished with warp
loops (no heading cord), the other with nine
7-strand braids.

Iconography: geometric forms.
   **This extremely long belt would have been
worn wrapped several times around the
waist to hold up aksu (Q.) or overskirt (AF).**

84–18 G
Adelson and Takami 1978:32–35
See **371, 372, 375–378** Female Costume

almilla (Q.)

Dress ∗

371

Potosi:
Quechua
GH 1950s 1984
53" x 23"   (138cm x 23cm)
Commercial wool cloth, embroidered with
couched threads, possibly by machine, on the
wide sleeves and at the hem.

Iconography: floral patterns.
   **Part of a woman's costume acquired in
La Paz. The costume is ceremonial (GH).
European-influenced, cut-and-sew tailoring
example.**

84–18 A
See **370, 372, 375–378** Female Costume

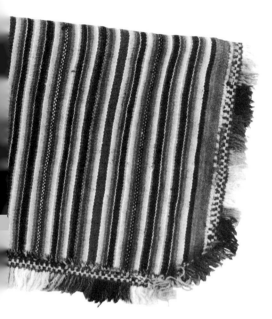

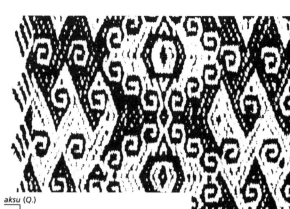

Poncho *

373
Potosi: Calcha
Quechua
GH   1950–70   1980
26½" x 51½"   (67cm x 129cm)
• *warp*: sheepswool, 2-ply handspun; multicolored; 90 epi (36 epc)
• *weft*: camelid, 2-ply handspun; tan; 22½ ppi (9 ppc)
Warp-faced plain weave, warp ikat, and warp stripes; 2-color complementary warp patterning. Woven as two 4-selvedge cloths and seamed together with brightly colored satin-stitched embroidery. Edges bound with warp-faced band with weft fringes.

This is a very fine example of warp ikat used along with other types of patterning. The design in the ikat stripes is a simpler variation of the zigzag patterns seen frequently in complementary warp bands. This pattern is sometimes referred to as *mayo k'enko* or meandering river (EF). Although the stripes in each half of the poncho are not identical, they are balanced and give the impression of a perfect symmetry (AF).

80–86
Wasserman and Hill 1981:pl. 21
Yorke 1980:32
Rowe 1977a:20
See **374**

Poncho *

374
Potosi: Calcha
Quechua
GH   1950–1970   1980
27½" x 55½"   (70cm x 136cm)
• *warp*: alpaca, 2-ply handspun; multicolored, primarily deep reds; 26 epi (10.5 epc)
• *weft*: alpaca, 2-ply handspun; dark brown; 7 ppi (3 ppc)
Warp-faced plain weave, warp stripes, ikat patterning and 2-color complementary warp weave. Woven as two 4-selvedge cloths, sewn together with satin stitch. Bound with plain woven strip with weft fringe.

The two halves are perfectly symmetrical and have internal bands of symmetry around the complementary warp stripes (EF). The ikat patterns are smaller than those in 372.

80–88
Wasserman and Hill 1981:pl. 21
See **373**

aksu (Q.)
Overskirt, half

375
Potosi: Calcha
Quechua
GH   late 19th cent.   1980
44½" x 25½"   (112cm x 64cm)
• *warp*: alpaca, 2-ply handspun; overdyed black; 125 epi (50 epc)
• *weft*: alpaca, 2-ply handspun; black; 20 ppi (8 ppc)
Warp-faced plain weave, 2-color complementary warp weave. Uses counter-spun yarn near selvedge.

Iconography: small geometric forms.
This is an extremely fine piece of Andean weaving. Not only is the design band incredibly intricate, but the color selection within the design is especially graceful. The piece was originally sewn to another piece of cloth to make a complete *aksu* (Q.) (the needle holes from that seam are still visible) (EF).

80–98
Adelson and Takami 1978:32–33
Adelson and Tracht 1983:102–109
See **370–372, 376–378**   Female Costume

aksu (Q.)
Overskirt

376
Potosi: Calcha
Quechua
GH   1970s   1984
47" x 53"   (120cm x 134cm)
• *warp*: alpaca, 2-ply handspun; black overdyed black and multicolored; primarily reds; 78 epi (36 epc)
• *weft*: alpaca, 2-ply handspun; tan; 20 ppi (8 ppc)
Warp-faced plain weave, warp stripes and 2-color complementary warp weave. Woven as two different 4-selvedge panels and seamed together by hand. One edge finished with decorative embroidery.

Iconography: small geometric forms.
One half of this piece has a wider pattern band than the other (EF).

84–18 C
See **370–372, 375, 377, 378**   Female Costume

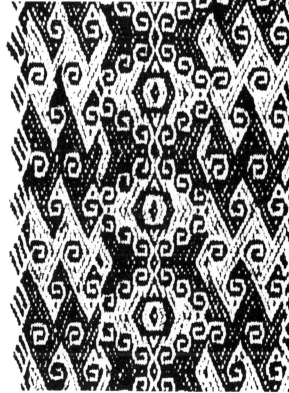

Detail 375

montera
Hat

372
Potosi: Calcha
Quechua
GH   1960s   1984
4½" x 12½"   (11cm x 32cm)
Orange felt hat, decorated with grosgrain and velvet ribbons, rickrack, wool tassels, and *golon* strips.

84–18 E
See **370, 371, 375–378**   Female Costume

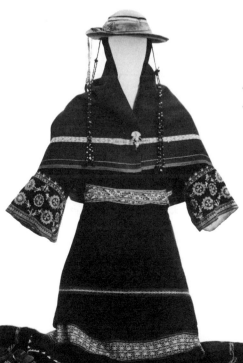

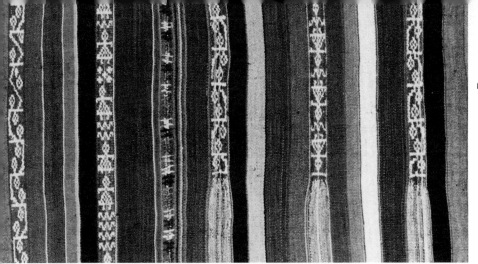

Detail 381

llijlla (Q.)

Shawl

377

    Potosi: Calcha
    Quechua
    GH 1960s 1984
36" x 42"   (92cm x 106cm)

- *warp*: alpaca, 2-ply handspun; black and multi-colored; 89 epi (40 epc)
- *weft*: alpaca, 2-ply handspun; tan; 20 ppi (8 ppc)

Warp-faced plain weave, warp stripes and 2-color complementary warp weave. Woven as two identical 4-selvedge pieces and seamed with decorative embroidery at center.

84–18 B

    See **370–372, 375, 376, 378** Female Costume

tulma (Q.)

Tie, hair *

378

    Potosi: Calcha
    Quechua
    GH 1970s 1984
34" x ¼"   (88cm x .5cm)

sheepswool, single handspun; black and multi-colored.

One 3-strand braid, split at the end into 2 smaller braids, and then those two split into 4 braids at each end. Decorated with yarn wrappings and tassels.

    Used by women to tie braids together in the back, and keep them from falling over the shoulders and getting in the way (EF).

84–18 D
See **370–372, 375–377** Female Costume

aksu (Q.)

Overskirt

379

    Potosi: Macha
    Quechua/Aymara
    GH 1960s 1984
31½" x 43"   (78cm x 109cm)

- *warp*: alpaca, 2-ply handspun; multicolored, primarily overdyed black and deep maroon; 90 epi (36 epc)
- *weft*: alpaca, 2-ply handspun; dark brown; 20 ppc (8 ppi)

Warp-faced plain weave, warp stripes, and 2- and 3-color complementary warp weave. Woven as two different 4-selvedge panels, seamed together by hand. Both panels use counter-spun yarns.

    Iconography: blocks and zigzags.
    The techniques used in each panel are the same, but the design bands vary. Used for special occasions (EF).

84–22
Cason and Cahlander 1976:108–112

llijlla (Q.)

Shawl

380

    Potosi: Macha
    Quechua/Aymara
    DH 1960s 1966
34" x 41"   (86.5cm x 104cm)

- *warp*: alpaca, sheepswool; 2-ply handspun; black overdyed black and multicolored; 42 epi (17 epc)
- *weft*: alpaca, 2-ply handspun; tan; 16 ppi (6.5 ppc)

Warp-faced plain weave, warp stripes and 2-color complementary warp weave. Woven as two identical 4-selvedge panels, seamed down center with decorative embroidery. Bound with tubular complementary warp strip.

    Iconography: lozenges.
    An excellent example of tightly woven Aymara work, with natural color predominating and geometric patterns smaller and less brightly colored than is typical of Quechuan weaving. This type of weaving was commonplace until the 1930s but is rapidly disappearing as inexpensive cloth and plastics gain popularity (DH).

66–4060

llijlla (Q.)

Shawl

381

    Potosi: Toropalca
    Quechua
    GH 1940s 1985
40" x 55"   (102cm x 140cm)

- *warp*: alpaca, 2-ply handspun; multicolored; 78 epi (31 epc)
- *weft*: alpaca, 2-ply handspun; dark brown; 22 ppi (8.5 ppc)

Warp-faced plain weave, warp stripes, and 2-color complementary warp weave. Woven as two 4-selvedge panels and seamed with zigzag embroidery.

    Iconography: female figures and geometric forms.
    No real *pampa* section in this piece, only color striping; some brown dyes may be vegetal; large needlework finishing sections (EF).

85–5

383

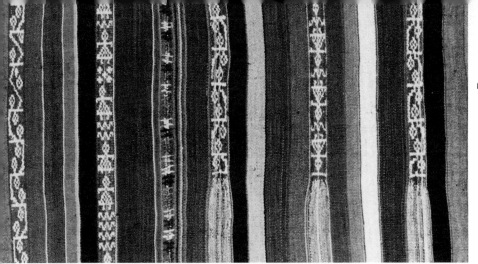

chuspa (Q.)

Bag, coca

382

    Potosi: Uncia (JA)
    Aymara
    Musuem purchase 1950s 1980
5" x 4½"   (12.5cm x 11cm)

- *warp*: alpaca, 2-ply handspun; multicolored; 46 epi (18.5 epc)
- *weft*: alpaca, 2-ply handspun; tan; 18 ppi (7 ppc)

Warp-faced plain weave, warp stripes and double cloth. Woven as one 4-selvedge cloth, folded and seamed into bag. Bound on sides with tubular edging with applied fringe. Complementary warp-woven strap of synthetic yarn is much newer than bag.

    Iconography: on strap; *tanka ch'oro* (Q.) or forked diagonal.
    This bag is very faded. The bright original colors can be seen on the inside of the bag (AF).

80–104
Cason and Cahlander 1976:77–81
Cahlander 1985

unkhu (Q.) *ccahua* (A.)

Tunic

383

    Potosi: Yura
    Aymara
    GH early 20th cent. 1984
32" x 32"   (81cm x 80cm)

- *warp*: alpaca, 2-ply handspun; natural dyed of indigo and cochineal; 59 epi (23.5 epc)
- *weft*: alpaca, 2-ply handspun; dark brown; 13 ppi (5 ppc)

Warp-faced plain weave, warp stripes. Woven as one 4-selvedge cloth. Neck slit woven in with two wefts and reinforced. Sides seamed together by hand. Bound at hem and armholes with tubular crossed-warp weave band.

    Worn by Aymara males during ceremonies in the early part of this century (GH). A pre-Columbian dress form survival.

84–21
Adelson and Tracht 1983:50–59

chumpi (Q.)

Belt

384

    Potosi: Exact location unknown
    Quechua
    DH 1960s 1966
73½" x 2"   (184cm x 4cm)

- *warp*: sheepswool, 2-ply handspun; multi-colored, primarily orange; 20 epi (8 epc)
- *weft*: sheepswool, 2-ply handspun; blue; 8 ppi (3 ppc)

Warp-faced plain weave, warp striping, finished one end with two 8-strand braids, other end with loops left by pulling out the heading cord.

66–4266

montera

Hat

385

Potosi: Exact location unknown
Quechua
DH 1960s 1966
6½" x 16½"   (16cm x 42cm)
Felt, with brown commercial ribbon trim, and colored oil cloth inside the brim.

"Pilgrim style" or stove pipe hats such as this one are worn by women in the area around Potosi. The colors are always dark (brown, green, blue, black), with no distinguishing marks from town to town (DH).

66–4048

CHUQUISACA

aksu (Q.)

Overskirt, half

386

Chuquisaca: Potolo
Quechua
GH 1970s 1980
25" x 21"   (63cm x 52cm)
• *warp*: sheepswool, 2-ply handspun; black overdyed black, deep red, purple, and green; 52 epi (21 epc)
• *weft*: alpaca, 2-ply handspun; dark brown; 18 ppi (7 ppc)
Warp-faced plain weave, warp stripes and 2-color complementary warp weave. One 4-selvedge panel. Edge finished with multicolored crochet stitch.

Iconography: fantastic animal and bird motifs with zigzag border.
Extremely wide pattern area with figurative motifs. Single white warps separate pattern area from *pampa* section (EF).

80–101
Wasserman and Hill 1981:pls. 22, 23, 24
Adelson and Takami 1978:44–46
See **387**

aksu (Q.)

Overskirt, half

387

Chuquisaca: Potolo
Quechua
GH 1970s 1980
25" x 21"   (62cm x 52cm)
• *warp*: sheepswool, 2-ply handspun; black overdyed black, deep red, purple, and green; 44 epi (17.5 epc)
• *weft*: alpaca, 2-ply handspun; tan; 15 ppi (6 ppc)
Warp-faced plain weave, warp stripes and 2-color complementary warp weave. One 4-selvedge panel.

Iconography: see 386.
Nothing is known about animal motifs; imagined menagerie (EF).

80–102
Rowe 1977a:76
See **386**

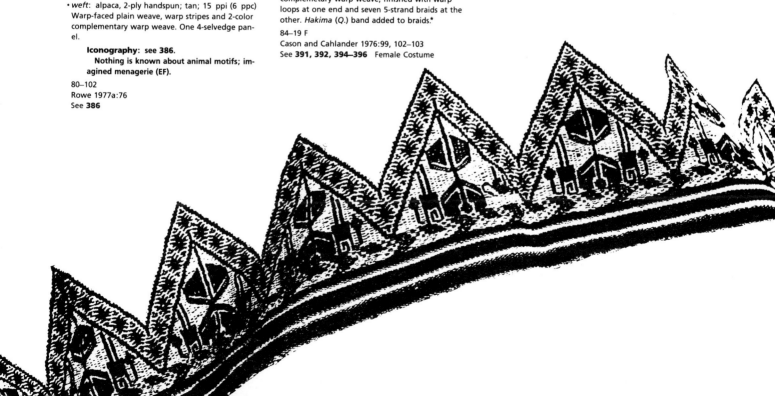

Detail 387

awayo (Q.)

Shawl

388

Chuquisaca: San Lucas
Quechua
GH early 20th cent. 1980
42½" x 33"   (106cm x 82cm)
• *warp*: alpaca, 2-ply handspun; tans and natural dyed red and blue; 75 epi (30 epc)
• *weft*: alpaca, 2-ply handspun; dark brown; 20 ppi (8 ppc)
Warp-faced plain weave, warp stripes, 2-color complementary warp weave. Woven as two 4-selvedge pieces, seamed with decorative zigzag embroidery. Bound with machine-made edging.

Iconography: diamond and zigzag forms.
Uses counter-spinning near side selvedges to prevent curling (AF).

80–99

montera

Hat *

389

Chuquisaca:
Quechua
DH 1950s 1966
17½" x 14"   (44cm x 34cm)
Factory-made black cloth, over a cardboard form. Decorated with beads, sequins, embroidery, metal foil, rickrack, tassels, and coins in geometric, floral, and random designs. Tassel on soft crown includes colored wool yarn, gold-colored metal thread, and coins.

Coins reflect galloping inflation; made in 1956; coins have disappeared, replaced by paper bills. This elaborately decorated hat was worn by Quechuan women near Sucre on festive occasions (DH).

66–4176
See **392**

chumpi (Q.)

Belt

390

Chuquisaca: Tarabuco
Quechua
GH 1980s 1984
61½" x 1½"   (154cm x 4cm)
• *warp*: sheepswool, 2-ply handspun; pink, yellow, green; 16 epi (22 epc)
• *weft*: sheepswool, 2-ply handspun; white; 9 ppi (3.5 ppc)
Warp-faced plain weave and 3-color complementary warp weave, finished with warp loops at one end and seven 5-strand braids at the other. *Hakima* (Q.) band added to braids.*

84–19 F
Cason and Cahlander 1976:99, 102–103
See **391, 392, 394–396** Female Costume

almilla (Q.)

Dress *

391

Chuquisaca : Tarabuco
Quechua
GH 1960s 1984
46" x 25"   (118cm x 63cm)
Treadle-woven bayeta of dyed black sheepswool sewn into long-sleeved dress. Completely covered with black wool embroidery, in a twill-like pattern. Finished with crochet border at sleeves, and plain woven tubular band at hem.

Part of a woman's costume from the town of Candelaria, near Tarabuco. This costume would have been used for special occasions. Acquired in La Paz (GH). The embroidery on this dress, which appears at first glance to be a woven twill pattern, is quite extraordinary. When cloth wears out, women embroider on cloth with twill effect patterns (Frame, pers. com. 1984). Because this dress has a very small neck opening, it must have been made for use by an older woman, as there is no way to nurse a baby (EF). The styling reflects European cut-and-sew tailoring.

84–19 A
Adelson and Takami 1978:19
Meisch 1986
See **390, 392, 394–396** Female Costume

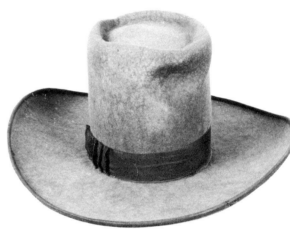

385

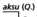

montera

| Hat *

392

    Chuquisaca: Tarabuco
    Quechua
    GH 1930s 1984
17" x 13½" (43cm x 34cm)
See **389**. Date on coin 1939.

84–19 D
See **390, 391, 394–396** Female Costume and **389**

montera

| Hat

393

    Chuquisaca: Tarabuco
    Quechua
    DH 1960s 1966
9" x 8" (23cm x 20.5cm)
Leather, straw, lined with moss, and decorated with ribbon and sequins.

    This style of hat, presumably modeled after the helmet worn by *Conquistadores* is now worn by both sexes in the region of Tarabuco, Bolivia. This example is of excellent quality and was made by a specialist (DH).

66–4046
Wasserman and Hill 1981:16
Adelson and Takami 1978:48–50
Meisch 1986

aksu (Q.)

| Overskirt *

394

    Chuquisaca: Tarabuco
    Quechua
    GH 1970s 1984
37½" x 31" (94cm x 78cm)
• *warp*: sheepswool, 2-ply handspun; cotton, 2-ply machine-spun; multicolored, primarily deep red and black; 45 epi (18 epc)
• *weft*: alpaca, 2-ply handspun; brown; 15 ppi (6 ppc)
Warp-faced plain weave, warp stripes and 2-color complementary warp weave."

    Iconography: horses, llamas, large zigzags. The half with patterning has an internal axis of symmetry, with one central abstract design band, surrounded on either side by an identical band of horse motifs. This weave technique which uses cotton threads and handspun colored wool in the pattern bands is distinctive of Tarabuco (EF, AF).

84–19 C
Wasserman and Hill 1981:16, pl. 28
See **390–392, 395, 396** Female Costume

llijlla (Q.)

| Shawl

395

    Chuquisaca: Tarabuco
    Quechua
    GH 1965 1984
36" x 42½" (92cm x 106cm)
• *warp*: sheepswool, 2-ply handspun; acrylic, cotton, machine-spun; multicolored, primarily deep red; 46 epi (18.5 epc)
• *weft*: alpaca, 2-ply handspun; dark brown; 15 ppi (6 ppc)
Warp-faced plain weave, warp stripes. Woven as two identical 4-selvedge pieces, seamed together with decorative buttonhole embroidery. Bound with tubular warp substitution band.

84–19 B
Cason and Cahlander 1976:129
Meisch 1986
Adelson and Takami 1978:19
See **390–392, 394, 396** Female Costume

llijlla (Q.)

| Shawl

396

    Chuquisaca: Tarabuco
    Quechua
    GH 1970s 1984
34" x 47" (86cm x 120cm)
• *warp*: sheepswool, 2-ply handspun; multicolored, primarily deep red; 56 epi (26 epc)
• *weft*: sheepswool, 2-ply handspun; red; 16 ppi (6 ppc)
Warp-faced plain weave, warp stripes. Woven as two 4-selvedge pieces, seamed together by hand. Bound with tubular warp substitution *ribete*.

84–19 G
See **390–392, 394, 395** Female Costume

sombrero chapaco (DH) *montera*

| Hat, friar style

397

    Tarija: Entrerios
    Guarani
    DH 1960s 1966
3" x 14" (8cm x 35.5cm)
Yellow felt with ribbon band around brim. Trimmed with a ribbon, tasselled cords, and a plastic buckle.

    This style of hat is worn by "Chapaco" women. "Chapacos" are Guarani-speaking tenant farmers and sheepherders. The men wear western dress, women wear urban Andean dress (*polleras*, sweaters, *llijllas* [Q.]) except for this distinctive hat, which may be modelled on a colonial friar's hat (DH).

66–4051

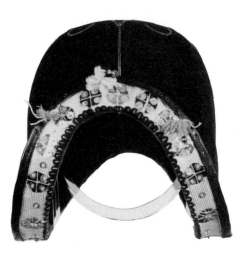

Detail 394

Female Costume 390–392, 394–396

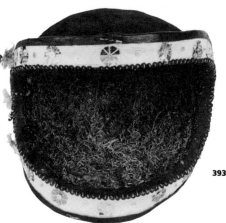

393

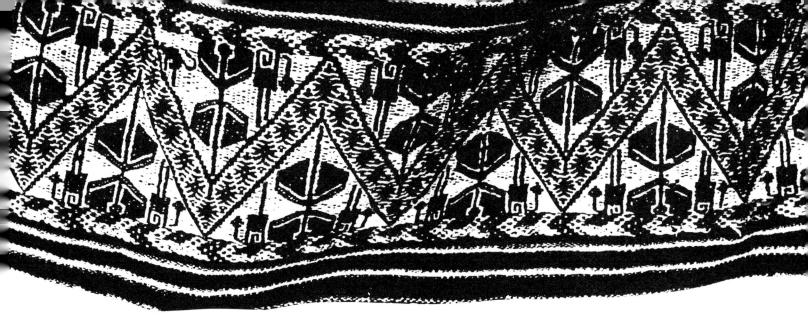

BOLIVIA

EXACT LOCATION UNKNOWN

bolsa

Bag ★

398

Bolivia: Exact location unknown
Quechua/Aymara
DH   1960s   1966
20½" x 19"   (51cm x 48cm)
• *warp*: camelid, 2-ply handspun; tan and brown;
28 epi (11 epc)
• *weft*: camelid, 2-ply handspun; tan; 9 ppi
(3.5 ppc)
Warp-faced plain weave, warp stripes, woven as
one 4-selvedge piece, folded and seamed at sides.

Used to carry small items such as herbs. Similar to a potato sack, but a quarter the size
(DH). Lots of repairs (EF).

66–4262
See **307, 308, 352, 399**

costalito

Bag, market ★

399

Exact location unknown
Quechua/Aymara
DH   1960s   1966
12½" x 9"   (31cm x 23cm)
• *warp*: alpaca, 2-ply handspun; various natural colors; 54 epi (21.6 epc)
• *weft*: alpaca, 2-ply handspun; various natural colors; 12 ppi (5 ppc)
Warp-faced plain weave, warp color patterning,
woven as one 4-selvedge cloth, folded and
seamed at side to make bag.

This miniature potato sack serves the purpose
of pockets, rare in Quechuan and Aymara
clothing. Bags of this sort are carried throughout the highlands (DH).

66–4244
See **307, 308, 352, 398**

blusa

Blouse

400

Exact location unknown
Quechua/Aymara/Spanish
DH   1960s   1966
22½" x 19"   (56cm x 47cm)
Machine-woven orange satin rayon, sewn into
blouse with muslin lining, ornamental embroidery
and smocking.

Satin blouses of this style are found throughout the Andes and are worn by women for
festive occasions and never tucked into skirts.
They are made by specialists and sold in markets (DH).

66–4170
See **246**

blusa

Blouse

401

Exact location unknown
Quechua/Aymara/Spanish
DH   1960s   1966
23" x 18½"   (58cm x 46cm)
Commercial cotton cloth, sewn into blouse with
lace and ribbon decoration.

This blouse is typical of the style worn
throughout the Andes by women. The cotton
cloth, called *imperial*, and decoration are of
exceptional quality (DH).

66–4177

llucho (A.)   *chullo* (Q.)

Cap

402

Exact location unknown
Quechua/Aymara
DH   1960s   1966
13" x 9"   (33cm x 20cm)
sheepswool, 2-ply handspun; beige; 8 spi (3 spc)
Knit: stockinette, rib, garter, and shell stitches,
with complex patterns, knit on straight needles in
the round to create one piece.

Ear flaps were knitted first (IS).

66–4255
See **403, 404**

llucho (A.)   *chullo* (Q.)

Cap

403

Exact location unknown
Quechua/Aymara
DH   1960s   1966
13" x 8"   (33cm x 21cm)
sheepswool, 2-ply handspun; multicolored, solid
areas yellow; 6 spi (2.5 spc)
Knit: stockinette, garter stitches, color patterning.
Ear flaps knitted separately, and knit into main
body of cap. Small tassel at peak. Knit on straight
needles in the round. Single chain crochet around
edge (IS).

Iconography: human figures.
Knit for a baby (DH). The design of the ear
flaps is especially lovely (AF).

66–4281
See **402, 404**

llucho (A.)   *chullo* (Q.)

Cap

404

Exact location unknown
Quechua/Aymara
DH   1960s   1966
13" x 3½"   (33cm x 21cm)
sheepswool, 2-ply handspun; white and blue;
6.5 spi (2.5 spc)
Knit: stockinette and garter stitch, color striping.
Knit on straight needles, flaps knit from stitches
picked up off cap. Edge finished with crochet
stitch in blue yarn. Added tassel (IS).

Knit for a school boy in his school's colors
(DH).

66–4282
See **402, 403**

pasamontaña

Cap, face

405

Exact location unknown
Quechua/Aymara
DH   1960s   1966
12" x 8½"   (31cm x 22.5cm)
alpaca, 2-ply handspun; brown; 8.5 spi (3.5 spc)
Knit: straight needles, stockinette and garter
stitches, color patterning in black alpaca (IS).

Worn by Quechuan and Aymara men in highlands, where nights are bitter cold. Knitted
by women (DH). A virtuoso knitting feat.★

66–4022 A
See **406**

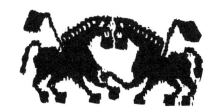

pasamontaña

Cap, face

406

Exact location unknown
Quechua/Aymara
DH 1960s 1966
15" x 7½"   (38cm x 18cm)
sheepswool, 2-ply handspun; brown; 4.5 spi
(2 spc)
Knit: straight needles, garter and ribbing stitches
(IS).
66–4022 B
See **405**

cinturon guaguita   wat'ana (Q.)

Cloth, swaddling

407

Exact location unknown
Quechua
DH 1960s 1966
106" x 4½"   (265cm x 11.5cm)
• *warp*: sheepswool, 2-ply handspun; white; 23 epi
(9 epc)
• *weft*: sheepswool, 2-ply handspun; white; 7 ppi
(3 ppc)
Warp-faced plain weave, warp ends formed into
twisted fringe.

Long strip used to bind Quechuan babies.
Swaddling is thought to make children grow
up "tall, strong, and industrious" and failure
to do so "explains" why others grow up
weak and lazy. Sash is woven by mother in
the last month of pregnancy, and the second
of twins may be abandoned because "he
couldn't turn out right without a swaddling
cloth" (DH). It is intended for first child (EF).

66–4265

Collar, llama

408

Exact location unknown
Quechua
GH 1960s 1984
26½" x 1"   (66cm x 3cm)
• *warp*: llama, 2-ply handspun; white and brown;
7 epi (3 epc)
• *weft*: llama, 2-ply handspun; tan; 8 ppi (3 ppc)
Crossed-warp weave collar band. Ends finished as
long 4-strand braids. Button constructed out of
knotted yarn.

Used to decorate llamas during festivals. Usually these collars have a bell (GH).

84–20
Cahlander 1980:16, pl. 15

aksu (Q.)

Overskirt

409

Exact location unknown.
Quechua/Aymara
GH late 19th cent. 1980
43½" x 51½"   (109cm x 129cm)
• *warp*: alpaca, 2-ply handspun; black, and natural
dyed multicolored; 50 epi (20 epc)
• *weft*: alpaca, 2-ply handspun; dark brown;
22.5 ppi (9 ppc)
Warp-faced plain weave, warp stripes and 3-color
complementary warp weave. Woven as 2 different
panels, one with complementary warp patterning,
the other with only warp striping, sewn together
by hand. Bound with plain woven indigo dyed
band.

Iconography: design areas called *chuupi pallay (Q.)* (EF).

Aksus typically are not symmetrical as are
llijllas (Q.) and *awayos (Q.)*, but instead, like
this one, have two different halves. They are
worn folded with the warp horizontal (AF).

80–85

guardaplata

Purse, coin

410

Exact location unknown
Quechua/Aymara
DH 1960s 1966
12" x 7"   (30cm x 18cm)
sheepswool, 2-ply handspun; black, tan, white;
7 spi (3 spc)
Knit: stockinette and garter stitches, color patterning, 2 large pockets on each side knit separately
and attatched. Tassels of single sheepswool sewn
on.

Iconography: human and animal forms,
stars, geometrics.
Small bags are carried tucked in the waistband or belt by women throughout the
Andes to carry small items since traditional
clothing does not have pockets (DH). This bag
may be from the Puno area, as a similar one
was purchased there in 1985.

66–4256
See **256, 299, 327**

rebozo

Shawl

411

Exact location unknown
Aymara/Spanish
DH 1960s 1966
62" x 33½"   (155cm x 84cm)
• *warp*: alpaca, 2-ply machine-spun; deep blue;
20 epi (8 epc)
• *weft*: alpaca, 2-ply machine-spun; deep purple;
22 ppi (9 ppc)
Machine made of *castillo* cloth; twill weave,
brushed to create a deep nap on one side. Bound
with matching machine-woven band.

This is an extremely luxurious factory-made
shawl. It would have been worn either by an
urban Andean, or wealthy Aymara woman.
The *Chola* retains the Indian style of dress (in
terms of shape and combination of items of
clothing) but generally uses finer materials,
i.e velvets, satins, *castillo* cloth, instead of
handspun and woven wool (DH).

66–4203

pollera

Skirt

412

Exact location unknown
Quechua/Aymara
DH 1960s 1966
30" x 78"   (75cm x 200cm)
• *warp*: sheepswool, single handspun; orange;
20 epi (8 epc)
• *weft*: sheepswool, single handspun; orange;
20 ppi (8 ppc)
Balanced warp-faced plain weave woven on a
treadle loom (*bayeta*) gathered into a full skirt
with 3 tucks. Hemmed with cotton twill tape, and
smocked at waistband.

This is a well-made example of the full skirts
worn layered one on top of the other, by
both Quechuan and Aymara women throughout the Andean highlands (DH,AF).

66–4187
See **325, 413**

pollera

Skirt

413

Exact location unknown
Quechua/Aymara
DH 1960s 1966
28½" x 76"   (73cm x 194cm)
• *warp*: sheepswool, single handspun; yellow;
16 epi (6.5 epc)
• *weft*: sheepswool, single handspun; yellow;
14 ppi (5.5 ppc)
Balanced plain weave, woven on a treadle loom
(*bayeta*) and sewn into a full gathered skirt.

66–4260
See **325, 412**

Skirt, half

414

Exact location unknown
Aymara
DH 1960s 1965–66
22½" x 76"   (57cm x 194cm)
• *warp*: sheepswool, single handspun; yellow;
20 epi (8 epc)
• *weft*: sheepswool, single handspun; yellow;
20 ppi (8 ppc)
Balanced plain weave woven on a treadle loom,
sewn into gathered skirt with factory-made cotton
cloth top. Decorated with rows of tucks.

Full width half-skirts such as this one are
worn by Aymara women under an outer skirt
of similar cut, except all wool; the cotton upper portion is a significant economy on use of
the more valuable wool (DH).

66–4037
See **248, 415**

Skirt, half

415

Exact location unknown
Aymara
DH 1960s 1966
23½" x 79"   (60cm x 200cm)
• *warp*: sheepswool, single handspun; orange;
20 epi (8 epc)
• *weft*: sheepswool, single handspun; orange;
20 ppi (8 ppc)
Balanced plain weave, woven on a treadle loom
gathered into panel made from a flour sack. Decorated with horizontal tucks and lined with flour
sacking.

In 1985 yardage for skirts included floral cotton and velveteen.

66–4038
See **248, 414**

Spindle

416

Exact location unknown
Quechua/Aymara
DH 1960s 66
13¾" x ½"   (35cm x 0.8cm)
Hand-held spindle, lathe-turned wooden whorl
with some alpaca yarn on it.
66–4023

pantalón

Trousers

417

Exact location unknown
Quechua/Aymara
DH 1960s 1966
39½" x 12½"   (99cm x 31cm)
• *warp*: sheepswool, single handspun; tan; 27 epi
(11 epc)
• *weft*: sheepswool, single handspun; tan; 19 ppi
(7.5 ppc)
Balanced twill woven on a treadle loom, cut and
tailored into trousers. Machine-stitched.

Trousers made of coarse handspun wool such
as these used to be worn throughout the
Andes by Quechuan and Aymara men. This
piece is unusual in having belt loops (DH).

66–4205

408

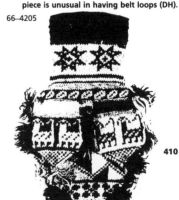

410

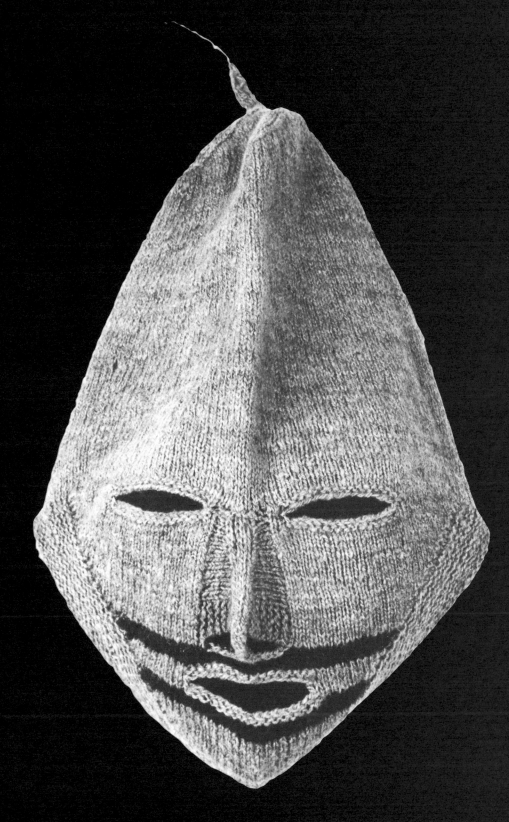

405

chuspa (Q.)

| Bag, coca

418

Exact location unknown
Quechua/Aymara
Museum purchase   mid 20th cent.   1980
4½" x 5"   (11.5cm x 12cm)
• *warp*: sheepswool and alpaca, 2-ply handspun; reds and purples; 24 epc (9.6 epc)
• *weft*: alpaca, 2-ply handspun; brown; 8 ppi (3 ppc)
Warp-faced plain weave, warp stripes and 3-color complementary warp weave. Woven as one 4-selvedge cloth, folded and seamed to make bag. Bound with tubular band with applied fringe. The complementary warp weave strap, made of synthetic yarn, was probably added at the sale of the bag to replace the original, either missing or broken.

Iconography: *hayka sisan* (Q.) or fertile flowers; strap, *tanka ch'oro* or forked diagonal (EF).

Although faded, this is a nice example of the complex double sided 3-color complementary warp weave (AF).

80–103

chaqueta

| Jacket

419

Exact location unknown
Quechua/Aymara
DH   1960s   1966
19" x 17½"   (49cm x 44cm)
Factory-made acrylic velvet, appliqued and embroidered with brightly colored yarn.

Part of dance costume worn by *Misti* dancers, men who burlesque actions of white men in dances during Carnival. Unlike other kinds of Aymara dancers, they do not perform in a troupe or follow any strict pattern of steps, rather they improvise as clowns on the sidelines while troupes of other dancers perform ceremonially. Elaborate embroidery portrays peacocks and eagles, as well as more abstract designs. Wire-mesh mask of white men and similarly embroidered trousers complete the costume (DH). *Misti* refers to Mestizo-Spanish culture people (EF).

66–4044
See **422**

awayo (Q.) *k'eparina* (Q.)

| Cloth, carrying

420

Exact location unknown
Quechua/Aymara
DH   1960s   1966
48½" x 50½"   (123cm x 128cm)
• *warp*: cotton, acrylic, 2-ply machine-spun; multicolored, primarily red; 36 epi (14.5 epc)
• *weft*: cotton, 2-ply machine-spun, red; 23 ppi (9 ppc)
Warp-faced plain weave and simple complementary-warp weave, woven on a treadle loom. Warp stripes.

This type of cotton carrying cloth, woven on a European-style floor loom, is typically used by urban Andeans (DH). It was probably woven by a professional weaver (EF).

66–4039
See **243, 244, 245**

hakima (Q.)

| Tie

421

Exact location unknown
Quechua/Aymara
unknown source
41" x ½"   (104cm x 1cm)
• *warp*: sheepswool, 2-ply machine-spun; multicolored; 24 epi (9.5 epc)
• *weft*: sheepswool, 2-ply, machine-spun, tan; 9 ppi (3.5 ppc)
Warp-faced plain weave, warp striping to create vertical and horizontal stripes, 2-color complementary-warp weave. Three *hakimas* (Q.) woven separately and sewn together by hand. Tassels added to finished *hakima* (Q.).

62–825

pantalón

| Trousers

422

Exact location unknown
Quechua/Aymara
DH   1960s   1966
34½" x 26"   (86cm x 65cm)
See **419**

66–4045

COSTUME AS COMMUNICATION: ANDEAN CATALOG SECTION ADDENDUM:*

After the Symposium, Costume as Communication, held at the Haffenreffer Museum in March, 1987, Lynn Meisch, Elayne Zorn, and Mary Ann Medlin added information and corrections to the catalog citations. We are grateful for their expertise and include their comments in the following addendum. An * has been placed within the citation to direct the reader to this section.

327. *monedero.*

330. In Bolivia the distinctions between neighboring groups are frequently very subtle and hard for outsiders to recognize, but residents of a general area can instantly recognize the particular *ayllu* (clan group) or hamlet of a person by fine details of his or her costumes such as certain motifs, techniques, layouts, colors, and combinations of these (Lynn Meisch).

332. *capachu* (Q. and A.).

335. *urku* (Q.), literally mountain.

345. *phullu* (Q. and A.).

357. *phullu* (Q. and A.).

359. Also supplementary warp weave. The loom bars are usually lashed to two vertical poles which are leaned against the wall at an angle (Lynn Meisch).

367. *Kunka* (neck) *unku* (tunic); a tiny poncho-like garment derived from the Inca worn over the shoulders for daily use by the Quechuan men of the Tarabuco region (Lynn Meisch).

368. Lynn Meisch and Elayne Zorn agree that they have only seen these *chalinas* or *bufadas* worn over the shoulder or around the neck as a scarf-like garment by a *jilicata* or Aymara leader.

371. San Lucas.

373. *Boliviano,* flag-colored poncho.

374. *panti listado* poncho; wine-colored poncho.

378. Not unlike those worn in Calcha but undeniably Tarabuco because of its colors (yellow, orange, red) and their sequence (Lynn Meisch).

389. *Quilla* (Q.), moon hat, from Tarabuco.

390. Bands also called *watu* (Q.).

391. *K'inku* (Q.) *almilla* (A.), dress with zig-zags; also people embroider brand new *almillas* simply for decorative effect (Lynn Meisch).

392. *Quilla* (Q.), moon hat.

394. Half *aksu* (Q.); a complete *aksu* consists of two four-selvedge panels joined together at the black, plain weave sections. This piece consists of one four-selvedge panel which has a plain weave section and a *pallay* section (Lynn Meisch).

398. *Wayakata* (Q.), *wayaka* or *tolega* (S.).

399. The same as 398.

405. For fiestas (Lynn Meisch).

Appendix

The Use of Costume and Textiles in the Haffenreffer Museum of Anthropology Education Program

by Barbara A. Hail

As a museum of anthropology, the Haffenreffer Museum follows a distinct philosophy in the use of its collections for education. Our goal is to interpret human cultures worldwide in a way that excites the imagination of young people. Through our experiential education programs, geared to elementary school-age children, we recreate the lifeways of other peoples and other times. We emphasize the basic similarities in all humans: everyone needs love, a home, and a family; everyone needs enough to eat, clothing for warmth and protection, an opportunity to be useful within the society, and an opportunity to create and enjoy other people's creations of beautiful things.

In order to explain the wide diversity of material culture that has been produced among different peoples, we discuss the many avenues that people have explored for meeting these basic human needs, and the differing cultural preferences and living patterns which have resulted from the unfolding of history and from the resource capabilities of each environment.

In interpreting the culture of the native people of Middle America and the Central Andes of South America, the Museum's education department has selected specific moments in time as settings for the programs. For the study of Andean culture, our program is set in the Inca period at the time of contact with the Spanish, around 1532. Contrastingly, in Middle America, the Museum's interpretation is of present-day life of various cultural groups, including *Mestizos*, indigenous peoples, and Spanish Americans.

The format of the programs follows a general pattern. School classes of about thirty chidren each, representing grades 3–6, reserve in advance for their morning at the Museum. Upon entering the Education Annex they are welcomed by docents wearing costume replications representative of the culture under study, and the children are each given a costume or partial costume to wear. A general activity, usually dancing to drum, flute, or taped music, helps to relax the children and open their minds to an unselfconscious involvement in another culture. All adults present – docents, teachers, and parents – dance with the children so that there will be no division of participants vs. observers. In the Middle American program one young couple dressed in the costume of the *Jerabe Tapatio*, (see fig. 33) dances around a very large *sombrero* placed on the ground. This serves as an opportunity for docents to explain the history of the costume and to get the children into the spirit of role-playing in the day's drama. Background information is provided by means of a slide presentation. This is followed by a division into smaller groups, each under the charge of a docent who takes the groups to separate learning centers: (1) a simulated household unit; (2) an area in which economic subsistence is explained, and farming tools, hunting weapons, cloth-making equipment, and the like are demonstrated; (3) the Museum proper, to view the formal exhibits on the Central Andes or Middle America. The groups reassemble for a craft activity during which the children make something to take home. This helps later in recalling the museum experience in the classroom. Finally, indigenous games and festival activities bring the programs to an exciting climax.

Middle America

In the Middle American program, after the entire class dances the *Jerabe Tapatio* they are divided into two groups. One enters the Museum for a guided tour of the Middle American exhibits which include both modern Mexican and Guatemalan costumes and articles of daily use, and pre-Columbian sculpture and ornaments. They move on to a hands-on display area for supervised handling of everyday objects and for a question-and-answer period.

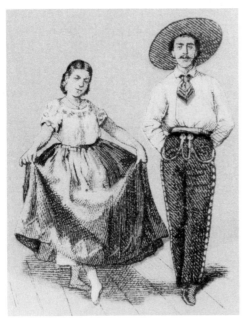

Fig. 33
Jerabe Tapatio. Plate by Antonio Garcia Cubas. 1876. Courtesy of the John Hay Library, Brown University, Church Collection.

The second group visits a walled patio outside of the education activity room, in which an open air market has been set up, with a canopy and tables. The children play-act at bargaining for items, handling clothing and other objects "for sale," exchanging Mexican coinage and purchasing foodstuffs, woven articles, household and farming equipment. There is also a food corner in which they prepare a chocolate drink, grind *masa* on a *metate* with a *mano*, cook tortillas on a *comal*, and grind garlic and chili peppers in a stone mortar with a pestle.

All of the children make a "god's eye" of yarn and sticks to take home. The day ends with the class gathering around a tree-hung *piñata*, hitting it with a stick, and joyously sharing the wrapped hard candy which falls to the ground.

The costumes which are used in this program are of wide variety, representing a range from the Tarahumara of the north to the *Mestizo* peoples of Chalco, Mexico, to the Guatemalan highland wear of the Maya. Fiesta dress is featured, such as the *China Poblana* costume of Mexico. Hats in a variety of styles representing different villages are passed around and tried on by the children.

An effort is made to identify both native traditional clothing styles derived from the past and European introductions since the time of the Spanish Conquest. The introduction of domestic animals, such as sheep, and the changes this caused in clothing materials and styles is emphasized. Also discussed is the mountainous terrain, which isolates and insulates many of the indigenous peoples living in Mexico from one another and reinforces traditional custom and costume.

The Central Andes

The educational focus reflects both the Museum's archaeological and ethnographic collections. As Franquemont has discussed (VI), weaving is an ancient and still vital art in the Andes. Great imagination in the use of every known kind of weaving technique, combined with vivid colors and complex designs, created changing styles throughout the long history of Andean clothmaking. Thus, although the education program time period is 1532, a base is established for the development of weaving since that time, and the ethnographic collection of the Museum can be interpreted as a recent phase in the evolution of Andean style and technique. For instance, it is pointed out that during the Inca Empire everyone was required to wear headgear and clothing that designated a person's rank and home village, or *ayllu*, so that the officials of government could identify the movement of populations. Even today, Andean people carry on the tradition of wearing colorful hats, shoulder cloths, and ponchos which are unique to specific villages or locales.

Cloth was of economic importance. Newly married couples within the Inca state system were given gifts of clothing and headbands (*llautu*); the latter were tailored to indicate rank. Each household of a comman man (*puric*) was expected to produce some woven cloth for the common storehouse; as with the stored common grain, these goods were redistributed by the government to those who were most needy during years of want.

The honored position of weavers during Inca times is emphasized through the example of the "chosen women," or "daughters of the Sun." These young women, selected from the ordinary population of the *ayllus* for their intelligence and grace, were brought to convents throughout the empire. They processed alpaca and vicuña wool, and wove garments for his royal highness, the Inca, as well as for his family and the court nobility. Such a young woman might serve for several years in a kind of religious and state seclusion, and then be chosen as wife for a member of the nobility or for a high-ranking military man. Thus, clothmaking figures as a means of social mobility within a basically static society.

The important role of cloth in the Inca Empire is made clear through role-playing and play-acting. The use of costume in the education program may be considered as an extension of Barthes' categories (1983:3–5) as discussed earlier by Schevill, by adding to "image," "written," and "real," a fourth division – "trans-formational." For example, the child dressed as a "chosen woman" in the

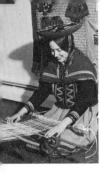

Fig. 34
Docent dressed in contemporary Cuzco costume demonstrating weaving on a backstrap loom. Haffenreffer Museum Photo Archives.

Inca Temple of the Sun truly becomes one for the period of the class and in her memory of the day's experience long afterward. Other role-playing activities might include the characters of the "Inca" or ruler, his sister-wife, the high priest of the Sun, newlywed couples from common or *puric* families, or a government courier or *chasqui*, carrier of the knotted records or *quipus*.

Actual recent ethnographic costumes are worn by both docents and students in addition to replications of pre-Columbian costumes. The Museum's acquisitions policy includes funds for costumes that can be worn, touched, and enjoyed as one's regular clothing, not as one "appreciates" a museum costume. Among these "touchable" objects are recently woven and knitted wool ponchos, as well as full costumes including hat, jacket, skirt, and shawl (277, 280, 287, 286). Also purchased "for touch" are knitted dolls (309–311) and embroidered *biyettas* (257–262). These are made by Quechuan children and depict scenes of everyday life such as ploughing, religious processions, school, home, church, and also mythic events.

Demonstrations of clothmaking techniques are performed by volunteer museum docents (see fig. 34). Children are instructed in carding, spinning with a drop spindle, and weaving. A typical Andean backstrap loom is demonstrated. Braiding is explained and each child is given a small hank of prepared yarn to try their hand at this craft. Very popular is the instruction in weaving on a toe-loom. The students take off their shoes and socks and attach one end of the loom around their big toe and the other end around their waists, using their body for tension while they weave. Each child makes for himself a narrow decorative band or *hakima* such as was used to ornament hats, jackets, and skirts in Colonial times (see fig. 35).

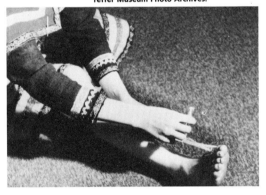

Fig. 35
Docent demonstrating the toe loom. Haffenreffer Museum Photo Archives.

Children love this activity. Its lessons are twofold: (1) in other times and places people have learned to use their own bodies as tools — that is, the foot braced against the hands and arms to create the proper tension for weaving — so that they can work without benefit of other equipment; (2) in other times and places even small children were economically productive in the manufacture of necessities such as cloth.

Summary

This experiential education program has been in existence for seventeen years. Through it, thousands of Rhode Island schoolchildren have been introduced to the life-styles, customs, and beliefs of people other than themselves, through donning their costumes, tasting their foods, learning their craft skills, and playing their games. The program has created a deep impression on the participants. As one child reported to us by letter, "After I was dressed up in that beautiful skirt I really wished I could be a little Mexican girl." Former students return to the Museum as adults, looking again for the excitement of cultures recreated. One of the current graduate students in the Department of Anthropology stated in her application to Brown University that her interest in anthropology as a career was initiated as a result of her experiences in the Museum's educational programs in elementary school. This was indeed proof that costume and cloth, through their use in the Museum's education programs as an aid to role-playing, have had affective as well as communicative powers which have vividly enhanced anthropological learning.

Among the textiles used in the Andean and Middle American education programs which are described in this catalogue are the following:

1. saddle bag for carrying loads of coca leaves or fruits on a mule (**352**)
2. hat (**277**), skirt (**287**), jacket (**280**), shawl (**286**) for ten-year-old Quechuan girl; jacket (**279**), shawl (**285**), skirt (**289**) for Quechuan woman; vest (**290**) for Quechuan man
3. ponchos (**282, 360**)
4. dolls, animals, knitted (**319–321**)
5. *biyettas*, woven and embroidered (**257–262**)
6. coca bags (**298, 304**)
7. braided sling (**253**)
8. "Pizarro helmet" (**393**)
9. fiesta jacket (**419**) and trousers (**422**)
10. male and female costumes of Sololá, Guatemala (**175, 179–182, 185, 187** male; **177, 178, 184, 188** female)
11. *China Poblana* costume of Mexico (**21–24**)

Glossary

The following definitions have been gleaned from sources listed in the Bibliography. Unless otherwise indicated, italicized words are in Spanish. Abbreviations are as follows: Q., Quechua; A., Aymara; Q.M., Quiché Maya; N., Nahuatl; T., Tzotzil.

Agave A species of monocotyledonous plants with fibrous leaves; includes several varieties producing fibers with either smooth or harsh, prickly characteristics.

Aksu (*Q.*) Woman's wrap skirt.

Alforjas Woven saddle bags.

Almilla (*Q.*) Shirt worn by men and women, also a dress.

Alpaca Domesticated animal, native to the Andes, with long and lustrous hair used for weaving cloth; member of the camelid family.

Appliqué A technique for decorating cloth by stitching pieces of cut and shaped material onto the ground fabric.

Artisela Artificial silk.

Atole A corn drink used to stiffen warp threads.

Awana (*Q.*) A loom.

Awasqa (*Q.*) The median level cloth woven by Inca commoners for their own daily clothing, probably warp-patterned cloth.

Awayo (*Q.*) Term used in Bolivia for a woman's shoulder wrap and/or a carrying cloth for food, babies, or firewood. See *llijlla*.

Ayllu (*Q.*) A social unit within a town or village, formed by geographic and geneological rules.

Backstrap loom A weaving apparatus with a continuous warp supported by two bars; a front bar tied to a support, and a back bar attached to a strap around the weaver's waist. Tension is controlled by the movement backward or forward of the weaver's body.

Balanced plain weave The equal spacing of either identical or approximately equal warp and weft yarns in size and flexibility.

Bast The stem fibers of dicotyledonous plants, such as *apocynum* and milkweed, also fibers extracted from beneath the bark of certain shrubs or trees such as willow.

Bayeta Yardage woven on European treadle looms by Quechuan and Aymara men.

Beat The movement of forcibly pressing the last-inserted shot of weft into position before passing the next shot of weft in a newly-formed shed. Most often done with a batten or sword.

Belt loom A smaller version of a backstrap or staked loom used for producing narrow textiles.

Biyetta A term used to describe embroidered *bayeta* cloths.

Blusa A European-style blouse.

Bolsa A bag or shoulder bag.

Bordado Embroidery.

Brocado A term used for supplementary weft brocading on a backstrap loom, sometimes confused with *bordado*.

Camelid Any of several South American animals related to the camel, but without a hump: alpaca, llama, vicuña, guanaco.

Camisa Shirt worn by men and women, European style.

Capacho A large bag used to carry almost anything.

Capixay An element of male costume used in Middle America; a long overgarment resembling a cape or tunic, sometimes with sleeves.

Cargador A large cloth used to carry children, firewood, and other material.

Ccahua (*A.*) Man's tunic constructed from a one-piece cloth which is folded in half and sewn up the sides, leaving openings for the arms at the top and an opening in the middle for the head. See *unkhu*.

Cinchon Girth for pack mule.

Cinta A narrow belt or hair ribbon.

Cinturon guaguito walt'ana (*Q.*) A combination of Spanish and Quechuan terms used to describe a swaddling cloth.

Coca (*A.* & *Q.*) The plant, *Erythroxylon coca*, E.; the leaf is chewed daily by Andean Indians and is an important element in social and ceremonial life.

Cochineal An insect which lives on the back of the cacti *Opuntia* and *Nopalea* and which is used to obtain a vast range of red dyes; used throughout Middle America and the Central Andes in the nineteenth and early twentieth centuries.

Cofradia Religious organization requiring special costume and accessories.

Colera A short tunic or *ehuatl*.

Comal Flat skillet for cooking.

Complementary-warp weave A compound fabric structure with two sets of warp (interlacing with the weft) that are complementary to each other. The two sets of elements play equivalent and reciprocal parts on each face of the fabric. The weave is double-faced with complementary sets of warp. Two and three colors can be utilized.

Corte A wraparound skirt.

Costal An all-purpose bag, woven in many sizes;

costalito refers to a small version.

Cotón A man's jacket, cut in the European manner; also refers to a woman's underblouse.

Counter-spinning S- and Z-spun threads are placed side by side as warp; when woven a subtle herringbone effect is created.

Crochet A single-element technique in which a single hooked needle is used to interloop the yarn vertically and horizontally through two previously made loops.

Crossing The movement of an element or group of elements across a textile, as a step in upward braiding; warps can be crossed to create tubes as in slings.

Cuyuscate Tawny, brown cotton, native to Guatemala; also called *ixcaco*.

Chaleco Man's vest, worn on fiestas.

Chalina A shawl, also called *rebozo* or *perraje*. In the Andes it refers to a neck scarf worn by headmen.

Chamarro Short tunic, open on the sides like an *ehuatl*.

Chaqueta A man's jacket, European style.

Chola An urban Andean.

Chullo (*Q.*) Man's knit earflap hat.

Chumpi (*Q.*) A belt, worn by men and women; varies in length, width, and motifs.

Chuspa (*Q.*) Pouch for *coca* leaves, carried by virtually all Indian men.

Delantal An apron, European-style.

Departamento A term used for state in Middle America and the Central Andes.

Double cloth A compound fabric in which the two separate weave structures (usually plain weave) are interconnected only where they exchange faces.

Double-faced Term used for compound weaves whose faces are structurally identical, as contrasted with two or single faced.

Dralon Term used for synthetic yarn in the Central Andes.

Draw loom A treadle loom with extra harnesses which allow for lifting groups of warps separately from other warps and for lifting them in any order required for a design.

Eccentric weft weave A pattern created by

wefts that deviate from the horizontal and from their normal right-angled relation to the warps; achieved by the use of tapestry technique.

Ehuatl (*N.*) A tunic; a pre-Columbian dress form; see *chamarro* and *colera* and *unkhu*.

Enagua Women's skirt with waistband of European origin.

Encomienda System whereby Indians were entrusted after the Conquest to Spanish settlers, or *encomenderos.*

Estera y rodera Pad and crupper for a pack animal.

Faja Wide belt used by men and women.

Falda See *corte.*

Falseria See draw loom.

Finca A large farm, ranch, or plantation.

Float A warp or weft thread which passes over or under more than two threads of the opposite element.

Frazada A blanket.

Frame loom A simple loom in which the loom bars are secured to a wooden frame in any of a variety of shapes.

Gabán Small *sarape* with head opening for men.

Gauze weave One in which the odd-numbered warps are crossed over the even numbered warps and held in this position by a passage of the weft, thus creating a line of openwork.

Golon A strip of complex balanced weave used as a trim for Andean costume.

Gorra A baby's cap.

Ground weave Any weave, but usually plain weave, on which supplementary warps and/or wefts float to provide a pattern.

Guardaplata A woman's purse.

Hakima A narrow strip of cloth used as a strap or for tying.

Heading cord One that is inserted in the end-loops of the warp. The loom bar is then lashed to this cord, rather than to the warps, making possible a 4-selvedge textile.

Heddle The device used to lift chosen warp threads together, in order to produce the shed, or space for the weft to pass through.

Heddle stick or rod One with heddle loops attached and used when a warp is too wide or closely spaced for it to be practical to use the loops bound together in a bunch.

Herringbone pattern A type of weave with zig-zag lines running horizontally from side to side of the cloth.

Honda A sling. See *waraka.*

Horizontal ground loom One that is staked-out in the ground with four posts; warp bars are

bound near the top of the stakes; warps are fastened to a heading cord and then to the warp bars; string heddles are attached.

Huata (*Q.*) Hair tie.

Huipil A blouse made of rectangular pieces of backstrap- or treadle-loomed cloth without sleeves.

Ikat A word of Malay origin; describes a method of resist or tie-dyeing done by binding warps or wefts at designated intervals then immersing them in dye. When bindings are removed, patterns result from areas of yarns not penetrated by dye. Four kinds of ikat patternings are possible: warp, weft, double, and complex.

Indigo A dark-blue dye obtained from plants of the *indigofera* genus.

Ixtle A plant with fibrous leaves of the agave species.

Jabón A waist length jacket.

Jacquard loom A mechanized weaving apparatus; patterning is controlled by a series of punched cards that succeed one another with each treadling.

Jaspe Warp and weft yarns dyed using ikat techniques. See ikat.

Jaspeado Cloth woven with ikat patterns. See ikat.

Jerga Broken twill weave.

Jilacata (*A.*) Headman.

Joronga See *gabán.*

Kelim Slits or openings created by discontinuous wefts.

K'eparina (*Q.*) An all-purpose carrying cloth.

Knitting An interlooping technique using a single element in a series of loops. Pointed rods or needles are utilized.

Ladino, Ladina A Guatemalan person of mixed Indian and Spanish ancestry who does not belong to one of the indigenous cultural groups. See *Mestizo.*

Loom bar One of the two bars of the simple two-bar loom, such as the backstrap or horizontal loom, between which the continuous warp is stretched.

Lustrina Mercerized cotton embroidery yarn having shinier texture and more brilliant colors than ordinary mercerized cotton yarn.

Llacota (*A.*) In pre-Columbian times and through the nineteenth century, a man's mantle; presently said to be worn by women.

Llajqa (*A.*) A baby blanket.

Llama A member of the camelid family, see camelid.

Llautu (*Q.*) A term used in Inca times for headband.

Llijlla (*Q.*) See *awayo.*

Lloq'e (*Q.*) S-twist yarn; meaning left; associated with magical practices.

Llucho (*A.*) See *chullo.*

Macramé Fringe or trimming of knotted thread.

Mankancha (*A.*) An underskirt; a woolen half-skirt.

Mano Tool for grinding.

Manta A shawl.

Masa Tortilla dough.

Mestizo See *Ladino.* Term used in Mexico, Peru, and Bolivia.

Metate A stone used for grinding.

Milpa A field used to grow corn, beans, and squash.

Mish A Guatemalan brand of mercerized cotton esteemed by weavers for its strength, fine color, and low cost.

Misti A term for *Mestizo.*

Montera A hat worn by both men and women.

Morga A type of wraparound skirt; see *corte.*

Muñeca Doll.

Multiloop heddle A group of heddles tied together without a stick to support them.

Nagua See *corte.*

Ñawi (*Q.*) Eye; used to describe the dots of opposite color that appear in a complementary float weave.

Oblique loom A frame loom used in a semivertical position in Bolivia; similar to the horizontal ground loom but the loom bars are lashed to two long poles and propped against a roof, wall, or ceiling beam.

Off-loom Those techniques such as knitting, netting, or twining that don't require a loom.

Open weave See gauze weave.

Overdyed A process of redyeing a natural or already dyed textile in the same color; i.e. black overdyed black.

Pallay (*Q.*) To pick up; either an object, or threads to create warp patterns.

Pampa A plain, or an empty, unoccupied space. Also refers to areas of single color plain weave in textiles.

Pantalónes Men's knee or full-length pants.

Pasamontaña Means literally to pass the montain; a face cap.

Pepenado A supplementary weft brocading pattern used in Guatemalan weaving.

Pepita See *pepenado.*

Perraje A shawl.

Phullu (*A.*) A rectangular woman's shoulder cloth, usually worn over an *awayo.*

Pick A term for wefts per inch or centimeter.

Pica-pica A knitting stitch used in casting on for caps.

Pickup Use of fingers or a pickup stick to select warps or wefts for a pattern.

Pickup stick A small pointed stick used to aid in picking up warp or weft yarns; could be made of bone or wood.

Plain weave The simplest possible interlacing of warp and weft in unvarying alternation, over and under. It may be balanced, warp-faced, or weft-faced.

Ply A verb meaning to twist; in 2-ply, two single threads have been twisted together.

Poc (*T.*) Head or shoulder cloth.

Pollera A full gathered skirt.

Poncho Square or rectangular overgarment worn by men, usually consisting of two pieces of hand-woven cloth sewn together with a slit in the center for the head.

Ponchito A small poncho; see *rodillera*.

Pot (*Q.M.*) See *huipil*.

Puric (*Q.*) Common person

Q'ompi (*Q.*) Pre-Columbian tapestry woven cloth.

Quechquémitl (*N.*) Woman's cape-like shoulder garment; a pre-Columbian dress form survival.

Quipu (*Q.*) A device used for calculations.

Quetzal (*N.*) A bird with iridescent green plumage and long tail feathers; the national symbol of Guatemala; also a unit of national currency.

Randa A hand-stitched joining with embroidery yarn of two pieces of cloth.

Rebozo See *perraje*.

Ribbon loom A four-harness counterbalance treadle loom with a backstrap apparatus used for making belts.

Ribete A tubular edging used to trim *llijillas*, *ponchos*, *unkhuñas*, and *aksus*.

Rigid heddle loom Also known as the hole and slot heddle; used in a backstrap arrangement; warps are threaded in the holes of the heddle set in the reed; slot threads are free to slide up and down; the rigid heddle reed is also used as a beater.

Rodillera A woolen blanket that men wear over their trousers; also called a *poncho*; a pre-Columbian dress survival.

S-twist yarn Composed of two or more plies that are twisted together so as to trend in the same direction as the diagonal center bar of the letter S when the yarn is held in vertical position.

Saco Tailored jacket worn by women.

Sarape A blanket, often with an opening for the head.

Seda Silk.

Sedalina Silk-like yarn; pearl cotton with a high gloss due to heavy mercerizing.

Selvedge The self-finished edge of a fabric, formed by the threads of one element turning around the thread of the other element.

Servilleta A multi-purpose cloth.

Sett Weaver's term for warp and weft count.

Shed The space created by separating the warp into two parts: one part to lie over and one part to lie under the weft.

Shedding device Any of various devices used to separate warps to make a shed such as a rigid heddle reed, a batten or sword, or a shed rod.

Shuttle A device to hold the weft and carry it through the shed.

Single A single-ply thread, sometimes used in un-plied pairs or multiples when doing supplementary weft brocading.

Single-faced In supplementary weft brocading, this term applies to the patterning that appears on one side of the textile only.

Slit See *kelim*.

Sobre-huipil A special *huipil* worn over the every-day one.

Sombrero The male hat.

Space-dyed Yarn is dyed in blocks of color creating a thread of many shades.

Spindle A straight shaft used for spinning. The spindle is weighted with a round whorl and is rotated rapidly to twist aligned fibers into thread, which is then wound around the spindle.

Spindle whorl The round weight on the bottom of a spindle, used to steady the rotating motion of the spindle while spinning thread.

Substitution A simple technique in which two or more sets of elements exchange interlacing and floating functions to create a pattern.

Supplementary warp weave Extra warps in a compound weave are used for adding a supplementary pattern to a ground weave; these warps are not essential to the structure of the cloth.

Supplementary weft weave Extra wefts used for patterning in addition to the ground weave; these wefts are not essential to the structure of the cloth.

Sword A weaving implement of wood used to create sheds and for beating; also called a batten.

Tablera A coat with tails worn by men.

Telar de palitos See backstrap loom.

Tension Tightness or looseness of warp yarns.

Tenter A device to help maintain an even width in the finished cloth. It is a stick placed crosswise on or under the fabric being woven, and has pegs, thorns, or nails at the ends which are pushed through the edges of the cloth.

Terminal zone The area of a 4-selvedge cloth which is woven last. Weaving becomes difficult in this area because there is not enough unwoven warp slack to produce a shed. The weft is inserted on bobbins of decreasing size, finally on a needle. This area is visible on a textile for patterning is usually abandoned and the texture of the cloth changes.

Tie-dye See ikat.

Típica A term used for traditional clothing in Guatemala, also known as *traje*.

Toe loom A backstrap loom in which the toe becomes the support to which the loom is attached.

Treadle loom An upright, stationary wooden structure for weaving, introduced by the Spaniards. Warps extend over back and front beams and are held at a rigid tension.

Tupu (*Q.*) Silver or nickel shawl pin used to pin a *llijlla* over a woman's shoulders.

Tulma (*Q.*) Braid ties worn by women.

Twill weave Twill weaves are float weaves characterized by a diagonal alignment of floats for which a minimum of three warp groupings is essential.

Twining A technique similar to basketry, used to produce fabrics; an off-loom technique.

Two-faced In supplementary weft brocading, this term applies to patterning that floats on the reverse side between pattern areas forming an inverse of the design on the other side.

Tzute A head or shoulder cloth, used by both men and women; see *poc*.

Unkhuña (*Q.*) A small cloth used for a woman's coca leaves and food stuffs; also used as a groundcloth for ceremonial offerings.

Unkhu (*Q.*) A tunic; see *ccahua*.

Vara Roughly three feet.

Vicuña A member of the camelid family; see camelid.

Waraka (*Q.*) See *honda*.

Warp Vertical threads that form the web.

Warp-faced A fabric structure characterized by the close set of the warps, completely covering the wefts.

Warp-predominant A fabric in which warps outnumber the wefts but do not entirely conceal them.

Web The basic structure of the textile created by unwoven warps and wefts.

Weft Horizontal threads that form the web.

Weft-faced A fabric structure that results when wefts are closely compacted over more widely spaced warps and warps are not visible.

Wincha See *llautu*.

Xicolli (*N.*) A sleeveless male garment described as a front-opening jacket and a closed tunic; a pre-Columbian dress survival.

Z-twist yarn Composed of two or more plies that are twisted together so as to trend in the same direction as the diagonal center bar of the letter Z when the yarn is held in vertical position.

Bibliography

Adams, Richard E.W.

1986 Archaeologists Explore Guatemala's Lost City of the Maya, Rio Azul. *National Geographic*, vol. 169, no. 4, April:420–451.

Adelson, Laurie and Bruce Takami

1978 *Weaving Traditions of Highland Bolivia*. Los Angeles: The Craft and Folk Art Museum.

Adelson, Laurie and Arthur Tracht

1983 *Aymara Weavings*. Washington D.C.: The Smithsonian Institution.

Anawalt, Patricia Rieff

1974 An Experiment in Cultural Reconstruction: Guatemalan Costume. Paper delivered at the 73rd Annual Meeting of the American Anthropological Association, Mexico City, November 19–24.

1980 Costume and Control: Aztec Sumptuary Laws. *Archaeology*, January/February, vol. 33, no. 1:33–43.

1981 *Indian Clothing before Cortes*. Norman: University of Oklahoma Press.

1984 Prehispanic Survivals in Guatemalan Dress. In *Beyond Boundaries*, ed. Nora Fisher, pp. 12–19. Santa Fe: Museum of New Mexico.

Anderson, Marilyn

1978 *Guatemalan Textiles Today*. New York: Watson-Guptil Publications.

1983 Guatemala: Traditional Weaving Is a Life and Death Struggle. *Craft International*, October–December 1983:24–26.

Arriola Geng, Olga

n.d. *Téchnicas de Bordados en Los Trajes Indígenas de Guatemala*. Guatemala City: Museo Ixchel del Traje Indígena de Guatemala.

Astúrias, Miguel Angel

1974 Leyenda de la Mujer de Ceníza, *Americás*, 26(1):2–7.

Badner, Mino

1972 A Possible Focus of Andean Artistic Influence in Mesoamerica. In *Studies in Pre-Columbian Art and Archaeology*, no. 9. Washington, D.C.: Dumbarton Oaks.

Baizerman, Suzanne and Karen Searle

1978 *Finishes in the Ethnic Tradition*. St. Paul: Dos Tejedoras.

Barrios, Lina E.

1983 *Hierba, Montañas y El Arbol de la Vida en San Pedro Sacatepéquez, Guatemala*. Guatemala: Ediciones del Museo Ixchel.

Barrios, Linda Astúrias de

1985 *Comalapa: Native Dress and Its Significance*. Guatemala City, Guatemala: The Ixchel Museum of Indian Dress of Guatemala.

Barthes, Roland

1983 *The Fashion System*. Trans: Mathew Ward and Richard Howard. New York: Hill and Wang.

Bastien, Joseph W.

1978 *Mountain of the Condor: Metaphor and Ritual in an Andean Ayllu*. St. Paul: West Publishing Co.

Beardsley, Grace

1985 Design Development in Tarahumara and Pueblo Sashes. *American Indian Art*, Autumn:39–73.

Berlo, Janet Catherine and Raymond E. Senuk

1985 Caveat Emptor: The Misrepresentation of Historic Maya Textiles. *Archaeology*, vol. 38, no. 2:84.

Bird, Junius B.

1979 Fibers and Spinning, Procedures in the Andean Area. In *The Junius B. Bird Textile Conference*, ed. Ann P. Rowe et al., pp. 13–17. Washington D.C.: The Textile Museum.

Bird, Junius B., John Hyslop, and Milica D. Skinner

1985 *The Preceramic Excavations at the Huaca Prieta Chicama Valley, Peru*. Anthropological Papers of the American Museum of Natural History, vol. 62, part I. New York: American Museum of Natural History.

Bjerregaard, Lena

1977 *Techniques of Guatemalan Weaving.* New York: Van Nostrand, Reinhold Co.

Bogatyrev, Petr

1971 *Function of Folk Costume in Moravian Slovakia.* The Hague, Paris: Mouton Publishers.

Bunch, Roland and Roger Bunch

1977 *The Highland Maya.* Visalia, Calif.: Josten's Publications.

Burgos-Debray, Elizabeth

1984 *I. . . Rigoberta Menchú: An Indian Woman in Guatemala.* Trans: Ann Wright. London and New York: Verso Editions.

Cahlander, Adele et al.

1978 *Bolivian Tubular Edging and Crossed Warp Techniques.* The Weaver's Journal, Monograph One. Boulder, Colo.: Colorado Fiber Center.

Cahlander, Adele with Elayne Zorn and Ann Pollard Rowe

1980 *Sling Braiding of the Andes.* Boulder, Colo.: Colorado Fiber Center.

Cahlander, Adele, E.M. Franquemont, and Barbara Bergman

1981 A Special Andean Tubular Trim – Woven Without Heddles. *The Weaver's Journal*, vol. VI, no. 3, issue 23:54–58.

Cahlander, Adele with Suzanne Baizerman

1985 *Double-Woven Treasures from Old Peru.* St. Paul: Dos Tejedoras.

Casagrande, Louis B.

1984 The Textile Art of the Chiapas Maya. In *Arte Vivo: Living Traditions in Mexican Folk Art*, ed. James R. Ramsey, pp. 75–82. Memphis, Tennessee: Memphis State University.

Cason, Marjorie and Adele Cahlander

1976 *The Art of Bolivian Highland Weaving.* New York: Watson Guptil.

Casteñeda Leon, Luisa

1981 *Traditional Dress of Peru.* Lima, Peru: Museo Nacional de la Cultura Peruana.

Cereceda, Veronica

1978 Semiologie des Tissus Andins: Les Talegas D'Isluga. *Annales*, 33rd Année, no. 5–6, Sept.–Dec.:1017–1035.

Cerny, Charlene

1984 Thoughts on Anonymity and Signature in Folk Art. In *Beyond Boundaries*, ed. Nora Fisher, pp. 34–37. Santa Fe: Museum of New Mexico.

Chonay, Dionisio José and Delia Goetz

1953 *Title of the Lords of Totonicapán.* Norman: University of Oklahoma Press.

Codex Mendoza

1673 In *Histoire de L'Empire Mexicain representée par figures. Relation de Mexique, ou de la Nouvelle Espagne.* Thomas Gage. Traduite par Melchisedec Thevenot. Paris: André Cramoisy.

Coggins, Clemency Chase and Orrin C. Shane II, eds.

1984 *Cenote of Sacrifice.* Austin: University of Texas Press.

Cohen, John

1957 *An Investigation of Contemporary Weaving of the Peruvian Indians.* MFA thesis, Yale University.

Collier, George A., Rosa Mendoza de Rick, and Steve Berger

1981 *Aymara Weavings from Highland Bolivia.* Unpublished catalogue text. Stanford, Calif.: The Stanford University Museum of Art.

Conklin, William J.

1983 Pucara and Tiahuanaco Tapestry: Time and Style in a Sierra Weaving Tradition. *Ñawpa Pacha* 21:1–45

n.d. Structure as Meaning in Ancient Andean Textiles. In *La Tecnología en el Mundo Andino*, ed. H. Lechtman and A.M. Soldi. Mexico City: Instítuto de Investigaciónes Antropológicas, Universidad Nacionál Autonoma de Mexico, vol. II.

Conte, Christine

1984   *Maya Culture & Costume.* A catalogue of the Taylor Museum's E.B. Ricketson Collection of
       Guatemalan Textiles. Colorado Springs, Colo.: The Taylor Museum of the Colorado Springs Fine
       Arts Center.

Cordry, Donald and Dorothy Cordry

1968   *Mexican Indian Costumes.* Austin and London: University of Texas Press.

Delgado, Hildegard Schmidt de

1963   *Aboriginal Guatemalan Handweaving and Costume.* Ph.D. dissertation, Department of
       Anthropology, Indiana University. University Microfilm, Ann Arbor.

Deuss, Krystyna

1981   *Indian Costumes from Guatemala.* Twickenham, Great Britain: CTD Printers LTD.

D'Harcourt, Raoul

1962   *Textiles of Ancient Peru and their Techniques.* Seattle: University of Washington Press.

Dieseldorff, Dr. Herbert Quirín

1984   *X Balám Q'eu, El Pájaro Sol: El Traje Regional de Cobán.* Guatemala City: Museo Ixchel del Traje
       Indígena de Guatemala.

Dieterich, Mary G., Jon T. Erickson, and Erin Younger

1979   *Guatemalan Costumes: The Heard Museum Collection.* Phoenix, Arizona: The Heard Museum.

Drooker, Penelope

1981   *Hammock Making Techniques.* Sanbornville, New Hampshire: published by Penelope Drooker.

Durán, Fray Diego

1971   *Book of the Gods and Rites of the Ancient Calendar.* Ed. and trans. D. Heyden and F. Horcacitas.
       Norman, Oklahoma: University of Oklahoma Press.

Edmonson, Munro S.

1971   *The Book of Counsel: The Popol Vuh of the Quiché Maya of Guatemala.* Middle American Research
       Institute, publication 35. New Orleans: Tulane University.

Emery, Irene

1966   *Primary Structures of Fabric.* Washington D.C.: The Textile Museum.

Femenias, Blenda

1984   Peruvian Costume and European Perceptions in the Eighteenth Century. *Dress: the Annual Journal
       of the Costume Society of America,* vol. 10:52–63.

Fisher, Abby Sue

1986   Clothing Change Through Contact: Traditional Guatemalan Dress. *The Weaver's Journal,* Winter,
       vol. X, no. 3, issue 39:60–64.

Fontana, Bernard L., Edmond J. B. Faubert, and Barney T. Burns

1977   *The Other Southwest.* Phoenix, Arizona: The Heard Museum.

Foppa, Alaída

1976   *Arte Popular de Guatemala.* Exposición-venta a beneficio de los artesanos damnificadas por el
       terremoto de febrero. Mexico City: Museo Nacional de Artes e Industrias Populares.

Frame, Mary

1986   The Visual Images of Fabric Structures in Ancient Peruvian Art. In *The Junius B. Bird Second
       Conference on Andean Textiles,* ed. Ann P. Rowe. Washington D.C.: The Textile Museum.

Franquemont, Christine

1986   Chinchero Pallays: an Ethnic Code. In *The Junius B. Bird Second Conference on Andean Textiles,* ed.
       Ann P. Rowe. Washington D.C.: The Textile Museum.

Franquemont, Christine and Edward M. Franquemont

n.d.   Learning to Weave in Chinchero. In *La Tecnología en el Mundo Andino,* ed. H. Lechtman and A.M.
       Soldi, vol. II. Mexico City: Instituto de Investigaciónes Antropologícas, Universidad Nacional
       Autonoma de Mexico.

Franquemont, Edward M.

1983 Reserved Shed Pebble Weave in Peru. In *In Celebration of the Curious Mind*, ed. Nora Rogers and Martha Stanley, pp. 21–34. Loveland, Colo.: Interweave Press.

1984 Change in Chinchero Textiles. Paper given at the Annual Meeting of the Institute for Andean Studies, Berkeley, Calif.

1986 Cloth Production Rates in Chinchero, Peru. In *The Junius B. Bird Second Conference on Andean Textiles*, ed. Ann P. Rowe. Washington D.C.: The Textile Museum.

García Cubas, Antonio

1876 *The Republic of Mexico in 1876*. Trans. G.F. Henderson. Mexico D.F.: La Enseñanza Printing Office.

Gastelow, Mary

1979 *A World of Embroidery*. New York: Charles Scribner's Sons.

Gayton, Anna H.

1961 The Cultural Significance of Peruvian Textiles: Production, Function, Aesthetics. In *The Kroeber Anthropological Society Papers*, no. 25, Fall 1961:111–128.

Girault, Louis

1969 *Textiles Boliviens*: *Region de Charazani*. Paris: Catalogues du Musée de L'Homme.

Glassman, Paul

1977 *Guatemala Guide*. Dallas: Passport Press.

Goodell, Grace

1969 The Cloth of the Quechuas. *Natural History*, vol. 78, no. 10, Dec.: 48–55, 64–65.

Goodman, Frances Schaill

1976 *The Embroidery of Mexico and Guatemala*. New York: Charles Scribner's Sons.

Guaman Poma de Ayala, Felipe

1980 *El Primer Nueva Corónica y Buen Gobierno*. Ed. John V. Murra and Rolena Adorno. Mexico D.F.: Siglo Veintiuno de España editores.

Hansen, H.H.

1956 *Histoire du Costume*. Paris: Flammarion.

Harris, Alex and Margaret Sartor, eds.

1984 *Gertrude Blom Bearing Witness*. Chapel Hill and London: The University of North Carolina Press.

Hearne, Pamela

1985 The Silent Language of Guatemalan Textiles. *Archaeology*, July/August:54–57.

Helms, Mary W.

1975 *Middle America*: *A Culture History of the Heartland and Frontiers*. Englewood Cliffs, New Jersey: Prentice-Hall Inc.

Hendrickson, Carol

1985 Indian Dress in Contemporary Highland Guatemala. Paper given at meeting of American Anthropological Association, Washington, D.C., December.

Johnson, Irmgard W.

1967 Miniature garments found in Mixteca Alta caves, Mexico. *Folk* (Dansk Etnografisk Tidsskrift) 8/9:179–190.

Johnston, Bernice

1970 *The Seri Indians of Sonora Mexico*. Tuscon, Arizona: The University of Arizona Press.

Jopling, Carol F.

1975 Yalalag Weaving: Aesthetic, Technological and Economic Nexus. *American Ethnologist Society Journal*, 211–236.

Kaufman, Terrence

1973–74 Meso-American Indian Languages. In *The New Encyclopedia Britannica*, 15th edition, vol. 8:956–963. Chicago, London, Toronto, Geneva, Sydney, Tokyo, Manila, Seoul: William Benton Publisher.

Keleman, Paul

1942 *Medieval American Art, a Survey in Two Volumes*. New York: The Macmillan Co.

Kent, Kate Peck

1983 *Prehistoric Textiles of the Southwest*. Santa Fe and Albuquerque: University of New Mexico Press.

1985 *Navajo Weaving*: Three Centuries of Change. Santa Fe: School of American Research Press.

King, Mary Elizabeth

1986 **Paracas Period Costume: A Semiotic View from Ocucaje. In** *The Junius B. Bird Second Conference on Andean Textiles*, **ed. Ann P. Rowe. Washington D.C.: The Textile Museum.**

Lathbury, Virginia Locke

1974 *Textiles as an Expression of an Expanding World View*: San Antonio Aguas Calientes, Guatemala. **MA thesis, Department of Anthropology, University of Pennsylvania.**

Lathrap, Donald W.

1966 **Relationships between Mesoamerica and the Andean Areas. In** *Handbook of Middle American Indians*, **ed. Wauchope, Ekholm, and Willey, vol. 4, pp. 265–276. Austin: University of Texas Press.**

Laver, J.

1949 *Style in Costume*. **London: Oxford University Press.**

Lechuga, Ruth D.

1982 *El Traje Indígena de México*. **Mexico D.F.: Panorama Editorial, S.A.**

López, Agustín López

1982 *Tejeduría Artesanal* (*Manual*). **Guatemala City: Sub-Centro Regional de Artesanías y Artes Populares.**

Lothrop, Joy Mahler

n.d. **Textiles from the Sacred Cenote. In** *Artifacts from the Cenote of Sacrifice, Chichen Itza: Textiles, Wood, Ceramics, Stone, Bone, Shell, Copal, and Other Vegetal Materials*. **ed. Clemency Coggins, Memoirs of the Peabody Museum, Harvard University, vol. 10, no. 3. Cambridge, Mass.**

Mahler, Joy

1965 **Garments and Textiles of the Maya Lowlands. In** *Handbook of Middle American Indians*, **ed. Wauchope, Ekholm and Willey, vol. 31 pp. 581–593. Austin: University of Texas Press.**

Maudslay, Alfred P. and Anne Maudslay

1899 *A Glimpse at Guatemala*. **London: John Murray.**

McEldowney, Margaret Ross

1982 *An Analysis of Change in Highland Guatemalan Tapestry Hairribbons*. **MA thesis, Department of Nutritional Sciences and Textiles, University of Washington.**

Medlin, Mary Ann

1983 *Awayqa Sumaj Calchapi*: Weaving, Social Organization, and Identity in Calcha, Bolivia. **Ph.D. dissertation, University of North Carolina. University Microfilms, Ann Arbor.**

Meisch, Lynn

1984 *A Traveler's Guide to El Dorado and the Inca Empire*. **New York: Viking Penguin Inc.**

1986 **Weaving Styles in Tarabuco, Bolivia. In** *The Junius B. Bird Second Conference on Andean Textiles*, **ed. Ann P. Rowe. Washington D.C.: The Textile Museum.**

Miller, Mary Ellen

1986 *The Murals of Bonampak*. **Princeton: Princeton University Press.**

Morales Hidalgo, Italo

1982 *U Cayibal Atziak: Imágenes en los Tejidos Guatemaltécos*. **Guatemala, Centroamerica: Four Ahau Press.**

Morley, Sylvanus G.

1956 *The Ancient Maya*. **Ed. Rev. George W. Brainerd. Stanford, Calif.: Stanford University Press.**

Morris, Walter F., Jr.

1980 *Luchetik: The Woven Word from Highland Chiapas*. **San Cristóbal de las Casas, Chiapas, Mexico: Publicaciónes Pokok de La Cooperativo de Artesanas Indigenas, Sna Jolobil.**

1984 *A Millennium of Weaving*. **Privately published by the author, distributed by Sna Jolobil, San Cristóbal de las Casas, Chiapas, Mexico.**

1985 *Flowers, Saints, and Toads: Ancient and Modern Maya Textile Design Symbolism*. *National Geographic Research Journal*, **Winter:63–79.**

1986   Maya Time Warps. *Archaeology*, May/June, vol. 39, no. 3:53–59.

Murra, John V.

1962   Cloth and Its Functions in the Inca State. *American Anthropologist*, vol. 64, no. 4, Aug.:710–728.

Murray, John A.H.

1893   *A New English Dictionary on Historical Principles.* Oxford and New York: Clarendon Press and Macmillan & Co.

Nebel, Carlos

1836   *Voyage pittoresque et archéologique dans la partie la plus intéressant du Mexique.* Paris.

Nicholson, H.B.

1967   The Efflorescence of Mesoamerican Civilization: A Resume. In *Indian Mexico Past and Present*, ed. Betty Bell, pp. 46–71. Los Angeles: University of California, Latin American Center.

O'Neale, Lila M.

1942   Early Textiles from Chiapas, Mexico. In *Middle American Research Records*, Middle America Research Institute, vol. 1, no. 1:1–6. New Orleans: Tulane University.

1945   *Textiles of Highland Guatemala.* Washington D.C.: Carnegie Institution of Washington.

1946   Weaving. In *Handbook of South American Indians*, ed. J.H. Steward, bulletin 143, vol. 5, pp. 97–137. Austin: University of Texas Press.

O'Neale, Lila M. and A.L. Kroeber

1930   Textile Periods in Ancient Peru: I. *Publications in American Archaeology and Ethnology*, vol. 28. Berkeley: University of California.

Osborne, Lilly de Jongh

1935   *Guatemalan Textiles.* Middle American Research Series, publication no. 567. New Orleans: Tulane University.

1965   *Indian Crafts of Guatemala and El Salvador.* Norman: University of Oklahoma Press.

Pancake, Cherri M.

1976   *Costume of Rural Guatemala.* Guatemala City: Museo Ixchel del Traje Indígena.

1977   *Textile Traditions of the Highland Maya: Some Aspects of Development of Change.* Paper presented at International Symposium on Maya Art, Architecture, Archaeology, and Hieroglyphic Writing. Guatemala City, Guatemala.

Pancake, Cherri M. and Suzanne Baizerman

1982   Guatemalan Gauze Weaves. *Textile Museum Journal*, vols. 19–20, 1980–1981:1–26.

Pasztory, Esther

1984   The Function of Art in Mesoamerica. *Archaeology*, January/February: 18–25.

Pendergast, David M.

1969   *Altun Ha, British Honduras* (*Belize*): *The Sun God's Tomb.* Occasional Paper 19, Art and Archaeology. Toronto: Royal Ontario Museum Publications.

Perera, Victor and Robert D. Bruce

1982   *The Last Lords of Palenque.* Boston, Toronto: Little, Brown and Company.

Pettersen, Carmen L.

1976   *The Maya of Guatemala.* Seattle and London: University of Washington Press.

Pierce, Donna, ed.

1985   ¡Vivan las Fiestas! Santa Fe: Museum of New Mexico Press.

Recinos, Adrian and Delia Goetz

1953   *The Annals of the Cakchiquels.* Norman: University of Oklahoma Press.

Rodas, Flavio N. and Olvidio C. Rodas

1938   *Simbolismos* (*Maya Quiches*) *de Guatemala.* Guatemala: Tipográfica Nacional.

Rodas Flavio N., Olvidio C. Rodas, and Laurence F. Hawkins

1940   *Chichicastenango: The Kiche Indians.* Guatemala: Union Tipográfica.

Rowe, Ann Pollard

1975   Weaving Processes of the Cuzco Area of Peru. *The Textile Museum Journal*, vol. 4, no. 2:30–46.

1977a   *Warp Patterned Weaves of the Andes.* Washington D.C.: The Textile Museum.

1977b   Weaving Styles in the Cuzco Area. In *The Irene Emery Roundtable on Museum Textiles, 1976 Proceedings*, ed. Irene Emery and Patricia Fiske, pp. 61–84. Washington D.C.: The Textile Museum.

1981   *A Century of Change in Guatemalan Textiles.* New York: The Center for Inter-American Relations. Seattle: University of Washington Press.

Rowe, John Howland

1946   Inca Culture at the Time of the Spanish Conquest. In *Handbook of South American Indians*, ed. J.H. Stewart, bulletin 143, vol. 4:183–330. Washington D.C.: Smithsonian Institution, Bureau of American Ethnology.

1962   Stages and Periods in Archaeological Interpretation. *Southwestern Journal of Anthropology*, vol. 18, no. 1:40–54.

Roys, Ralph L.

1931   *The Ethno-Botany of the Maya.* New Orleans: The Department of Middle American Research, Tulane University.

Rugg, Carmen Neutze de

1974   *Designs in Guatemalan Textiles.* Guatemala City, Guatemala, C.A: Turismas Publications.

Sahagún, Fray Bernardino de

1950–69   *Florentine Codex: General History of the Things of New Spain.* Trans. and ed. Arthur J.O. Anderson and Charles E. Dibble. Monographs of the School of American Research, no. 14, pts. 2–13. Santa Fe: University of Utah and School of American Research Press.

Salvador, Mari Lyn

1978   *Yer Dailege! Kuna Women's Art.* Albuquerque: The Maxwell Museum of Anthropology, University of New Mexico.

Sayer, Chloë

1985   *Costumes of Mexico.* Austin: University of Texas Press.

Schele, Linda and Mary Ellen Miller

1986   *The Blood of Kings.* Fort Worth, Texas: The Kimbell Art Museum.

Schevill, Margot Blum

1980   *The Persistence of Maya Indian Backstrap Weaving in San Antonio Aguas Calientes, Sacatepéquez Guatemala.* MA thesis, Department of Anthropology, Brown University.

1983   The Art of Ixchel: Learning to Weave in Guatemala and Rhode Island. *Weaver's Journal*, Summer, vol. VIII, no. 1, issue 29:57–61.

1986   *Evolution in Textile Design from the Highlands of Guatemala.* Occasional Papers, no. 1. Berkeley: Lowie Museum of Anthropology, University of California.

1987   Backstrap Weaving in San Antonio Aguas Calientes, Sacatepéquez, Guatemala. *Threads*, issue 11.

Schneider, Jane and Annette B. Weiner

1986   Cloth and the Organization of Human Experience. *Current Anthropology*, April 1986:178–184.

Sherzer, Dina and Joel Sherzer

1976   Mormaknamaloe: The Cuna Mola. In *Ritual and Symbolism in Native Central America.* Ed. Philip Young and James Howe, pp. 23–42. Eugene: Department of Anthropology, University of Oregon.

Silverman-Proust, Gail

1986   Cuadro Motivos Inti de Q'ero. *Boletin de Lima*, numero 43, Enero:61–75.

Sperlich, Norbert and Elizabeth Katz Sperlich

1980   *Guatemalan Backstrap Weaving.* Norman: University of Oklahoma Press.

Start, Laura E.

1948   *The McDougall Collection of Indian Textiles from Guatemala and Mexico.* Occasional Papers on Technology, 2. Oxford: University of Oxford Press.

Tedlock, Barbara

1983   A Phenomenological Approach to Religious Change in Highland Guatemala. In *Heritage of Conquest: Thirty Years Later*, ed. Carl Kendall, John Hawkins, and Laurel Bossen, pp. 236–246. Albuquerque: University of New Mexico Press.

Tedlock, Barbara and Dennis Tedlock

1985   Text and Textile: Language and Technology in the Arts of the Quiché Maya. *Journal of Anthropological Research*, vol. 41, no. 2:121–146.

Tedlock, Dennis

1985   *Popol Vuh*. New York: Simon & Schuster, Inc.

Tozzer, Alfred M., ed.

1941   *Landa's Relación de las cosas de Yucatán*. Papers of the Peabody Museum, Harvard University, vol. 18. Cambridge, Mass.

Wasserman, Tamara E. and Jonathan S. Hill

1981   *Bolivian Indian Textiles*. New York: Dover Publications Inc.

Westphal, Katherine

1980   Wearable Art. Lecture given at the World Crafts Council, Vienna, Austria.

Wilkerson, S. Jeffrey K.

1985   The Usumacinta River: Troubles on a Wild Frontier. *National Geographic*, vol. 168, no. 4, October:514–543.

Yorke, Roger

1980   *Woven Images: Bolivian Weaving from the 19th and 20th Centuries*. Halifax, Nova-Scotia: Dalhousie Art Gallery.

Zorn, Elayne

1985   Analysis of Textiles in Andean Herders' Ritual Bundles. Paper given at the American Anthropological Association meeting, Washington, D.C., December.

1986   *Unkhuñas* in Herders' Ritual Bundles (*Senal Q'epi*) of Macusani, Peru. In *The Junius B. Bird Second Conference on Andean Textiles*, ed. Ann P. Rowe. Washington D.C.: The Textile Museum.

Zumbuhl, Hugo

1979   *Tinte Naturales*. Huancayo, Peru: Una Publicación de *Kamaz Maki* auspiciado por S.E.P.A.S.

Personal Communications

Arriola Geng, Olga	1985–86
Bainton, Barry	1986
Baizerman, Suzanne	1986
Bell, James	1978
Callañaupa, Nilda	1985
Casagrande, Louis	1984
Davis, John	1986
Feest, Christian	1986
Frame, Mary	1984
LeCount, Cynthia	1986
Menchú, Rigoberta	1985
Murra, John	1985
Morris, Walter F., Jr.	1985–86
Pancake, Cherri M.	1978, 1982
Plunkett, James	1986
Rowe, Ann P.	1985
Sakiestewa, Ramona	1985